Essentials of Terror Medicine

Shmuel C. Shapira, MD, MPH
Professor of Medical Administration, Director,
Hebrew University-Hadassah School of Public Health,
Deputy Director General, Hadassah University Hospital,
CEO, International Center of Terror Medicine, Jerusalem, Israel

Jeffrey S. Hammond, MD, MPH, FACS
Professor of Surgery, Section Chief, Trauma/Surgical Critical Care,
Robert Wood Johnson Medical School, New Brunswick, NJ, USA

Leonard A. Cole, PhD, DDS
Adjunct Professor, Department of Political Science and Division of Global Affairs,
Rutgers University, Newark, NJ, USA

Editors

Essentials of Terror Medicine

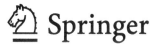 Springer

Shmuel C. Shapira
Professor of Medical Administration,
Director, Hebrew University-Hadassah
    School of Public Health,
Deputy Director General,
    Hadassah University Hospital,
CEO, International Center of Terror Medicine,
Jerusalem, Israel

Jeffrey S. Hammond
Professor of Surgery, Section Chief,
Trauma/Surgical Critical Care,
Robert Wood Johnson Medical School,
New Brunswick, NJ, USA

Leonard A. Cole
Adjunct Professor, Department of
    Political Science and Division of
    Global Affairs, Rutgers University,
Nework, NJ, USA

ISBN: 978-1-4614-9899-5   ISBN: 978-0-387-09412-0 (eBook)
DOI:10.1007/978-0-387-09412-0

9 8 7 6 5 4 3 2 1

springer.com

Dedication

Dedicated with love and gratitude to my parents Eli and Dora for teaching me the importance of education and modesty, to my wife Sarinha for ongoing support, and to my children Elad and Daniel for brightening my life.
Shmuel C. Shapira

Dedicated to the men and women on the front lines in the war on terror, who have sacrificed so much, both physically and emotionally, in the hopes that our children and grandchildren will not have to do so.
Jeffrey S. Hammond

Dedicated to the victims of terrorism and their loved ones, who, while suffering grievous injury and anguish, have strengthened the will of good people everywhere to defeat this wanton scourge.
Leonard A. Cole

Acknowledgments

The health care concerns of terror medicine are far-reaching, as evidenced by the variety of backgrounds and expertise of the contributors to this volume. They include physicians, dentists, nurses, psychologists, scientists, policy planners, and more – all distinguished and all engaged with demanding responsibilities in their own fields. But while attending to their customary obligations they have also managed to write extraordinarily thoughtful and informative chapters, and for their efforts we are deeply grateful.

In the course of developing this book, we have benefited from the ideas not only of the contributors but also of others including Richard Karlen, Jonathan Moreno, Kobi Peleg, Michael Stein, and our wives, Jill Brooks, Ruth Cole, and Sarinha Shapira. We are also indebted to our publisher, Springer, for encouraging this project and we thank especially Brian Belval, editor for clinical medicine, and Portia Bridges, developmental editor, for their patience and abundant wisdom. It is the fondest wish of all that this volume might help to mitigate the evils of terrorism.

Contents

Acknowledgments.. vii

Contributors xiii

PART I: INTRODUCTION

Chapter 1
Introduction to Terror Medicine.. 3
Shmuel C. Shapira, Jeffrey S. Hammond, and Leonard A. Cole

Chapter 2
Terrorism in the Twenty-First Century 13
Boaz Ganor

PART II: PREPARATION AND RESPONSE

Chapter 3
EMS and Pre-Hospital Issues.. 29
Ari Leppäniemi

Chapter 4
Effects of Terrorism on the Healthcare Community 45
David O'Reilly and Karim Brohi

Chapter 5
Terror Medicine: Education and Training.. 59
Yuri Millo

Chapter 6
Modeling and Simulation in Terror Medicine 79
Asher Hirshberg and Kenneth L. Mattox

Chapter 7
National Coordination and Integration 95
Shlomo Mor-Yosef and Shmuel C. Shapira

Chapter 8
Response Planning 111
Jorie D. Klein

Chapter 9
Technology Opportunities and Challenges 133
Annette L. Sobel

PART III: WEAPON ETIOLOGIES

Chapter 10
Epidemiology of Terrorism Injuries 149
Limor Aharonson-Daniel and Shmuel C. Shapira

Chapter 11
Explosions and Blast Injury 171
Eric R. Frykberg

Chapter 12
Biological Agents and Terror Medicine 195
Meir Oren

Chapter 13
Chemical Agents and Terror Medicine 223
Kristan Staudenmayer and William P. Schecter

Chapter 14
Radiological Agents and Terror Medicine 241
Jeffrey S. Hammond and Jill Lipoti

Chapter 15
Cyber-Terrorism: Preparation and Response 255
Abraham R. Wagner and Zvi Fisch

PART IV: TYPES OF INJURY

Chapter 16
Penetrating Injury in Terror Attacks 271
Gidon Almogy and Avraham I. Rivkind

Chapter 17
Orthopedic Injury in Urban Terrorism 287
Meir Liebergall and Rami Mosheiff

Chapter 18
Terror-Inflicted Burn Injury 299
Tomer Tzur and Arieh Eldad

Chapter 19
Neurosurgical Injury Related to Terror 313
Jeffrey V. Rosenfeld

Chapter 20
Crush Injury, Crush Syndrome 337
Moshe Michaelson

Chapter 21
Maxillofacial Injury Related to Terror 347
Eran Regev and Rephael Zeltser

Chapter 22
Pediatrics and Terrorism 365
David Markenson

PART V: AFTERMATH AND ETHICAL CONSIDERATIONS

Chapter 23
Forensic Investigation of Suicide Bombings 393
Jehuda Hiss and Tzipi Kahana

Chapter 24
Psychological Effects of Terror Attacks 405
Sara A. Freedman

Chapter 25
Ethics and Terror Medicine 425
Leonard A. Cole

Contributors

Limor Aharonson-Daniel, PhD
Leon and Mathilda Recanati School for Community Health Professions,
Ben Gurion University of the Negev, Beer-Sheva, Israel

Gidon Almogy, MD
Attending Surgeon, Department of Surgery, Hadassah Hebrew University
Medical Center, Jerusalem, Israel

Karim Brohi, FRCS, FRCA
Consultant in Trauma, Vascular & Critical Care Medicine, Department of Trauma
Surgery, Queen Mary, University of London, The Royal London Hospital,
London, UK

Leonard A. Cole, PhD, DDS
Adjunct Professor, Department of Political Science and Division of Global
Affairs, Rutgers University, Newark, NJ, USA

Arieh Eldad, MD
Associate Professor of Plastic Surgery, Department of Plastic Surgery, Hadassah
Hebrew University Medical Center, Jerusalem, Israel

Zvi Fisch
Information Systems Division, Hadassah Hebrew University Medical Center,
Jerusalem, Israel

Sara A. Freedman, PhD
Center for Traumatic Stress, Department of Psychiatry, Hadassah Hebrew
University Medical Center, Jerusalem, Israel

Eric R. Frykberg, MD, FACS
Professor of Surgery, Department of Surgery, University of Florida College
of Medicine, Jacksonville Medical Center; Chief, Division of Surgery, Shands
Jacksonville Medical Center, Jacksonville, FL, USA

Boaz Ganor, PhD
Executive Director, ICT – The International Institute for Counter-Terrorism,
Interdisciplinary Center, Herzliya, Israel

Jeffrey S. Hammond, MD, MPH, FACS
Professor of Surgery, Section Chief, Trauma/Surgical Critical Care, Robert Wood
Johnson Medical School, New Brunswick, NJ, USA

Asher Hirshberg, MD, FACS
Professor of Surgery, Department of Surgery, SUNY Downstate College
of Medicine, Brooklyn, NY, USA

Jehuda Hiss, MD
Professor, Chief Medical Examiner, Assaf Harofeh Medical Centre, National Centre of Forensic Medicine, Tel Aviv, Israel

Tzipi Kahana, PhD
Forensic Anthropologist, Israel National Police, Division of Identification and
Forensic Science – DVI, National Centre of Forensic Medicine, Tel Aviv, Israel

Jorie D. Klein, RN
Director, Trauma & Disaster Services, Parkland Health & Hospital
System, Dallas, TX, USA

Ari Leppäniemi, MD, PhD, DMCC
Associate Professor of Surgery, Chief of Emergency Surgery, Department
of Surgery, Meilahti Hospital, University of Helsinki, Helsinki, Finland

Meir Liebergall, MD
Professor of Orthopedic Surgery, Department of Orthopedic Surgery, Hadassah
Hebrew University Medical Center, Jerusalem, Israel

Jill Lipoti, PhD
Director, Division of Environmental Safety and Health, New Jersey Department of
Environmental Protection, Trenton, NJ, USA

David Markenson, MD, FAAP, EMT-P
Director, Center for Disaster Medicine, New York Medical College School
of Public Health; Department of Pediatric Emergency Medicine, Maria Fareri
Children's Hospital, Valhalla, NY, USA

Kenneth L. Mattox, MD, FACS
Professor and Vice Chairman, Michael E. DeBakey Department of Surgery,
Baylor College of Medicine; Chief of Staff & Chief of Surgery, Ben Taub
General Hospital, Houston, TX, USA

Moshe Michaelson, MD
Head of Emergency Department and Trauma Unit, Rambam Medical Center,
Haifa, Israel

Yuri Millo, MD
Director, Simulation and Training Environment Lab (SiTEL), Emergency Department, ER One Institute, Washington Hospital Center of MedStar Health, Washington, DC, USA

Shlomo Mor-Yosef, MD, MPA
Associate Professor, Department of Obstetrics and Gynecology, Hadassah Hebrew
University Medical Center, Director General, Hadassah University Hospital,
Jerusalem, Israel

Rami Mosheiff, MD
Associate Professor of Orthopedic Surgery, Department of Orthopedic Surgery,
Hadassah Hebrew University Medical Center, Jerusalem, Israel

David O'Reilly, MB, BCh, MRCS
Specialist Registrar in General Surgery, Royal Air Force; Research
Associate, Academic Department for Military Surgery and Trauma,
Royal Centre for Defence Medicine, Birmingham, UK

Meir Oren, MD, MSc, MPH
Director-General, The Hillel-Yaffe Medical Center, Hadera, Israel; Chairman, The
National Advisory Committee of Hospital Preparedness for Biological
Exceptional Scenario, (BW, Bioterrorism, Natural Outbreaks), The Ministry
of Health, Hadera, Israel

Eran Regev, DMD, MD
Clinical Senior Lecturer, Department of Oral and Maxillofacial Surgery,
Hadassah Hebrew University Medical Center, Jerusalem, Israel

Avraham I. Rivkind, MD, FACS
Associate Professor of Surgery, Director, Department of General
Surgery, Shock Trauma Unit, Hadassah Hebrew University Medical Center,
Jerusalem, Israel

Jeffrey V. Rosenfeld, MD, MS, FRACS, FRCS(Ed), FACS, FRCS(Glasg)Hon.
Professor and Head, Department of Surgery, Monash University; Director,
Department of Neurosurgery, The Alfred Hospital, Melbourne, Australia

William P. Schecter, MD
Professor of Clinical Surgery, Department of Surgery, University of California-
San Francisco, San Francisco General Hospital, San Francisco, CA, USA

Shmuel C. Shapira, MD, MPH
Professor of Medical Administration, Director, Hebrew University-Hadassah
School of Public Health, Deputy Director General, Hadassah University
Hospital, CEO, International Center of Terror Medicine, Jerusalem, Israel

Annette L. Sobel, MD, MS
Major General, USAF (Res.), Tijeras, NM, USA

Kristan Staudenmayer, MD
Trauma Fellow, Clinical Instructor in Surgery, Department of Surgery,
University of California-San Francisco, CA, USA

Tomer Tzur, MD
Department of Plastic and Reconstructive Surgery, Hadassah Hebrew University
Medical Center, Jerusalem, Israel

Abraham R. Wagner, MA, PhD, JD
Professor of International and Public Affairs, School of International and Public
Affairs, Columbia University, New York, NY, USA

Rephael Zeltser, DMD, DipOdOnt.
Associate Clinical Professor of Oral and Maxillofacial Surgery, Director,
Department of Oral and Maxillofacial Surgery, Hadassah Hebrew University
Medical Center, Jerusalem, Israel

Part I
INTRODUCTION

1
Introduction to Terror Medicine

Shmuel C. Shapira, Jeffrey S. Hammond, and Leonard A. Cole

In this era of global terrorism, the medical community has had to confront new and difficult challenges. In some regions of the world, the nature of terror attacks and the effects on victims have prompted novel approaches to rescue operations, diagnosis, treatment, and coordination of services. These measures and others, which collectively may be described as terror medicine, are the subject of this book. Although distinctive in its own right, terror medicine is related to the fields of emergency and disaster medicine. The principal mission of emergency medicine, which has been recognized as a specialty since the late 1960s, includes the evaluation, management, treatment, and prevention of unexpected illness and injury.[1] Subsequently, in the 1990s, disaster medicine was also seen as bearing singular characteristics that relate to the prevention, immediate response, and rehabilitation of the health problems arising from disaster.[2] Now the proliferation of terrorist attacks during the past decade has produced an understanding of the distinctive features of medical evaluation, treatment, and management associated with these assaults.

Whether a society has experienced many terrorism incidents or few, no part of the world remains free from the threat. The 35 contributors to this volume, all eminent specialists in areas related to the subject, understand that reality. Each chapter details a particular aspect of terror medicine. Some perspectives are framed by the authors' own country, but all speak to the unique responsibility of healthcare providers in the face of a terror attack. Many of the authors have personally helped save the lives of victims of such attacks. Most medical issues associated with terrorism are explored here with the benefit of these authors' tested knowledge. Taken as a whole, this volume can equip medical practitioners with a base of information that could prove invaluable in the event of an attack.

Role of the Medical Community

Emergency responders, physicians, nurses, and other health professionals are bound to serve in lead positions during and after a terror event. Engagement begins when paramedics and ambulances arrive at a scene and continues through the periods of acute and long-term care for victims and their families. Advance knowledge and preparation by providers are indispensable to highly effective medical responses.

S.C. Shapira et al. (eds.), *Essentials of Terror Medicine*,
DOI: 10.1007/978-0-387-09412-0_1, Springer Science+Business Media, LLC 2009

Every member of the healthcare community, from hospital director to psychological counselor, could play a crucial part during an event, and all have a responsibility to understand what their roles would be.

While certain principles about preparedness are universal, medical responses will vary according to the type of weapon used and the nature of injury. It is incumbent on practitioners to recognize the circumstances that would require their particular expertise. Thus, if a terrorist's weapons are conventional explosives, trauma surgeons and anesthesiologists are likely to be called to service. If chemical or radiological agents are dispersed, toxicologists, radiologists, and pulmonologists might be engaged. If biological agents are released, specialists in infectious disease and dermatology could be essential.

Beyond treating specific forms of injury, responders and emergency medicine physicians should anticipate handling large numbers of patients with multiple impairments. Victims of a suicide bombing may suffer from penetration wounds, inhalation injuries, blunt trauma, crush injuries, blast injuries, or burns. Under other conditions, combinations of these wounds are rarely seen in one patient, yet after a close-proximity terror bombing, scores of individuals often suffer from some or all of these injuries. Rapid determination of which injuries require priority attention can be a matter of life or death. Frequent experience with these attacks, most recently in Afghanistan and Iraq, but also for a longer period in Israel, has enabled medical personnel in those locations to respond with increased effectiveness. Clearly, there are lessons to be learned from those who have experience.

Some forms of terrorism pose particularly difficult challenges, including recognizing when biological or chemical weapons have been launched. Detection devices can sense the presence of some agents, though not all. Moreover, the apparatus would need to have been in the vicinity of a release. In fact, physicians are often better positioned than anyone else to make a determination. Whether diagnosing an individual case of anthrax, plague, or smallpox (all potentially caused by a bioattack), or through syndromic surveillance that identifies outbreaks of more familiar ailments, the role of the health professional can be pivotal. The difficulty in identifying such modes of attack is evident from past experience. Recognition that biological or chemical agents were deliberately released has often come long after the fact. In 1984, an outbreak of salmonella poisoning in Oregon was initially attributed to unsanitary food handling in some restaurants. But nearly a year later, Rajneesh cult members confessed to having laced local salad bars with salmonella bacteria.[3]

In 1994, seven people in Matsumoto, Japan, died, presumably from accidental exposure to an unidentified toxic material. The following year, Aum Shinrikyo cult members released sarin nerve agent in the Tokyo subway and later admitted having dispersed that same lethal agent in Matsumoto.[4] Similarly, in the fall of 2001, letters containing anthrax spores were leaking the deadly bacteria throughout the US postal system. Early victims of the disease were unaware that they had been exposed to the organisms, nor did their doctors realize their illness was due to anthrax bacteria. Widespread contamination of buildings with spores was not recognized until a month after the mailings had begun.[5] The perpetrator of the anthrax attacks was not identified until seven years later.

In all three cases, physicians were among the first professionals to see the victims. Although some were suspicious of the cause of illness, most were oblivious to the possibility of any connection to terrorism. Had they been aware of the causal mechanisms, symptoms, and relationship to terrorism of agents like these, medical responses could have been quicker and lives might have been saved. While biological and chemical attacks have been infrequent, their potential to cause great damage cannot be ignored. Concerns about their threat can only be heightened by the fact that Al-Qaeda and other terrorist organizations have sought to develop and use such weapons.[6]

Terrorism and Medicine

Terrorism has been variously defined, but it commonly refers to deliberate violence against innocent individuals to instill fear and influence political outcomes.[7] Murderous attacks against innocent people, especially by suicide bombers, increased dramatically toward the end of the twentieth century and into the twenty-first. The targets were in countries with diverse populations and political systems including Egypt, India, Indonesia, Iraq, Israel, Kenya, Pakistan, Russia, Saudi Arabia, Spain, Sri Lanka, Tanzania, Turkey, the United Kingdom, and the United States.[8]

Repeated terror attacks in India, Russia, Sri Lanka, and Turkey have cumulatively resulted in thousands of casualties. The jetliner assaults on the World Trade Center and the Pentagon in the United States on September 11, 2001, killed nearly 3,000 people. In the West, subsequent terror bombings were launched on a Madrid train in 2004 and in the London metro in 2005, though they caused fewer fatalities than in the US incident. Meanwhile, between 2000 and 2006, Palestinians attempted some 20,000 terror attacks against Israelis.[9] More than 95% of these efforts were thwarted; still, about 1,100 Israelis were killed and 6,500 injured during that period. Israel's response and medical systems were sometimes strained, but the repeated attacks, including 150 suicide bombings, enabled Israelis to continually improve their techniques of rescue and treatment. Several concepts of terror medicine arose from Israel's experiences and the remainder of this introductory chapter makes reference to a number of them. Not all Israeli medical practices may be applicable elsewhere, but many are. The distinctive qualities of terror medicine, burnished by the Israeli experience, lie in four broad areas: preparedness, incident management, mechanisms of injuries and responses, and psychological consequences.

Preparedness[10*]

Preparedness ranges from the development of standard operating procedures to the stockpiling of supplies in accessible locations. These stored materials should match the needs of casualties, not only casualties caused by explosives but also those caused

---

*The following discussion derives in part from Ref. 10.

by other potential weapons including chemical, biological, and radiological agents. These include smallpox vaccine and the antibiotics ciprofloxacin and doxycycline to treat anthrax and other illnesses associated with select biological agents; atropine and pyridostigmine bromide to counter the effects of sarin or soman nerve agents; and potassium iodide to mitigate damage from exposure to certain types of radiation.[11]

The United States is well positioned in this regard. Its Strategic National Stockpile (formerly called the National Pharmaceutical Stockpile) includes 50-ton packets of medical supplies and equipment stored at eight secret locations around the country. Within 12 hours, a packet can be flown to any site in the country to enhance local stockpiles.[12]

In addition to drug supplies, preparedness requires quick access by hospitals to equipment such as extra ventilators, vital-sign monitors, emergency mobile carts, communications apparatus like portable radios and walkie-talkies, and decontamination and toxic sewage facilities.[13] Hospitals commonly have shower facilities available for decontamination, but they should also have reserve wash-down capabilities in case of mass exposures to chemical or radiological materials.

Preparedness requires the ability to address sharp increases in the number of casualties. The government of Israel mandates that every hospital be able to handle at least 20% more emergencies than its usual capacity. Several Israeli hospitals have developed surge capacities that greatly exceed the minimal requirement. In 2005, a newly built Center for Emergency Medicine was opened at Hadassah University Hospital in Jerusalem. In minutes, the emergency bed capacity can be doubled to more than 100. The center's 4-ft-thick stone and cement walls can withstand massive explosive impact. Two sets of shatterproof glass for each window can prevent outside air from entering the hospital. A room adjacent to the emergency area is filled with ducts and filters that can recirculate the indoor air. This self-contained system can function for more than a week.

Other hospitals, including Tel Hashomer in Tel Aviv and the Western Galilee Hospital in Nahariya, have large underground rooms with hundreds of empty beds and IV stands at the ready. During the summer of 2006, Hezbollah militants in Lebanon launched 4,000 missiles into northern Israel. At the outset of the month-long conflict, every patient in the Western Galilee Hospital was moved underground. As a result, a missile that later destroyed the fourth floor ophthalmology department failed to cause even one human casualty.

Finally, preparedness requires educating healthcare workers about the various conventional and nonconventional agents, their clinical effects, and their implications for medical and administrative management. This is accomplished through lectures, seminars, and simulation exercises. Hospitals should participate in periodic citywide and regional exercises that build on lessons from actual events. A practice drill may involve hundreds of mock "casualties" from a variety of weapons.[14] In the end, drills and exercises that simulate conditions of an actual event are indispensable to proper preparedness.

Incident Management

A second defining area of terror medicine relates to incident management. Distinctive procedures begin when emergency medical responders arrive at a scene and a pre-assigned triage commander assesses the condition of individual victims. Since the modus operandi is *scoop and run*, only minimal treatment is provided at the attack site: maintenance of an airway, needle drainage of tension pneumothorax, and local pressure to stop external bleeding. The most severely injured survivors are triaged to a "level 1 trauma center," a hospital with advanced equipment and special expertise in trauma therapy. The less seriously injured may be sent to level 2 or 3 trauma centers with efforts not to overload any single hospital. On the basis of the experience of recent years, Israeli ambulances begin to arrive at hospitals within minutes of an attack. By the end of the first hour, 90% of the victims are in a hospital.[15]

A second triage occurs at each hospital where patients may be arriving as often as one every 20 seconds. At the emergency area entrance, the designated surgeon-in-charge assesses each new patient. Patients are triaged to one of three admission sites according to severity of injury: (1) severe and critical, (2) moderate, and (3) mild. The frequency of recent events has prompted hospitals to refine triage and hasten the admissions process.[16]

Incident management also includes wariness that a second attack may be attempted soon after the first. Thus, *scoop and run* means not only quicker hospital care for victims, but a rapid clearing of the target area, which simplifies the security efforts at that location. Massive numbers of casualties could also prompt another deviation from conventional rescue. Rather than trying to provide optimal care for each patient, the philosophy shifts to providing help to those most likely to benefit. Thus, if resources are limited, priority attention goes not necessarily to those most gravely ill, but to those with the best chance of recovery if given timely care.

Protocols should also be in place for a variety of communication requirements that connect hospitals with each other and with law enforcement authorities and inquiring families. With computer assistance, hospitals should be able to quickly share information about their patients so that family members can find each other.[17] This need was highlighted by news reports in August 2003, when a young mother and her baby were among scores of victims of a suicide bombing of a Jerusalem bus. She was pulled from the carnage and awoke in Shaare Zedick Hospital without her baby. At first frantic, her distress was eased after hospital-to-hospital inquiries located the unidentified baby at Hadassah, where he was being treated for noncritical injuries.[18]

Terrorists have also sought to exploit the medical system. Since the discovery in 2003 of weapons and gunmen in some Palestinian ambulances that were ostensibly carrying patients, all ambulances, even if conveying critically injured victims, must pause for brief inspection at the perimeter of a hospital's ground.[19]

Injuries and Responses

The third area of terror medicine encompasses the nature of injuries and manner of treatment. The worldwide spate of attacks with explosives has signaled the need for physicians and other healthcare providers to become familiar with the effects of blast devices.[20–22] Analysts have divided the cumulative information about blast effects into four categories.[23] Primary blast injuries arise from rapid changes in air pressure that can rupture the tympanic membrane (ear drum) and severely disrupt the lungs and other organs. Secondary blast injuries include penetrating wounds from fragments and other uneven projectiles. Tertiary blast injuries arise from compression caused by the collapse of buildings and the hurling of victims or surrounding objects. The quaternary category covers all other injuries from blast, including burns, crush injuries, and damage from the inhalation of toxic particles.

Accepted forms of treatment for each type of injury generally predated contemporary terrorism. But novel features of terror attacks include their frequency, the likelihood of finding multiple mechanisms of injury, the deliberate targeting of children and other innocents, and the consequent need for treatment strategies to address these conditions. A close-quarter bombing generates a combination of injuries that is otherwise rarely seen in a single individual: numerous penetration wounds from small projectiles (nails, screws, etc.) that damage soft tissues and vital organs; fractured bone and severed arteries and nerves; blast effects on the lungs, the tympanic membrane, and other organs; and severe burns.

This expansive list of injuries suffered by large numbers of victims prompted Israeli trauma surgeons to modify their response protocols. For example, multiple penetration wounds are now simply packed to avoid excessive loss of blood and loss of heat, while the patient is operated on for more serious injuries. Experience also showed that patients who seemed stable were in fact suffering from severe injury that was not initially obvious, such as internal bleeding from a severed blood vessel. Thus, repeated reassessments are warranted, which increases the likelihood of discovering critical injuries that were not first apparent.[24]

Beyond injuries generated by explosives, terror medicine includes effects of nonconventional agents—chemical, biological, radiological, and nuclear. If recognized in time, infection from bacterial agents like *Bacillus anthracis* and *Yersinia pestis* (the cause of plague) can be treated with antibiotics. In the case of smallpox, vaccination may offer protection even if administered a few days after exposure to the virus. Similarly, antidotes, if administered in time, can neutralize the effects of certain chemical agents and some forms of radiation. Terrorist groups have shown interest in delivering lethal combinations of conventional and nonconventional agents. Organizations including Hamas and al-Fatah sought to detonate explosives mixed with the anticoagulant rat poison warfarin, with AIDS-tainted blood, and with the chemical hydrogen cyanide.[25-27]

Psychological Consequences

The fourth component of terror medicine relates to the psychological effects of terror assaults. Terror incidents are recognized as a new kind of traumatic event that combines features of criminal assaults, disasters, acts of war, homicide, and political violence. As manifested by survivors of the 9/11 jetliner attacks, the sense of rage, grief, and despair becomes compounded.[28] Experience elsewhere has also shown that initial psychological reactions after a terror attack are more intense than from other traumatic events like road accidents. Accordingly, early psychological intervention is essential. If not appropriately treated during the first 6 months after an incident, patients may suffer irreversible stress disorders.[29–31]

Israelis have undertaken a community response to the psychological effects of terrorism. Teams of psychologists and social workers visit day-care centers and schools to interview teachers about the behavior of youngsters in their care. They have been able to identify and help children who have been traumatized by terror incidents but whose parents had not previously sought psychological assistance for them.[32,33]

The psychological aspects of terror medicine also encompass the heightened emotional effects prompted by certain weapons. Biological weapons in particular can generate frightening reactions. People experiencing common forms of attack, such as the bombing of a bus or building, tend to act rationally because their sensory cues enable them to assess the threat and plan the rescue. But lethal bacteria and viruses might not produce symptoms for days or weeks after exposure. The insidiousness of a bioattack and the extended period of uncertainty after exposure can elevate anxiety. Treatment of these heightened emotional states can be more difficult.[34]

The anthrax attacks in the United States in the fall of 2001 underscored the widespread anxiety that can be caused by a bioattack. Perhaps a half-dozen letters containing spores of *B. anthracis* were mailed to government and media offices. Because of leakage from the letters, some 30,000 people were considered at risk of exposure and were treated with prophylactic antibiotics. But anxiety reached far beyond those directly at risk. Pharmacists and physicians were inundated by demands for antibiotics by fearful customers and patients who were in no particular danger. People in all parts of the country became afraid to open mail.[35]

Stress in the general population prompted by the anthrax attacks may have exceeded that generated by the jetliner attacks on September 11, 2001. One study suggested that the more time a person spent watching television coverage of the jetliner attacks, the more likely he was to have a stress reaction.[36] But another study found that media exposure to the anthrax attacks predicted distress, while media exposure to 9/11 did not.[37] The particularly stressful effect of deliberately released biological agents is attributable to their being invisible, potentially lethal, and hard to avoid and control. Addressing the emotional reaction to such events may be enhanced through an understanding of "terror management theory," which includes consideration of an individual's worldview and awareness of one's own mortality.[38]

Conclusion

The constellation of medical issues related to terror attacks can be understood as comprising terror medicine. Although aspects of terror medicine overlap with emergency and disaster medicine, several characteristics, as shown here, are distinctive. Besides preparedness, management, nature of injuries, and psychological effects, these include the intentionality behind an attack, the threat to healthcare providers, and the need for special security measures. The uniqueness of terror medicine as a field derives from features beyond the usual scope of trauma surgery, clinical microbiology, infectious disease, internal medicine, and psychotherapy. The field integrates knowledge relevant to the medical management of terror victims and the spectrum and pattern of their injuries. It serves as a basis for developing curricula and standard operating procedures toward prevention, treatment, and rehabilitation both of individuals and of communities.

Efforts to discourage and prevent terrorist attacks should be among a society's highest priorities. No less important are the requirements to prepare for, respond to, and recover from these events. Not only do these capabilities enhance the rates of survival, but they also strengthen a society's overall resilience and ability to cope. Describing the features of terror medicine broadens understanding of the subject and can help develop its systematic study. The more that individuals and institutions become familiar with the essentials of terror medicine, the greater the protection they can provide to others.

The vast majority of physicians, nurses, and other health practitioners in the United States and elsewhere have had no exposure to terror medicine. The purpose of this book is to provide a coherent structure to the lessons both from past experiences and those posed by anticipated future events.

References

1. Schneider SM, et al. Definition of emergency medicine. *Acad Emerg Med.* 1998; 5:348.
2. Gunn SWA, Masellis M. The scientific basis of disaster medicine. *Ann MBC.* 1992; 5:1.
3. Torok TJ, Tauxe RV, Wise, RP, Livengood JR, Sokolow R, Mauvais S, Birkness KA, Skeels MR, Horan JM, Foster LR. A large community outbreak of salmonellosis caused by intentional contamination of restaurant salad bars. *JAMA.* 1997; 278:389–395.
4. Olson KB. Aum Shinrikyo: once and future threat? *Emerg Infect Dis.* 1999; 5:513–516.
5. Cole LA. *The Anthrax Letters: A Medical Detective Story.* Washington, DC: Joseph Henry Press/National Academies Press; 2003: 72–94.
6. National Commission on Terrorist Attacks upon the United States. *The 9/11 Commission Report.* NY: W.W. Norton; 2004: 151.
7. Hoffman B. *Inside Terrorism* (rev.). New York: Columbia University Press; 2006: 1–20.
8. Pape RA. *Dying to Win: The Strategic Logic of Suicide Terrorism.* New York: Random House; 2005: 3–5.
9. Address by Israeli Prime Minister Ehud Olmert to the U.S. Congress. *Wash Post.* May 24, 2006. http://www.washingtonpost.com/wp-dyn/content/article/2006/05/24/AR2006052401420.html. Accessed Oct. 10, 2007.
10. Shapira S, Cole, LA. Terror medicine: birth of a discipline. *J Homeland Security Emerg Manage.* 2006; 3. http://www.bepress.com/jhsem/vol3/iss2/9/. Accessed December 7, 2007.
11. Cole LA. *The Eleventh Plague: The Politics of Biological and Chemical Warfare.* New York: W.H. Freeman; 1998: 134–139.
12. Centers for Disease Control and Prevention. April 14, 2005. http://www.bt.cdc.gov/stockpile/. Accessed Aug. 5, 2005.
13. Shapira SC, Shemer J. Medical management of terrorist attacks. *Israel Med Assoc J.* 2002; 4:489–492.

14. Gofrit ON, Leibovici D, Shemer J, Henig A, Shapira SC. The efficacy of integrating "smart simulated casualties" in hospital disaster drills. *Prehospital Disaster Med.* 1997; 12:26–30.

15. Aschkenasy-Steuer G, Shamir M, Rivkind A, Mosheiff R, Shushan Y, Rosenthal G, Mintz Y, Weissman, C, Sprung CL, Weiss YG. Clinical review: the Israel experience: conventional terrorism and critical care. *Crit Care.* 2005; 9.

16. Leibovici D, Gofrit ON, Heruti RJ, Shapira SC, Shemer J, Stein M. Interhospital patient transfer: a quality improvement indicator for prehospital triage. *Am J Emerg Med.* 1997; 15:341–344.

17. Shapira SC, Mor-Yosef S. Terror politics and medicine: the role of leadership. *Studies in Conflict Terrorism.* 2004; 27:65–71.

18. Matza M. Family separated in bus bombing reunited through nurse's work. Knight Ridder Newspapers, August 20, 2003. http://static.highbeam.com/k/knightriddertrib-unenewsservice/august202003/familyseparatedinbusbombingreunitedthroughnurseswo/. Accessed July 20, 2005.

19. Israel Ministry of Foreign Affairs. The Palestinian use of ambulances and medical materials for terror. Dec. 22, 2003. http://www.mfa.gov.il/MFA/MFAArchive/2000_2009/2003/12/The+Palestinian+use+of+ambulances+and+medical+mate.htm. Accessed July 25, 2005.

20. Gutierrez deCeballos JP, Turegano Fuentes F, Perez Diaz D, Sanz Sanchez M, Martin Llorente C, Guerrero Sanz JE. Casualties treated at the closest hospital in Madrid, March 11, terrorist bombings. *Crit Care Med.* 2005; 33:107–112.

21. Roduplu U, Arnold JL, Tokyay R, Ersoy G, Cetiner S, Yucel T. Mass-casualty terrorist bombings in Istanbul, Turkey, November 2003: report of the events and the prehospital emergency response. *Prehospital Disaster Med.* 2004; 2:133–145.

22. Stein M, Hirshberg A. Medical consequences of terrorism: the conventional weapon threat. *Surg Clin North Am.* 1999; 79:1537–1552.

23. DePalma RG, Burris DG, Champion HR, Hodgson MJ. Blast injuries. *N Engl J Med.* 2005; 352:1335–1345.

24. Almogy G, Belzberg H, Mintz Y, Pikarsky AK, Zamir G, Rivkind AI. Suicide bombing attacks: update and modification to the protocol. *Ann Surg.* 2004; 239:295–303.

25. Bryen SD. Poison multiplies terror. *Baltimore Sun*, December 13, 2001; reprinted as "Bio-Terrorism in Israel" at http://cryptome.org/bio-terr-il.htm. Accessed June 15, 2005.

26. Hamas threatens to use chemical weapons against Israel. *World Tribune.com*, June 17, 2002, http://216.26.163.62/2002/me_palestinians_06_17.html. Accessed June 15, 2005.

27. Terrorists attempted bio-warfare attack. *Maariv*, April 13, 2004, http://maarivenglish.com/index.cfm?fuseaction=article&articleID=5889. Accessed June 15, 2005.

28. Miller L. Psychotherapeutic interventions for survivors of terrorism. *Am J Psychother.* 2004; 58:1–16.

29. Kroll J. Posttraumatic symptoms and the complexity of responses to trauma. *JAMA.* 2003; 290:667–670.

30. Bleich A, Gelkopf M, Solomon Z. Exposure to terrorism, stress-related mental health symptoms, and coping behaviors among a nationally representative sample in Israel. *JAMA.* 2003; 290:612–620.

31. Shalev A, Galili-Weisstub E. Panel on Terror Medicine and Domestic Security, Jerusalem, May 30, 2005.

32. Brom D. Panel on Terror Medicine and Domestic Security, Jerusalem, May 30, 2005.

33. Baum NL. Building resilience: a school-based intervention for children exposed to ongoing trauma and stress, in Danieli Y, Brom D, Sills J, eds. *The Trauma of Terrorism.* Binghamton, NY: Haworth Press, 2005: 487–498.

34. Kron S, Mendlovic, S. Mental health consequences of bioterrorism. *Israel Med Assoc J.* 2002; 4:526.
35. Cole. *The Anthrax Letters*: 70–71.
36. Schuster MA, Stein BD, Jaycox LH, Collins RL, Marshall GN, Elliott MN, Zhou AJ, Kanouse DE, Morrison JL, Berry SH. A national survey of stress reactions after the September 11, 2001, terrorist attacks. *N Engl J Med.* 2001; 345:1507–1512.
37. Dougall AL, Hayward MC, Baum A. Media exposure to bioterrorism: stress and the anthrax attacks. *Psychiatry.* 2005; 68:28–43.
38. Pyszcynski TA, Solomon S, Greenberg J. *In the Wake of 9/11: The Psychology of Terror.* Washington, DC: American Psychological Association; 2003.

2
Terrorism in the Twenty-First Century

Boaz Ganor

Terrorism is not a new phenomenon; it has long been a method of violent action by organizations and individuals attempting to achieve political goals. Indeed, terrorism is not an end but rather a modus operandi. According to Bruce Hoffman, all terrorists share one common denominator: they "live" in the future, and are convinced that they will defeat their enemies and achieve their political goals.[1]

There are perhaps hundreds of different definitions of terrorism, all of which tend to reflect the political world-view of the definer. The same act of violence can be classified differently, depending on the identities of the perpetrators. Groups that engage in identical behavior might be considered by their sympathizers as *freedom fighters*, and by their enemies as *terrorists*. For the purposes of this chapter, the working assumption is that terrorism is a modus operandi in which deliberate violence against civilians is used for the purpose of achieving political goals. In this respect, it is the intentional harming of civilians, which is at the core of terrorism, that makes this modus operandi illegitimate, even if it is meant, prima facie, to achieve justified objectives. This definition makes a distinction between an action intended to harm civilians and one intended to harm military and security personnel. The latter is defined as a guerilla or insurgency action, even though the perpetrator might use the same modus operandi (shooting, suicide bombing, or rocket fire). Thus, in seeking to achieve the same political objectives, an organization or perpetrator might carry out a "terrorist" attack on one occasion and a "guerilla" attack on another. Furthermore, even the political goal of an organization may change as it engages in acts of terrorism or guerilla warfare. Sometimes attacks are executed for the purpose of achieving social, economic, or national goals, such as a separate state or national liberation.

In yet other contexts, attacks are carried out in the service of a certain extreme ideology, such as communism, fascism, and anarchism. However, it is when terrorists are motivated by what they identify as a religious mission – when they regard themselves as the messengers of god – that the highest level of danger is introduced. When motivated by a religious purpose, such terrorist operatives do not perceive room for compromise; their objective is served only by an all-out war. At most, cease-fire agreements can be negotiated for limited time periods.

S.C. Shapira et al. (eds.), *Essentials of Terror Medicine*,
DOI: 10.1007/978-0-387-09412-0_2, Springer Science+Business Media, LLC 2009

Modern Terrorism

Modern history has seen the rise of terrorist organizations, diverse in their political objectives and geographic origins. All these organizations, however, share one, unifying variable – their reliance on the use of violence against civilians to achieve their goals. The decision to embrace terrorism as their preferred modus operandi is the outcome of a rational decision-making process, based on a cost–benefit analysis that leaves terrorism outweighing any other alternative. The decision to conduct a terrorist act does not necessarily mean that the perpetrators are "abnormal" or that they suffer from severe personality disorders. Rather, a rational calculation of the costs and benefits leads them to adopt the modus operandi,[2] which they perceive as being the most effective method to achieve their political objectives and make a mark in their theater of operations.[3]

The dynamic nature of terrorism further exacerbates the threat such actors pose to security officials. Even if they achieve success in foiling terrorist plots, security agencies cannot rest on their accomplishments as terrorist organizations constantly change their tactics, organizational structure, and even their tactical objectives. As such, terrorist groups and those who work to counter them are constantly competing strategically in an attempt to stay one step ahead of each other, whether via new technologies or operational tactics. In this manner, the phenomenon of terrorism has evolved over the years, with each stage emerging more dangerous and lethal than the preceding stage.

As opposed to targeting state leaders or political rivals for assassination, modern terrorism does not necessarily aim to change a political reality through the direct removal of a leader. Instead, terrorists seek to achieve their political goals indirectly, using psychological warfare as their weapon. The anxiety that terrorism creates in the target population translates into political pressure, intended to coerce decision-makers into changing their policies according to the interests of the terrorist organization.

As the term implies, terrorism does in fact aim to "terrorize" its target population. While terrorist attacks are ordinarily limited in terms of resulting fatalities, their effect does not stop with the physically harmed crowd.[4] A message of intimidation and fear is passed to the general public through the terrorist act itself and the resulting media coverage. Video cassettes edited by terrorist organizations, false alarms of possible follow-up attacks, and other methods adopted by terrorist groups, all contribute to a general sense of anxiety and fear.

One of the most crucial elements in this campaign of psychological warfare is mass media. Terrorist groups rely on mass media to transfer their messages of fear and intimidation to the public.[5,6] This fear can be understood in two different spheres: rational fear and irrational anxiety. Rational fear is a natural response to the perceived risk of getting physically injured in a terrorist attack, no matter how remote the probability. To a certain degree, such "rational fear" is actually positive in that it encourages public vigilance and awareness of one's immediate surroundings, thus allowing citizens themselves to help in thwarting attacks.[7] A vigilant civilian is an important arm of the security apparatus.

However, modern terrorism is aimed primarily at heightening the public's fear of terrorism to a level of irrational and uncontrolled anxiety. The random nature of terrorist attacks actually personalizes the threat: anybody, including one's self or a loved one, could be the next victim. Such irrational fear translates into political pressure on leaders to fulfill terrorist demands, as people feel they must do whatever it takes to halt a terrorist campaign. This is essentially the method of modern terrorism, which has come to characterize the activities of all terrorist organizations in the second half of the twentieth century and the beginning of the twenty-first century.

Modern Terrorism at the End of the Twentieth Century

Modern terrorism became common toward the end of the twentieth century due to, among other things, advances in technology, the development of new weapons, and the activities of some governments after World War II. In the period of the cold war and nuclear deterrence, the phenomenon of state-sponsored terrorism developed as an alternative to traditional warfare. Terrorist organizations were utilized within a framework of local conflicts and used as tools to expand the global influence of a superpower, for example, the Soviets.

While terrorism sponsored by states such as Libya, Syria, Iraq, and Sudan decreased at the end of the twentieth century, other states, including Afghanistan and Pakistan, became more involved with terrorist groups.

The intervention of "big powers" in regional disputes, as in Bosnia, Kosovo, Chechnya, and the Gulf War, may have led sub-state groups and third world countries to turn to terrorism or other low intensity measures as a means of fighting for their causes in the face of disproportionate military power. In the past, political goals could be achieved only through the use of armies in a conventional war setting; today, it requires only a handful of determined individuals. By engaging in terrorist activities, these attackers can achieve the same aims without putting the burden of blame on a state sponsor. Examples can be drawn from attacks executed in Dhahran in Saudi Arabia in June 1996 and against the American military training facility in Riyadh in November 1995.

Terrorism is a form of asymmetric warfare in which a non-state actor fights a state. However, contrary to the popular understanding of the term, the balance of power between the two actors does not necessarily favor the state. Even though, prima facie, the state has stronger military, intelligence, and economic capabilities than the terrorist organization, a modern liberal-democratic state is subject to the rules of war and harboring of values, which, in effect, restrict its ability to operate and maneuver. A form of reverse asymmetry is established as a result: in a conflict portrayed as a war between David and Goliath, Goliath (the state) is bound hand and foot, while David (the substate actor) is exempt from all moral or legal restraints.

At the end of the twentieth century, the phenomenon of modern terrorism experienced another shift in terms of geography. Terrorist activity increased in central and south Asia, shifting focus from the traditional epicenter of the Middle

East. This shift can be largely attributed to the emergence of Wahhabist-Salafist fundamentalist terrorist groups founded by Afghan "veterans." Afghanistan had additionally become the central base for international terrorist organization training camps, headquarters, and offices, some of which had formerly been based in Lebanon.[8]

One of the most important developments in the 1990s was the creation in February 1998 of Osama Bin Laden's "World Islamic Front for Jihad against the Jews and the Crusaders."[9] Bin Laden had identified terrorism as a tool for achieving the group's goal of bringing Islamic rule to Muslim lands and "cleansing" them of Western influence and corruption. He established operational connections with Islamic fundamentalist groups in Egypt, Algeria, Yemen, Tunisia, Indonesia, Jordan, and other countries. He also inspired and instigated Islamist groups worldwide to wage war against their own governments and internationally against the United States and its allies.[10]

When Bin Laden initiated his "World Islamic Front for Jihad against the Jews and Crusaders," he issued a Fatwa (Islamic legal ruling) proclaiming it a religious duty for all Muslims to wage war on US citizens, whether military personnel or civilians, anywhere in the world. Soon after, his organization took responsibility for the violent terrorist attacks against the US embassies in Kenya and Tanzania.

One of the most important terrorist events at the end of the twentieth century was the chemical attack by the Japanese cult Aum Shinrikyo in Tokyo in 1995. Aum members released the nerve agent sarin in the Tokyo subway with the aim of inflicting mass casualties. That attack resulted in 12 deaths and a limited number of injured. The organization's earlier releases of anthrax from the roof of its headquarters building failed to cause any casualties.[11] In the wake of the sarin attack, the Japanese government initiated a severe crackdown on the doomsday cult, which was founded on a fusion of religious, spiritual, and supernatural doctrines. Amidst increasing public pressure, the government established legal restrictions against Aum Shinrikyo.

Even so, security officials and academics warned that Aum Shinrikyo's introduction of unconventional weapons into the arena of terrorism was a kind of "crossing the Rubicon," and would be followed by similar attempts at causing mass casualties. After the attack in Tokyo and the cult's attempted biological assaults, other terrorist organizations were expected to follow the lead of the Japanese group. This prediction, however, is yet to be realized.

Terrorism at the Beginning of the Twenty-First Century

Instead, on September 11, 2001, the world awakened to a new danger – global jihadi terrorism of unanticipated magnitude. The attacks represented a transformation in international terrorism, both on the scale and the motive: these attacks were motivated by religious grievances. The message conveyed to the public through the attacks was that no place is safe. No state is immune – not even a superpower like the United States.

The September 11 attacks represented a new reality in international terrorism. The world community, in the wake of these attacks, found itself seemingly in unprecedented peril. The face of international terrorism had changed. But the phenomenon of global jihadi terrorism has roots and ramifications that reach back several years.

Before 9/11, it was convenient for many states and world leaders to turn a blind eye to the unfolding threat, as long as they were not its direct victims or its central focus. Indeed, the radical Islamic movement originally focused not on attacking western targets, but on conquering the hearts and minds of Muslim communities all over the world through educational, religious, and welfare activities, known as "*dawah*" activities. These activities were based on the dogmatic radical perspectives of the movement, which praised the use of violence in "defense of Islam." Still, in most cases, the principle remained theoretical, and the call to violence never manifested itself as a concrete act of violent terrorist activity. This made it possible – and even convenient – for world leaders to underestimate the threat. The death of nearly 3,000 civilians, the collapse of the World Trade Center buildings, and the destruction of parts of the Pentagon building on September 11th, forced the international community – and especially the American people and US administration – to acknowledge the imminent threat of terrorism.[12]

Since then, members of the global jihadi network have not hesitated to utilize a method of modern terrorism that has proved more effective than any other, namely, suicide attacks.

The Suicide Attack Phenomenon

A suicide attack is an "operational method in which the very act of the attack is dependent upon the death of the perpetrator."[13] A suicide attack is carried out by a terrorist operative who activates explosives worn or carried in the form of a portable explosive device, or planted in a vehicle he is driving. The terrorist is fully aware that if he does not kill himself, the planned attack will not be successful.

The suicide attack phenomenon is spreading; more and more terrorist organizations, primarily radical Islamic in nature, are finding this modus operandi very productive. Since a bomber can choose the time and place to launch the attack, and can consider the circumstances he encounters, suicide attacks maximize potential casualties and cause extensive damage. Other techniques, such as a timer-activated bomb or even a remote-controlled explosive, can be deactivated by security forces before causing any damage. But a suicide bomber is an unusually sophisticated smart bomb – a carrier who brings the explosive device to the right location and detonates it at the right time.

Because of the high number of casualties these cause, suicide attacks generally attract wide media coverage. A suicide attack is of news interest because it demonstrates extraordinary determination and self-sacrifice on the part of the terrorists. It is extremely difficult to thwart a suicide attack once the terrorist is on his way to the target location. Even if security forces succeed in stopping him before he reaches the intended target, he can still activate the explosive device and cause damage. Such attributes have made suicide attacks a very appealing option for jihadi organizations.

In addition, it is not only terrorist organizations that find suicide attacks appealing. The suicide attackers themselves also believe they will benefit personally by committing the "*istishad*" (martyrdom operation). Their extreme religious beliefs make them aspire to become "shahids" (martyrs), and they are thus happy to die for their cause. In fact, they believe that they will not really die at all, but will instead be guaranteed eternal life in paradise. In most cases of Muslim suicide bombers, among the perceived benefits are eternal life in paradise, the permission to see the face of Allah, and the loving kindness of 72 young virgins who will serve them in heaven. The *shahid* also takes altruistic motives into consideration: by committing a suicide attack, he earns the privilege to promise life in heaven to 70 of his relatives and friends.

All these factors create a substantial incentive for fundamentalist believers to adopt suicide attack tactics. As such, the growing phenomenon of suicide terrorism and the use of suicide attacks by global jihadi terrorists such as Al-Qaida should be considered a result of a rational decision-making process. It is a rational choice both by the terrorist organization that initiates, plans, prepares, and executes the attack; and by the perpetrators – the shahids – since, in their eyes, the benefits exceed all possible costs.

Global jihadi suicide attacks have proved to be the most effective and deadly method of modern terrorism. The only exception may be unconventional, CBRN (Chemical, Biological, Radiological, and Nuclear) terrorism.

Unconventional Terrorism

Despite some unsuccessful earlier attempts by terrorists to use unconventional weapons, the revival of international terrorism in the radical Islamic arena under the direction of Al-Qaida has renewed the threat of unconventional terrorism in the twenty-first century.

To determine what conditions must be in place for a terrorist organization to choose unconventional weapons, it is helpful to categorize the types of possible unconventional terrorism attacks. While it is customary to base such distinctions on the substance used – be it chemical, biological, nuclear, or radiological – one can also classify attacks by their intended result. One important distinction is that attacks using unconventional means can be "limited" or "unlimited" in nature.[14]

A limited unconventional attack differs from the standard terrorist bombing only in the means used. As in the case of a conventional assault, a limited unconventional attack aims to achieve political goals with both direct and indirect effects. By causing multiple casualties at the site of the attack it incites fear and anxiety among the larger public. A limited unconventional terrorist attack could be carried out by dispersing a chemical substance in an enclosed space, or by using explosives to disperse a radiological agent at a selected location. Another example of a limited unconventional attack would be a destructive assault on a facility containing dangerous substances, such as a military or industrial facility. In all these examples, the damage is of limited scope, although potentially more serious than a conventional attack on the same target.

As opposed to limited assaults, unlimited attacks are meant to cause damage or carnage not merely in a specific public area. Rather, they are designed to cause mass casualties in large areas (a town, a city, a specific geographical area, etc.). The conceptual basis of these two categories differs: while tactical, or limited, unconventional terrorism serves as leverage in altering a political reality indirectly through the use of intimidation, unlimited unconventional terrorism strives to change the political reality directly by annihilating large populations or contaminating extensive geographical regions. This type of attack may have a severe psychological impact on public morale. It may, in fact, completely undermine the population's confidence in government institutions and their values. Even without this effect though, the unlimited unconventional attack causes grave and prolonged damage to the target area.

In general, chemical attacks are mostly limited in scope, while biological attacks can be unlimited, especially if the bioagents are contagious. Nuclear attacks are unlimited, with far-reaching ecological impact, while radiological attacks are likely to be limited in scope. "The dirty bomb," for example, is an explosive device in the immediate vicinity of radiological material. When the explosives are detonated, the radiological material is spread across the target area.

By classifying unconventional terrorist attacks as limited or unlimited, counterterrorism experts and officials are better equipped to determine whether such attacks will likely be perpetrated in the foreseeable future. In general, the launching of "limited" unconventional terrorist attacks is within the capability of many organizations, but "unlimited" unconventional terrorism is less likely in the near future. As long as conventional, or limited unconventional, terrorist attacks remain an effective tactic of modern terrorist strategy – including the spread of fear and anxiety – terrorist groups are less likely to turn to the more extreme alternative of an unlimited unconventional attack, based on their rational calculation of cost and benefit. The extra costs, or challenges, associated with an unconventional attack – such as difficulty in obtaining materials, severe global reaction and response, justifying the act to their constituency, or the possibility of harming members of the population they identify with – may not be worth the perceived benefits – especially because fear and anxiety can effectively be created in the target population without engaging in an unlimited attack, which would cause more physical destruction.

Still, it is arguable that Islamic groups now active will usher in a new era in terrorism, launching a transition from conventional to unconventional terrorism. Organizations influenced or motivated by religious doctrine – a divine commandment, decree, or doomsday cult mentality – will calculate costs and benefits differently than their counterparts; their commands are nonnegotiable, influenced by an external force. Islamic radical spokesmen have already expressed their interest in using unconventional terrorism, and several plots have already been thwarted in

Europe and the Middle East, such as Islamic radical activists planning to launch attacks using ricin toxin and other poisons.

In addition to limited and unlimited attacks, the threat of unconventional terrorism will likely manifest itself in one of the following operational forms:

Threats to Use Unconventional Means

Individuals and organizations may threaten to use unconventional weapons if their demands are not met. This category can be divided into two sub-groups.

Attacks for the Purpose of Bargaining

Terrorist organizations may seize a certain installation – a structure or vehicle – threatening to unleash an unconventional weapon, which would kill hostages if their demands are not met. The terrorist operatives or hostage-takers might hold in their hands a device, box, or bottle, claiming it contains an unconventional material that, upon activation, would cause massive damage. The terrorists could be situated in a known location and surrounded by security forces. One challenge is to verify that the device in question actually contains unconventional material that could endanger the area.

Attacks for the Purpose of Extortion

In this case, the terrorist group or individual does not physically seize a defined installation, but rather sends a message to decision-makers threatening to carry out an attack with unconventional means if their demands are not met. This type of extortion will ordinarily be accompanied by an ultimatum that defines timetables. The first challenge facing decision-makers and security personnel is to determine whether the threat is genuine and whether those making the threat are capable of using unconventional means to cause casualties and damage. The target location for the attack may be unidentified, the number and location of terrorists unknown, and the ability of security forces to respond effectively unlikely. This subgroup can be further divided. Threats of "concrete extortion attacks" include a specific and defined target, such as a certain town and military installation. Threats of "general extortion attacks" do not specifically define the planned target. In determining the extent to which a threat is genuine, yet another classification is possible: a "tangible threat" occurs when there is indication that the terrorist organization is able to obtain unconventional means or carry out an attack using these means. An "intangible threat" occurs when there is no indication that the terrorist organization is able to carry out an attack using unconventional means. The level of concreteness and tangibility of extortion threats may gradually change, depending on the characteristics of the group making the threat.

Personal Terrorism Using Unconventional Means

This category includes attacks targeting specific figures using unconventional means. These attacks do not actually take advantage of the weapon's potential for mass damage, but are used because of other favorable characteristics such as ease of transport and concealment.

Scope of Damage

While deciding whether to carry out an unconventional assault, a terrorist organization will assess the scope of damage that may potentially be caused by the attack. Such a calculation involves four primary variables: The *number of direct casualties* caused during the attack and immediately after, the *direct economic damage* caused during the attack itself, the *area of damage* – the size of the geographic space affected by the unconventional attack – and no less important, *future damage* caused by the attack. Future damage can include long-term contamination of areas, physical injuries appearing at a later stage or in future generations, indirect economic damages due to loss of revenues from tourism, export, and more. Another variable could be added to this list: the *level of fear and anxiety* among the affected population because of the use of unconventional materials.

The potential damage caused by an unconventional terror attack is a result both of a specific *blueprint* for the attack designed by the organization, and the *type and quantity of unconventional material* used in the attack, whether chemical, biological, radiological, or nuclear.

The blueprint of an attack, whether conducted via conventional means (explosives, firearms, cold arms, etc.) or unconventional means (chemical, biological, radiological, or nuclear), consists of the following factors: *type of attack* – bargaining, mass killing, suicide; *target of attack* – civilian or military, crowded location, building, vehicle; and the *location of attack* – an open space, a closed facility, etc. In the unconventional terrorist attack, special significance is also given to the *method of attack* or the manner in which the unconventional material is released, whether through spraying, attacking a manufacturing or storage installation, poisoning, or a delay mechanism.

The terrorist organization can employ three operational methods in the execution of an unlimited attack.

Dispersal of Hazardous Materials

In this scenario, a terrorist organization may use chemical or biological materials that are generally limited in nature. To ensure that the attack is essentially unlimited, the perpetrators must maximize its effect through dispersal methods and the use of a sufficient quantity of unconventional materials.

Poisoning of Water and Food Sources

To achieve an unlimited effect through attacks in which water and food sources are poisoned, the terrorist organization must pollute large water sources or reservoirs and national or regional food depots, using chemical and/or biological materials.

Attack Involving Assault on an Installation

Terrorists can attack installations containing unconventional materials, causing contamination of the immediate surroundings (particularly when the installation is holding dangerous chemical materials). The scope may reach that of an unlimited threat when the targets are nuclear installations or facilities holding dangerous biological materials, and when these facilities are in the vicinity of large population centers. The assault may itself be executed by firing from a distance, causing a technical malfunction, or launching a ground or aerial suicide attack.

The Threat of Terrorism to the Healthcare System

As the phenomenon of international and domestic terrorism continues to develop, the healthcare system faces the challenge of providing effective medical attention for the casualties of attacks, and defending against assaults on the system itself.

Some of the challenges facing the healthcare system in dealing with terrorist attacks are described here.

Number of Casualties

The growing number of terrorist attacks, their global prevalence, and their severity in terms of fatalities, all constitute a growing challenge to health systems throughout the world. The aforementioned advantages of a suicide bomber – primarily the ability to maximize casualties by controlling the time and place of the attack – mean a large number of casualties are sent to the hospital after an attack.

Types of Injuries

In an attempt to maximize the number of casualties, terrorists often add metallic objects (nails, screws, ball bearings) to the explosives used in an attack. These efforts result in multisystem injuries that can complicate medical treatment.

Swiftness of the Transfer of Casualties to Hospitals

Efforts by emergency services to rapidly transfer casualties to hospitals after an attack can be complicated by several factors: A high number of casualties, location of the attack in a crowded civilian center, and the need for precautions against follow-up attacks in the same area. As a result, significant pressure is placed on the hospital nearest to an attack site, requiring an organized evacuation plan for victims and, if needed, for some patients to be sent to other hospitals nearby.

Treatment of Relatives

After a mass-casualty event, relatives of the victims will likely rush to the hospitals in search of loved ones. Some who have failed to locate family members will approach hospitals even when doubting that they were anywhere near the attack site. These inquiries, whether by telephone or in person, place a further burden on hospitals, following an attack.

Medication and Medical Instruments

The possibility of multiple-casualty attacks, sometimes reaching hundreds or even thousands, obligates the health system to maintain large reserves of medication, blood units, and other medical supplies. It also requires medical teams to stay on standby for long periods of time.

Some challenges are the same whether confronting conventional or unconventional terrorism. Many issues facing the healthcare system are identical whatever the mode of attack, such as summoning medical personnel for duty and handling a large influx of victims. Differences will depend on the nature of the agent of attack. However, challenges facing the health system that are specific to unconventional terrorist attacks are described below.

Rapid Detection and Identification of the Agent of Attack

In many unconventional attacks, especially those with biological weapons, healthcare staff treating victims may be exposed to dangerous materials – bacteria, viruses, toxins – within hours, or days, of the attack. Passage of time could even enhance the threat, as contagious diseases spread from the source to distant and widespread locations. It is therefore critical that emergency services rapidly identify the type of material used in the attack, both to properly treat victims and prevent the dispersion of harmful agents. Surveillance, monitoring, and rapid detection techniques are essential.

Quick Containment of the Attack Area

When harmful substances have been released, it is critical that the site of the attack be contained to prevent further dispersion. Only authorized people in protective gear should have access to the area, and contaminated individuals must be prevented from exiting. This mission is complicated by two contradictory goals: Maintaining, as much as possible, a normal lifestyle in the region of the attack, while attempting to isolate the area to prevent the spread of infectious agents.

Protection of Medical Teams

An unconventional attack, or even the suspicion of such an attack, obligates emergency and medical crews to take special precautions, including donning protective gear, before they treat casualties. Bulky outerwear presents an additional challenge to providing rapid and effective treatment.

Forestalling Panic

In cases of multiple-casualty, unconventional terrorist attacks, the possibility of widespread panic and extreme anxiety among the public needs to be taken into consideration. Staff and officials of the healthcare system play a major role in calming the public and enabling proper and organized treatment of casualties, while containing a conceivably contagious environment. As denying access to relatives could be resented, officials also need to address the possibility of disorder in the hospital grounds.

Given the current and future challenges to the healthcare system, it must be noted that hospitals and medical institutions have already been targeted in a variety of scenarios.

Direct Attack on Hospitals and Medical Institutions

Various terrorist organizations have attempted to execute attacks on hospitals in the past. For example, Hamas attempted to carry out a suicide attack in the Israeli Sheba Medical Center at Tel Hashomer in September 2002. In that same month, the Israeli Security Agency thwarted an attempt by the Islamic Jihad to poison the water in one of the hospitals in Jerusalem. In 1995, Chechen rebels seized a hospital in Budyonnovsk in southern Russia, holding more than 1,000 hostages. A direct attack on a medical institution helps terrorist groups spread fear and anxiety by sending a message that all locations are vulnerable to attack, even institutions that seek to save lives.

Sequential Conventional Attacks Against Health Systems

Attacks have been carried out simultaneously, or shortly after primary attacks, in which emergency and medical services have been targeted. Since the 1990s, Palestinian terrorist organizations have attempted to carry out secondary suicide attacks immediately following the first. The goal is to harm rescue forces and medical teams arriving at the scene of the attack, and disrupt the transfer and treatment of casualties. In this framework, two (or more) terrorists are sent on suicide missions, with the second one waiting to activate explosives until the arrival of rescue teams following the first attack.

Sequential Unconventional Attacks Against Health Systems

Considering the strategy of terrorist organizations over the past several years, officials should note the possibility that, following or during a mass conventional or unconventional attack, a terrorist group may execute a parallel attack on a nearby hospital, seeking to further disrupt the transfer and treatment of casualties.

Cyber-Terrorism Against Medical Institutions

Medical databases of hospital activities, patient records, medications, vaccines, or blood units are also potential terrorist targets. Disruption of this information by cyber-terrorists could severely impair the organization and functioning of the healthcare system. Moreover, terrorists could attempt to hack into databases to obtain information to help plan attacks and to ascertain the storage location of toxic chemical and biological materials.

These threats place the healthcare system – both its staff and its institutions – at the forefront of the modern terrorism phenomenon. The system must be prepared to both contain and thwart terrorist attacks against its facilities – hospitals, clinics, ambulances, emergency services, staff, storage facilities, and control centers. In the event of a large-scale attack, whether conventional or unconventional, the healthcare system must be able to provide care to large numbers who are suffering from physical injury as well as shock and trauma. It must also protect medical staff and relatives of victims from exposure to harmful agents carried by victims of an unconventional attack. These challenges are all complicated by the fact that there may be no early warnings of an impending attack.

Future Trends

At the dawn of the twenty-first century, the phenomenon of terrorism has exhibited distinctive characteristics and defining trends. Terrorism, while not unique to this century, has been recognized by scholars, experts, and political leaders as a growing and dynamic threat. This recognition arises from its increasingly deadly nature (e.g., the 9/11 attacks) and from its potential to cause serious psychological and physical damage from unconventional weapons.

Previous trends in terrorism, such as the increasing number of suicide bombings, have demonstrated the ability of modern terrorist organizations to adapt and respond to new challenges, in competition with the security agencies that seek to combat them. It is in this context that global jihadi terrorism has become a growing threat, as organizations that embrace it seek to sustain themselves and widen their impact.

This chapter has underscored the fact that a terrorist attack is commonly based on a rational cost–benefit assessment. A number of attempted attacks with unconventional weapons have been unsuccessful, which helps account for the infrequent use of these weapons. Yet when unconventional assaults resulted in deaths, as with the sarin attack in Tokyo and the anthrax letters in the United States, they generated massive anxiety and disruption. Such demonstrated effectiveness could prompt a trend toward greater interest in these weapons by terrorists, especially by organizations that harbor religious or doomsday ideologies.

In attempting to create fear and anxiety in a target population, terrorist organizations will continue to employ a range of methods. In response, national and international institutions and actors must prepare for a variety of threats. The underlying reality is that the threat of terrorism will not disappear in the near future.

References

1. Hoffman B. *Inside terrorism*. New York: Columbia University Press; 1988: p. 169.
2. Post J. Terrorism on trial: the context of political crime. In: Kushner HW, ed. *Political terrorism – analyses of problems and prospects for the 21ˢᵗ Century*. Lincoln, NE: Gordian Knot Books—University of Nebraska Press; 2002. p. 46.
3. Crenshaw M. The logic of terrorism: terrorist behavior as a product of strategic choice. In: Reich W, ed. *Origins of terrorism*. Washington, DC: Woodrow Wilson Center Press, 1998; pp. 7–11, 24.
4. Ganor B. Terrorism as a strategy of psychological warfare. In: Danieli Y, Brom D, and Sills J, eds. *The trauma of terrorism*. New York: Haworth Press; 2005. pp 38–40.
5. Hinckley RH. American opinion toward terrorism: the Reagan years. *Terrorism*. 1989;12(6):394–395.
6. Schmid AP and De Graaf J, eds. *Violence as Communication*. London: Sage Publications; 1982. p. 172.
7. Ganor B. *The counter terrorism puzzle – A guide for decision makers*. Herzliya, Israel: Interdisciplinary Center Publishing House; 2005. pp. 253-255.
8. Sageman, M. *Understanding terror networks*. Philadelphia: University of Pennsylvania Press; 2004.
9. Laqueur W. *Voices of terrorism*. Canada: Reed Press; 2004. p. 410.
10. Chandler M, Gunaratna R. *Countering terrorism – can we meet the threat of global violence?* London: Reaktion Books; 2007. p. 20.
11. Stern J. Getting and using the weapons. In: Howard R, Sawyer R, eds. *Terrorism and counterterrorism – understanding the new security environment*. New York: McGraw-Hill; 2004. p. 189–191.
12. Ganor B. The democratic dilemma in counter-terrorism: efficacy vs. democracy and individual rights. In: Ganor B, Azani A, eds. *Trends in international terrorism and counterterrorism*. Herzliya, Israel: Interdisciplinary Center Publishing House; 2007. p. 9.
13. Ganor B. Suicide attacks in Israel. In: Ganor B, ed. *Countering suicide terrorism*. Herzliya, Israel: Interdisciplinary Center Publishing House; 2001, p. 134.
14. Ganor B. The feasibility of post-modern terrorism. In: *Post modern terrorism*, Ganor B, ed. Herzliya, Israel: Interdisciplinary Center Publishing House; 2005. pp. 19–21.

Part II
PREPARATION AND RESPONSE

3
EMS and Pre-Hospital Issues

Ari Leppäniemi

Bombing attacks against civilians have become the primary weapon of terror groups worldwide, and they are likely to remain the primary instrument of terrorism because bombs are easily and inexpensively manufactured, are simple to activate, and require no more than a motivated and determined perpetrator. The explosive can be of military, commercial, or homemade origin. Metal particles of various shapes are often added to the explosive to increase its wounding potential; steel balls, nails, nuts, and the like are the most commonly used. The explosive is detonated by an electrical charge activated remotely or through a switch operated by a suicide bomber.[1] Especially, the new bomb compositions containing metal objects and the use of suicide bombers have characterized the terror attacks in Israel.[2]

The typical suicide bomber carries a vest of explosives around the torso with a typical charge of 5–12 kg of TNT-equivalent. Detonation results in fatal consequences to the bomber, and the damage to people and property in the immediate vicinity of the detonation is often devastating, especially when the explosion occurs in a confined space. Suicide bombers are trained to seek circumstances where the damage can be maximized, and target mass gathering sites such as public buses and bus stations, wedding halls, hotel dining rooms, restaurants, open markets, supermarkets, and discotheques.[3]

During a time period from September 2000 to December 2003 in Israel, a total of 19,948 terrorist incidents were reported; most victims were injured in explosions resulting from suicide bombers.[4] During a 3-year period in Jerusalem district only, 28 terror-related multiple casualty incidents occurred with a total of 2,328 victims and 273 deaths, with an overall fatality rate of 11.7%.[5]

In a retrospective analysis of a number of incidents, injuries, and deaths because of explosive, incendiary, premature, and attempted bombing in the United States from 1983 through 2002, a total of 36,110 bombing incidents, 5,931 injuries, and 699 deaths were reported.[6] Fifty-nine percent were explosive bombings, 17% incendiary bombings, 3% premature bombings, and 21% attempted bombings. In bombings with known materials, nitrate-based fertilizers accounted for 36% of injuries and 30% of deaths, and smokeless powder and black powder for 33% of injuries and 27% of deaths, respectively.

S.C. Shapira et al. (eds.), *Essentials of Terror Medicine*,
DOI: 10.1007/978-0-387-09412-0_3, Springer Science+Business Media, LLC 2009

Another characteristic, experienced in London and Madrid, is the occurrence of simultaneous multiple attacks targeting the transport system, which can pose a serious challenge to a medical system.[7,8]

Terrorist Bombings

How Terrorist Bombings Differ from Other Explosion Incidents

Although maximizing the number of casualties might be the main aim of the terrorist bomber, other motifs, such as intimidation, coercion, spreading of fear, creating panic in the public, and gaining wide media attention, could determine the way the bombing is planned. In addition to the magnitude and location of explosion, other factors that can influence the effect of the bomb have to be taken into account when planning a medical response to a terrorist bomb explosion.

The use of *spherical metal pellets* propelled by the explosion increase the severity of injuries, and the possibility of this type of penetrating injury, even in patients remote from the origin, should be kept in mind. Medical teams assessing and treating terrorist bomb victims should be trained to recognize these injuries.[9]

Dirty bomb is a mix of a conventional explosive with radioactive powder or pellets resulting in dispersion of radioactive material in the explosion plume. Although the major medical risk in a "dirty" bomb is blast injury caused by the conventional charge, the casualty profile of such a bomb will include a small group of casualties that may also be contaminated with radioactive material.[10] This may require implementation of decontamination procedures either in the field or at the receiving hospital. There will also be a much larger group of "worried well," presenting to the healthcare system for evaluation and decontamination, but only a small fraction of these patients will require decontamination.[10]

The effects of a potential *second hit* (a second bomb designed to explode in the vicinity of the first bomb after a short time period to injure helpers and bystanders) must be minimized by strict security procedures when approaching the accident scene and by establishing a secure perimeter as soon as possible, minimizing the number of people in the area under risk as determined by on-scene security and police officials. In two cases recorded from Israel, the second bombs exploded 10–30 minutes after the first detonation.[11] In addition, the discovery in Israel in 2003 of arms and gunmen in some ambulances led to the practice that all ambulances, even those conveying critically injured victims, had to pause for brief inspection at the perimeter of the hospital's grounds.[12] Another potential security risk for Emergency Medical Services (EMS) personnel entering a "hostile" area is the possibility of a sniper in the area.[13]

Finally, in addition to the conventional injury pattern associated with explosions (primary, secondary, tertiary, and quaternary blast injuries—see Chapter

11 and Table 19.1 for more information) the possibility of *biological foreign body implantation* from the suicide bombers or other victims has been recently reported.[14,15]

Casualty Patterns in Terrorist Bombings

Explosive agents are materials that undergo rapid exothermic reaction when appropriately stimulated. The degree to which this reaction occurs is dependent upon the characteristics of the explosive agent. Low-order explosives react by rapid burning and conflagration, whereas high-order explosives produce extreme heat and energy, and result in the formation of a pressure wave or "blast wave."[16] Pipe bombs, gun powder, and pure petroleum-based bombs ("Molotov Cocktail") are examples of low-energy explosives. The most common high-energy explosives are TNT, C-4, Semtex, nitroglycerine, dynamite, and ammonium nitrate fuel oil (ANFO).[17]

The blast wave produced by high-energy explosives is reflected and sustained by fixed structures and confined environments such as rooms and vehicles, and may portend the effects of blast-related injury. By the same mechanism, water, which is a relatively noncompressible medium, sustains more of the energy from the blast and as such blast waves in water have a greater injurious effect propagated over a greater distance.[16]

Explosion injuries present with great variation, and include classic manifestations of blunt, penetrating, and thermal trauma in addition to the unique blast injuries. Primary blast injury is induced by the blast wave itself, secondary blast injury is caused by projectiles, tertiary blast injury is caused by thrusting the victims against stationary objects, and quaternary blast injury results from fire and heat generated by the explosion.[18]

The type of injuries suffered by unprotected victims depends on the distance from a high-explosive detonation in the open air with inverted relation between severity and distance: total body disruption, burns and inhalation injuries, toxic inhalations, traumatic amputations, primary blast injury of the lung and bowel, tertiary blast injuries, blast injury of the ear, and secondary blast injuries.[19]

The most susceptible organs to primary blast injury are the ears, lungs, and gastrointestinal tract. The ears have been considered the most sensitive organs to blast injury and tympanic membrane rupture has been considered as a reliable marker of exposure to significant overpressure.[17,20] Eardrum perforation occurs at very low peak overpressure, with a 50% likelihood between 15 and 50 psi. However, because cerumen-filled auditory canals and eardrums of younger patients are relatively resistant to the blast, intact eardrums may not be indicative of the exposure and other signs of injury should be sought.[1] In the 2004 Madrid train bombings, tympanic perforation occurred in 41% of the 243 patients with moderate to severe trauma.[7]

The magnitude of the explosion and the number of people in the vicinity primarily determine the number of casualties, whereas indoor location and building collapse maximize lethality and the proportion of casualties killed.[18] The risk of death is strongly associated with the amount of blast loading (amount of overpressure depending on the distance from explosion). In an analysis of 828 servicemen killed or injured in Northern Ireland between 1970 and 1984 the victims were grouped according to the blast loading into four groups. Among the 52 patients with traumatic amputations, for example, only 3 out of 35 (9%) with overpressures over 550 kPa survived in contrast with 6 out of 17 (35%) with lower overpressures. Although most of the servicemen were wearing body armor that offers considerable protection from secondary missiles, it did not seem to protect from primary blast injury.[21]

The majority of deaths from terrorist bombings occur immediately or within the first few hours. Of the 273 deaths resulting from 2000–2003 terrorist attacks in Jerusalem, 83% occurred immediately, at the scene of the attack, and of the remaining 17% of the patients who died in the hospital, half died within 4 hours of arrival and one quarter within 5–24 hours.[5] In the 1996 Khobar Towers terrorist truck bombing in the Kingdom of Saudi Arabia, 19 out of 574 injured died; all were immediate deaths. Of the 420 persons injured directly by the bombing, 16% were hospitalized, 41% treated on an outpatient basis, and 39% self-treated. In contrast to the 1995 bombing of the Alfred P. Murrah Federal Building in Oklahoma City, the bomb detonated at Khobar Towers was five times larger but was associated with only one-fifth of the death rate (5% vs. 22%), primarily because there was no major building collapse.[22]

The incidence of critical injuries among survivors of terrorist bombings is 9–22%.[18] The mortality rate for those succumbing to late deaths despite medical care is 19% for abdominal injuries, 15% for chest injuries, and 11% for blast lung cases and traumatic amputations.[18]

Burns caused by terror attacks are often more severe compared with other burns. An analysis of 219 terror-related burns from Israel from 1997 through 2003 showed that large burns (20–80% total body surface area) are more common in terror casualties, with greater mortality (6.4% vs. 3.4%).[23]

Most injuries in bombing survivors are caused by secondary and tertiary blast effects causing noncritical soft tissue and skeletal injuries. Because of size and contamination, these may require subsequent debridement and multiple procedures. A smaller proportion of patients will have critical abdominal, head, and thoracic injuries that require urgent surgery emphasizing the importance of immediate availability of capable surgical services in the receiving hospital.[18] Because of the combination of blast, penetrating, blunt, and thermal injuries, some patients need prolonged care in the intensive care unit.[24]

The main feature of casualty patterns following most terrorist bombings, however, is characterized by a large number of minor and nonfatal injuries.[25–28] In these instances, efficiency of care can be degraded by overtriage (proportion of survivors assigned to immediate care, hospitalization, or evacuation who are not critically injured). In a compiled data analysis of 10 terrorist bombing incidents, Frykberg[18] showed a linear relationship between overtriage and critical mortality rate (proportion of immediate survivors with critical injuries who died) confirming that overtriage can result in loss of potentially salvageable lives in this setting. The analysis of the 2004 Madrid train bombings concluded that there was an overtriage to the closest hospital where the critical mortality rate was 17%.[7]

Aim of Pre-Hospital Response in Terrorist Bombings

From the trauma care perspective, it has been emphasized that successful coping with an urban bombing does not mean streamlining the flow of 80 casualties, but rather providing high-quality trauma care to very few critical (but salvageable) patients.[29] The set-up of minor injury assessment areas to treat the large number of patients with minor injuries was found to be useful in the 2005 London bombings.[8]

The special characteristics that have to be taken into account when planning for medical care of victims of terrorist bombings are summarized in Table 3.1. With these special characteristics applied to a general mass casualty plan, the single most important aim of the pre-hospital response is to reliably identify and provide lifesaving trauma life support to the few critically injured but not moribund patients, and transfer them with minimal delay to an adequately equipped and manned surgical hospital avoiding both overtriage and undertriage (assignment of critically injured casualties needing immediate care to a delayed category). To accomplish this, the preparation must include a comprehensive plan incorporating all players into a single command system, and specifically utilizing the resources of all appropriate medical assets in a pre-specified region.[11,30]

Preparation

Preparedness ranges from the development of standard operating procedures to educating healthcare workers about the specific requirements and stockpiling of supplies, with the ability to address sharp increases in the number of casualties

TABLE 3.1. Special Characteristics to Be Considered When Planning for Medical Care of Victims of Terrorist Bombings

Possibility of a
- Second bomb exploding near the original scene
- Radioactive or chemical contamination
- Presence of primary blast injury not immediately recognizable
- Biological foreign body implantation
- Building collapse and indoor explosion more lethal
- Most deaths occur immediately
- Large number of minor injuries and uninjured distressed victims
- Small but definitive proportion of patients with critical injuries

when needed.[12] There are some essential components to medical disaster planning. Strategic planning including establishment of authority and developing a coherent philosophy of regional health disaster management is the first one, followed by tactical plans, that is, specific written plans, establishing and maintaining funding, and operational capability.[31]

Previous experience shows that in most mass casualty incidents, victims will not be evenly distributed. Nineteen of the 22 injured survivors of the 1982 Metrorail crash in Washington, DC, went to one hospital, and the closest geographical hospital to the 1995 Oklahoma City bombing was swamped while most nearby emergency departments were idle.[32]

A regionalized mass casualty plan with integrated EMS response and involving multiple hospitals under one system is the best way to reach the main aim of any mass casualty: to reduce the critical mortality rate. Overwhelming a large university hospital with more than 3–5 critically injured at the same time can temporarily disrupt medical care even in the most advanced centers. Therefore, distributing casualties between several hospitals around the bombing site, some of which may be lower echelons of trauma care, is a much better option.[3] This has also been confirmed in a computed simulation model based on 223 patients from 22 bombing incidents showing that there is a sigmoid-shaped relationship between casualty load and level of care, with the upper flat portion of the curve corresponding to the surge capacity of the trauma assets of the hospital. This capacity is 4.6 critical patients per hour using immediately available assets, and a fully deployed disaster plan increase it to 7.1 Overtriage rates of 50% and 75% shift the curve to the left, decreasing the surge capacity to 3.8 and 2.7, respectively.[33]

Because of the almost identical requirements to mobilize the resources in any kind of terrorist or other mass casualty incident, a single plan should be in place for all types of terrorist attacks that can be modified to account for special characteristics and include preparedness for bioterrorism, for example.[34]

After the 1994 car bombing of the seven-story Argentine Israeli Mutual Association building in Buenos Aires, casualties started to arrive, brought in by volunteers, on foot or by ambulance, along a 150-m traffic-free route cleared all the way to the nearest hospital, the Clinicas University Hospital in Buenos Aires, which did not have a preexisting mass casualty plan at the time. Because of the proximity of the hospital, very few victims were transported to other hospitals in the city resulting in the rapid overcrowding of the emergency department with minor and moderate injuries. Of the total 86 victims arriving, 2 were dead on arrival, 41 were admitted, and 43 with minor injuries assisted and discharged.[35]

During the 2003 terrorist bombings in Istanbul, victims were distributed to 24 medical facilities including university hospitals, public hospitals, and private hospitals, but apparently there was no regional plan to stratify the patients according to the type or severity of their injuries.[36,37]

In preparation for the Centennial Olympic Games in Atlanta in 1996, extensive medical planning and preparation took place to care for all the athletes, other participants, staff, media, volunteers, and spectators. When a bomb exploded near a concert resulting in a multiple casualty incident, 96 of the 111 victims were triaged to four hospitals within 3 miles of the bombing. Only four minor operations were performed in 61 patients evacuated to the three community hospitals, whereas 35 out of 50 remaining victims were evaluated at the regional trauma center, and 10 out of 35 underwent emergency or urgent operations with no mortality.[38]

The greater Helsinki area in southern Finland with a population base of 1.4 million has a regional Helsinki Area Disaster Plan that contains a medical section with integrated EMS system and regionally structured plan comprising nine different hospitals. The key principle of the plan is to triage the most severely injured patients directly from the scene to the three university hospitals with minimal delay and avoiding overtriage by triaging patients with minor injuries to the other six hospitals in the region depending on the location of the incident. All three university hospitals have active emergency surgical departments but with different profiles, with one being mainly an orthopedic, plastic, and neurosurgical center, the other having general, cardiothoracic, and vascular services, and the third being a pediatric surgery center. All other six hospitals have an emergency surgical service with a varying and limited range of available surgical specialties.

The plan was put into use in October 2002 when a self-made explosive was detonated in a shopping center. Five people including the bomber died immediately, and 66 of the 161 immediate survivors requiring some kind of medical assistance were treated in six different hospitals triaged according to the severity and type of their injuries and the age of the patient (pediatric age group). The distances of the hospitals from the accident scene varied from 10 to 50 km, with the three university hospitals being 10–12 km away. Three of the 13 patients with severe injuries (Injury Severity Score > 15) were not initially triaged to the main three university hospitals with an undertriage rate of 23%, whereas the number of patients initially received by the three university hospitals was 5 (1 severe), 4 (all severe), and 9 (5 severe), respectively. Three regional hospitals received a total of 16 (none severe), 15 (2 severe), and 6 patients (1 severe), respectively. Overall, two of the immediate survivors died, both within 24 hours, for a critical mortality rate of 15%. Both nonsurvivors were initially triaged to the university hospitals, but died in spite of treatment from severe brain and thoracic injuries.[39,40]

Regional Mass Casualty Plan

A single regional mass casualty plan designed for all kinds of mass casualty types (conventional, unconventional, natural disasters, and major accidents) should be based on the day-to-day activities of the EMS system and hospitals in the region. Specifically, the following aspects should be assessed:

- location and distances of the different hospitals in the region
- emergency department capacities and diagnostic facilities in different hospitals

- surgical and intensive care specialties available for emergencies (especially neurosurgery, cardiothoracic surgery, pediatric surgery)
- facilities for decontamination and possession of certain antidotes

A plan should include a centralized medical command and control system utilizing the expertise of the major trauma center or university hospital in the region. The regional command center can be formed in the major trauma center, but should be in a different room from the hospital command center. The regional command center should have a good and safe communication capability with the nonmedical authorities in the field, the EMS system, all hospitals in the region, and government agencies and major hospitals neighboring the region. Cell phones and landlines may not be reliable and alternative means such as Internet, satellite phone, 800 mHz radio, amateur ("ham") radio, and CB Citizens' Band radio should be available.[32]

Principles of Triage

The large number of casualties, limited resources on the scene, and the critical time factor characterizing a mass casualty incident preclude a thorough evaluation and treatment of all injured patients according to standard practices. Therefore, the standard goal of providing the greatest good for each individual patient must change in a mass casualty setting to "the greatest good for the greatest number." The main instrument to achieve this is the application of sorting out the patients according to the severity of their injuries, or triage, and assigning those who are the most seriously injured to receiving priority care.[41]

The initial triage should not take place in or immediately outside of the hospital, but should be done at the scene utilizing multiple successive pre-hospital triage sites to improve triage accuracy through a progressive filtering process.[41]

Medical Management on the Scene

The medical management at the scene can be divided into four phases.[11] The first phase is the chaotic phase. It starts from the incident and lasts until the commanding EMS person and vehicles arrive, and typically lasts for 10–15 minutes in an urban setting. By this time, victims who can walk and usually with minor injuries only have evacuated themselves to the nearest hospital, sometimes with the help of civilian transportation. These victims seldom receive any treatment at the scene or en route.

The most important phase is the reorganization phase that begins when the leader, usually an EMS commander in close cooperation with the overall scene commander, usually a rescue commander, assumes control of the medical management, assigns other medical personnel to their duties, and organizes triage and evacuation. Depending on the scale of the incident, this may last as long as 60 minutes.

The subsequent site-clearing phase lasts one or more hours depending on the scope of the event and whether any victims need prolonged extrication and ends

TABLE 3.2. Principles of Pre-Hospital Triage in Terrorist Bombings

Attempts to control field chaos are futile
Secure location of the triage points
Multiple successive triage sites are preferable to one
Uniformly recognized triage categories (color codes)
Special awareness of
  − radioactive or chemical contamination
  − penetrating injuries from small metal fragments
Triage is a dynamic process
Avoid excessive procedures in the field (scoop and run)
Even and stratified distribution of patients to multiple hospitals according to severity and type of injuries

when the EMS commander leaves the site. It is important that before leaving, the whole area is scrutinized thoroughly for victims who were missed in the initial two phases. In the late phase (24–48 hours after the incident), some victims who have suffered slight wounds acknowledge their injuries many hours later and may seek medical help even in emergency departments that are remote from the place of explosion.

Although the organization of the pre-hospital medical management is subject to local circumstances, available resources, organization of emergency services during normal times, and many other variables, there are some main principle and characteristics of triage in the field listed in Table 3.2.

Scene Safety

In the chaotic phase, there might be some medical first aid given by bystanders or less injured victims, but the organized approach can be implemented after the arrival of one or more trained EMS personnel with a clear leader or commander. Scene safety is a major concern for rescuers, and in addition to the risk of secondary explosive devices, the risk of structural collapse, inhalation of airborne particulate material, and contamination should be taken into account. Wearing full personal protective equipment, and being familiar with this kind of environment and technical rescue skills, were found to be useful in the 2005 London bombings.[8]

Selection of Triage Site and Assigning Key Duties

The medical or EMS commander in the field, after consultation with the overall incident commander, should select the triage sites. The site should be safe and secured from a potential second hit on a dry and possibly sheltered area, upwind from the incident, and close to the evacuation route for the ambulances with a one-way traffic direction. After assigning the leaders of the initial key responsibilities (primary triage, secondary triage and treatment, and evacuation) with appropriate teams, and establishing communication with the overall regional medical commander who has the knowledge of the current situation and capabilities of each hospital in the region, the EMS commander directs and supervises the organized field triage process. It also includes the establishment of a place for deceased victims, separate from the treatment areas.

Primary Triage

The initial sorting of the victims by the primary triage officer can be based on the ability of the victims to walk and follow orders. Directing the "walking wounded" to another site for appropriate evaluation and treatment separates them from the more severely injured who are collected to the main secondary triage point to be evaluated by the secondary triage and treatment officer. Overtriage can be reduced by focusing on physiologic and anatomic criteria rather than on mechanism in selecting patients for transport to trauma centers, and this can be achieved without increasing undertriage.[41]

Triage Categories and Secondary Triage

The more severely injured are evaluated, sorted out, and treated by the secondary triage officer for immediately life-threatening problems (airway and breathing, external bleeding) and assigned a category for evacuation (Table 3.3).[41] It should be noted that triage is a dynamic process and the condition of the patient can change, either because the immediate life-threatening problem has been solved (by establishing a secure airway or stopping external bleeding, for example) or because the condition of a patient with an unrecognized severe injury, such as internal bleeding, has deteriorated. The triage category should reflect the urgency of evacuation to get the patient to the hospital for definitive treatment, not the initial condition.

An analysis of suicide bombers in Israel showed that penetrating head and torso wounds, burns >10%, traumatic amputation, skull fracture, and close space versus open air explosion were predictive of the risk of blast lung injury and the need for immediate care.[41]

Patients who need immediate evacuation (red code) should be transported first to the nearest appropriate medical facility that has the capability to deal with the suspected injuries. Typical injuries include conditions that might have been treated in the field initially but need subsequent definitive surgical treatment, such as airway compromise, open chest wounds, tension pneumothorax, and

TABLE 3.3. Field Triage Categories and Commonly used Color Codes

Immediate (red)
Delayed (yellow)
Minimal (green)
Expectant (violet)
Dead (black)

major external hemorrhage, or conditions that cannot be treated in the field, such as hypotension, intermediate burns, or unconscious patients with focal suggested. The receiving hospital is usually the major trauma center in the area, but under some circumstances it might be the hospital with special expertise, such as a burn unit, cardiothoracic surgery, or neurosurgery. If possible, no hospital should receive more than five severely injured patients during the first hour.

The delayed category (yellow code) includes patients who need definitive treatment that often includes surgery, such as hemodynamically stable patients with penetrating abdominal wounds, extremity vascular injuries, unconscious patients without airway compromise or lateralizing signs, pelvic, spinal, or extremity fractures, or major soft tissue wounds. They should be transported after the immediate category patients following the same stratification according to the potential injuries as the immediate category patients.

The minimally injured patients (green code) should be equally divided among the lower echelon or more distant hospitals in the area using mass transportation means, such as buses, if possible. The actual updated capacity situation of the receiving hospitals should be taken into account, and the EMS commander can obtain this information from the overall medical commander and pass that on to the evacuation officer.

In terrorist bombings, the recognition of severe blast injury can be challenging, and patients with primary blast injuries with little or no external injuries can easily be triaged to the minor injury category. Although otoscopic evaluation of a potential ruptured tympanic membrane can be used to screen for primary blast injury, it is more practical and useful in the emergency department, not in the field.[20] Because a significant number of patients with primary blast injury have no external injuries, the recognition of the potentially serious consequences and demand for ICU and ventilator care later on is crucial and patients with suspected primary blast injury should be evaluated in a hospital even if they have no or only minor injuries treatable at home.[21,42] They should not, however, be evacuated before the more severely injured.

Other patient groups that might present initially with minor findings but may require assessment in a hospital include patients with scalp lacerations or a concussion who often have an underlying skull fracture,[43] and patients who have been trapped and might develop a crush syndrome.[44]

The expectant category (violet code) refers to patients who are alive but with unsurvivable injuries or patients with such severe injuries that their rapid evacuation would unlikely lead to survival and might divert the limited resources away from patients with potentially more survivable injuries. Examples for this type of injuries could include severe head injuries with open skull fractures and unconsciousness, extensive deep burns, and imminent cardiac arrest with major torso trauma. This category is the most difficult to assign patients to and requires the necessary mindset and medical competence from the triage officer. These patients should be segregated from the others at least in the initial phase, and kept comfortable and monitored for any improvement in their condition that may warrant care later in the evolution of the incident response.[41]

Dead victims (black code) should be segregated from all others to decrease the possibility of resource-utilizing treatment efforts, and to facilitate later identification and communication of their outcome to families.[41]

The overall conduct and main points of field triage in terrorist bombings are summarized in an algorithm in Fig. 3.1.

Decontamination

Preparation for an adequate pre-hospital response to a radiological, chemical, or other additional contaminating hazards following a terrorist bombing is challenging. Not only will the number of casualties be potentially overwhelming, but there is the added risk for contamination from the patients and the environment. The current approach favors the management of any terrorist incident with chemical or biological substances as far as possible according to standard HAZMAT Hazardous Materials operating procedures because, although the agents might be unfamiliar, the protection, decontamination, and resuscitation procedures are identical to those used for normal civil HAZMAT incidents.[45]

For radiological contamination it should be remembered that patients who have been exposed to ionizing radiation are not contaminated and do not need decontamination. For those externally contaminated with radioactive material, the removal of clothes usually eliminates more than 90% of the contamination.[46]

For medical personnel working in the disaster area, some type of protective clothing including surgical masks or even a breathing apparatus might be necessary, although their use has been associated with claustrophobia, overheating, dehydration, failure to recognize danger, and anxiety.[47] However, at least in simulated situations the modern personal respiratory protection devices, especially the air-purifying respirators with panoramic visors, seem to have little effect in the efficiency of care.[48]

Even the detection of a potential contamination source might be difficult in the early stages of the disaster response while patients with serious life-threatening injuries are already being given medical attention. In the Tokyo sarin attack, very few of those exposed were decontaminated before seeking care. EMS personnel wore conventional clothing instead of protective equipment, and about 10% of the emergency medical technicians developed poisoning from secondary contamination.[49]

In general, decontamination is indicated if the substance is toxic and stays in the skin and clothes of the patient or could be transferred to medical personnel. Field decontamination is indicated only if without it there would be a considerable risk to the patient or others, and the establishment of a full decontamination line in the field should be assessed in view of the overall triage needs and situation.

Decontamination is started at the inner edge of the protected area by asking the patients to remove their clothes and put them into a tightly closed plastic bag. If possible, bags should be tagged and identified for later forensic or police anaysis. Patients unable to do it themselves need to be assisted by a person wearing protective clothing. Removal of outer layers of clothing may reduce up to 85% of

Terrorist bombing with multiple casualties

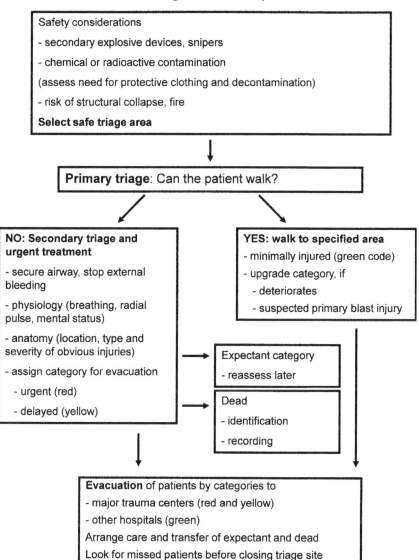

FIG. 3.1. Triage algorithm for terrorist bombings.

contamination. After removing clothes, the patients should be rinsed (including the hair) with lukewarm (about 30 °C) water to prevent both vasodilatation caused by too warm water and hypothermia caused by too cold water. Brushes or other equipment that might abrade or injure the skin should not be used. After rinsing, the patient will be transferred to the treatment area and provided with clothing.

Valuables can be stored in plastic bags and taken along to the hospital, whereas contaminated clothes should be left on the scene.

For the use of specific treatments and antidotes in the field, please see Parts III and IV. Specifically for radiation casualties, immediate life-threatening interventions may precede decontamination, and early closure of simple wounds is mandatory in irradiated casualties.[46]

Record Keeping

One important aspect of triage is the record keeping that prevents losing track of casualties and allowing a post-event analysis of triage decisions, casualty management, and casualty outcomes, from which important decisions can be derived to improve performance in future events.[41] A proposal has been made for tracking mass casualties utilizing the existing databases and creating a unique mass casualty code to be added to the patient codes.[50]

Conclusion

The essence of triage is to identify the critically injured rapidly and reliably, manage the immediately life-threatening but treatable problems (airway, external bleeding) and evacuate the patients as soon as possible to the most appropriate hospital while recognizing the potentially severely injured with initially benign clinical presentation who might deteriorate rapidly. Specifically in terrorist bombings, the recognition of severe blast injury can be challenging.

Utilizing a unified EMS system and a regional agreement of multiple hospitals within reasonable distances and stratified according to their trauma management capacity and resources, a rational plan can be developed to ensure that the most critically injured patients are sent directly to the right hospitals without overwhelming these hospitals with patients with minor injuries. Avoiding overtriage and not exceeding the surge capacity of the major trauma hospitals are the most efficient ways of decreasing the critical mortality rate, the hallmark of the efficiency of the medical response to a mass casualty incident.

References

1. Kluger Y, Kashuk J, Mayo A. Terror bombing—mechanisms, consequences and implications. *Scand J Surg*. 2004;93:11–14.
2. Aharonson-Daniel L, Peleg K, the ITG. The epidemiology of terrorism casualties. *Scand J Surg*. 2005;94:185–190.
3. Stein M. Urban bombing: a trauma surgeon's perspective. *Scand J Surg*. 2005;94:286–292.
4. Singer P, Cohen JD, Stein M. Conventional terrorism and critical care. *Crit Care Med*. 2005;33:S61–S65.
5. Shapira SC, Adatto-Levi R, Avitzour M, Rivkind AI, Gertsenshtein I, Mintz Y. Mortality in terrorist attacks: a unique modal of temporary death distribution. *World J Surg*. 2006;30:2071–2077.

6. Kapur GB, Hutson HR, Davis MA, Rice PL. The United States twenty-year experience with bombing incidents: implications for terrorism preparedness and medical response. *J Trauma.* 2005;59:1436–1444.

7. Peral Gutierrez de Ceballos J, Turegano Fuentes F, Perez Diaz D, Sanz Sanchez M, Martin Llorente C, Guerrero Sanz JE. Casualties treated at the closest hospital in the Madrid, March 11, terrorist bombings. *Crit Care Med.* 2005;33:S107–S112.

8. Lockey DJ, MacKenzie R, Redhead J, et al. London bombings July 2005: the immediate pre-hospital medical response. *Resuscitation.* 2005;66:ix–xii.

9. Kluger Y, Mayo A, Hiss J, et al. Medical consequences of terrorist bombs containing spherical metal pellets: analysis of a suicide terrorism event. *Eur J Emerg Med.* 2005;12:19–23.

10. Schecter WP. Nuclear, biological and chemical weapons: what the surgeon needs to know. *Scand J Surg.* 2005;94:293–299.

11. Stein M, Hirshberg A. Medical consequences of terrorism. The conventional weapon threat. *Surg Clin North Am.* 1999;79:1537–1552.

12. Shapira SC, Cole LA. Terror medicine: birth of a discipline. *JHSEM.* 2006;3:1–6.

13. Sullivan JP. Medical responses to terrorist incidents. Prehosp Disaster Med. 1990;5:151–153.

14. Eshkol Z, Katz K. Injuries from biologic material of suicide bombers. *Injury Int J Care Injured.* 2005;36:271–274.

15. Wong JM-L, Marsh D, Abu-Sitta G, et al. Biological foreign body implantation in victims of the London July 7th suicide bombings. *J Trauma.* 2006;60:402–404.

16. Eastridge BJ. Things that go boom: injuries from explosives. *J Trauma.* 2007;62:S38.

17. Born CT. Blast trauma: the fourth weapon of mass destruction. *Scand J Surg.* 2005;94:279–285.

18. Frykberg ER. Medical management of disasters and mass casualties from terrorist bombings: how can we cope? *J Trauma.* 2002;53:201–212.

19. Wightman JM, Gladish SL. Explosions and blast injuries. *Ann Emerg Med.* 2001;37:664–678.

20. DePalma RG, Burris DG, Champion HR, Hodgson MJ. Blast injuries. *N Engl J Med.* 2005;352:43–50.

21. Mellor SG, Cooper GJ. Analysis of 828 servicemen killed or injured by explosion in Northern Ireland 1970–84: the Hostile Action Casualty System. *Br J Surg.* 1989;76:1006–1010.

22. Thompson D, Brown S, Mallonee S, Sunshine D. Fatal and non-fatal injuries among U.S. Air Force personnel resulting from the terrorist bombing of the Khobar towers. *J Trauma.* 2004;57:208–215.

23. Haik J, Tessone A, Givon A, et al. Terror-inflicted thermal injury: a retrospective analysis of burns in the Israeli–Palestinian conflict between the years 1997 and 2003. *J Trauma.* 2006;61:1501–1505.

24. Shamir MY, Rivkind A, Weissman C, Sprung CL, Weiss YG. Conventional terrorist bomb incidents and the intensive care unit. *Curr Opin Crit Care.* 2005;11:580–584.

25. Hadden WA, Rutherford WH, Merrett JD. The injuries of terrorist bombing: a study of 1532 consecutive patients. *Br J Surg.* 1978;65:525–531.

26. Cooper GJ, Maynard RL, Cross NL, Hill JF. Casualties from terrorist bombings. *J Trauma.* 1983;23:955–967.

27. Rignault DP, Deligny MC. The 1986 terrorist bombing experience in Paris. *Ann Surg.* 1989;209:368–373.

28. Peleg K, Aharonson-Daniel L, Stein M, et al. Gunshot and explosion injuries. Characteristics, outcomes, and implications for care of terror-related injuries in Israel. *Ann Surg.* 2004;239:311–318.

29. Hirshberg A. Multiple casualty incidents. Lessons from the front line. *Ann Surg.* 2004;239:322–324.

30. Einav S, Feigenberg Z, Weissman C, et al. Evacuation priorities in mass casualty terror-related events. Implications for contingency planning. *Ann Surg.* 2004;239:304–310.
31. Epley E. Regional medical disaster planning: an integrated approach to ESF-8 planning. *J Trauma.* 2007;62:596.
32. Hammond J. Mass casualty incidents: planning implications for trauma care. *Scand J Surg.* 2005;94:267–271.
33. Hirshberg A, Scott BG, Granchi T, Wall MJ Jr., Mattox KL, Stein M. How does casualty load affect trauma care in urban bombing incidents? A quantitative analysis. *J Trauma.* 2005;58:686–695.
34. Jacobs L, Burns KJ, Gross RI. Terrorism: a public health threat with a trauma system response. *J Trauma.* 2003;55:1014–1021.
35. Biancolini CA, Del Bosco CG, Jorge MA. Argentine Jewish Community Institution bomb explosion. *J Trauma.* 1999;47:728–732.
36. Rodoplu U, Arnold JL, Yucel T, Tokyay R, Ersoy G, Cetiner S. Impact of the terrorist bombings of the Hong Kong Shanghai Bank Corporation headquarters and British consulate on two hospitals in Istanbul, Turkey, in November 2003. *J Trauma.* 2005;195–201.
37. Taviloglu K, Yanar H, Kavuncu A, Ertekin C, Guloglu R. 2003 terrorist bombings in Istanbul. *Int J Disaster Med.* 2005;4:45–49.
38. Feliciano DV, Anderson GV, Rozycki GS, et al. Management of casualties from the bombing at the centennial Olympics. *Am J Surg.* 1998;176(6):538–543.
39. Örtenwall P, Almgren O, Deverell E. The bomb explosion in Myyrmanni, Finland 2002. *Int J Disaster Med.* 2003;2:120–126.
40. Torkki M, Koljonen V, Sillanpää K, et al. Triage in bomb disaster with 166 casualties. *Eur J Trauma.* 2006;32:374–380.
41. Frykberg ER. Triage: principles and practice. *Scand J Surg.* 2005;94:272–278.
42. Avidan V, Hersch M, Spira RM, Einav S, Goldberg S, Schecter W. Civilian hospital response to a mass casualty event: the role of the intensive care unit. *J Trauma.* 2007;62:1234–1239.
43. Scott BA, Fletcher JR, Pulliam MW, Harris RD. The Beirut terrorist bombing. *Neurosurgery.* 1986;18:107–110.
44. Aoki N, Demsar J, Zupan B, et al. Predictive model for estimating risk of crush syndrome: a data mining approach. *J Trauma.* 2007;62:940–945.
45. Baker DJ. The management of casualties following terrorist release of chemical and biological agents: the current approach of the Paris Emergency Medical Service (SAMU). *Scand J Trauma Emerg Med.* 2002;10:164–165.
46. Briggs SM, Brinsfield KH. Radioactive agents. In: Briggs SM, Brinsfield KH, eds. *Advanced Disaster Medical Response. Manual for providers.* 1st ed. Boston, MA: Harvard Medical International Trauma & Disaster Institute; 2003:71–92.
47. Slater MS, Trunkey DD. Terrorism in America. An evolving threat. *Arch Surg.* 1997;132:1059–1066.
48. Brinker A, Gray SA, Schumacher J. Influence of air-purifying respirators on the simulated first response emergency treatment of CBRN victims. *Resuscitation.* 2007;74:310–316.
49. Tokuda Y, Kikuchi M, Takahashi O, Stein GH. Prehospital management of sarin nerve gas terrorism in urban settings: 10 years progress after the Tokyo subway sarin attack. *Resuscitation.* 2006;68:193–202.
50. Garthe E, Mango N. A method for tracking mass casualty or terrorism incidents in existing databases. *J Trauma.* 2002;53:793–795.

4
Effects of Terrorism on the Healthcare Community

DAVID O'REILLY and KARIM BROHI

Planning for medical response to terrorist incidents focuses almost exclusively on the early hours after the event. Once scenes have been cleared and all patients dispatched from the emergency department, the major incident is stood down. However, it may be many hours before the last patient leaves the operating room and critical care areas are only just beginning to absorb the impact of the event.[1] Further surgery will be required the next day and for several days to come. For many staff members these victims will dominate their workload for weeks or months. A terrorist incident will therefore affect the functioning of a hospital for a considerable period after the event. The hospital's response must go beyond the care of the patient to include handling of the media, police and public.

Other sectors of the healthcare community may be affected secondarily. Directly or indirectly a healthcare system itself suffers from the effects of terrorism. Finally, the political consequences of terrorism can bear heavily on healthcare funding.

The Aftermath

The medical response to a terrorist incident has several key phases which are useful to recognize.

Phase 1: Chaos. During the first minutes and hours of an incident there is a phase of chaos.[2] Information is minimal and unreliable. Communication is poor and the nature of the incident and the scale and severity of injured casualties is unknown. Hospitals begin to implement their disaster plans, deploy staff and reorganize resources. In the majority of cases these will have been previously activated only for practice drills and will be found wanting in several key areas.

This phase is unavoidable and must be incorporated into the emergency response plan. Under-triage of casualties will occur amidst the chaos and plans should incorporate reassessment and monitoring of all the injured. Attention to detail including meticulous documentation during this time will reduce errors, complications and workload during the later phases.

S.C. Shapira et al. (eds.), *Essentials of Terror Medicine*,
DOI: 10.1007/978-0-387-09412-0_4, Springer Science+Business Media, LLC 2009

Phase 2: Casualty receiving phase. During this phase, casualties are arriving at the designated receiving hospitals. There is limited information from the scene and there is overlap with Phase 1. Initially, hospitals have to depend on the resources immediately available. Blood stocks, diagnostic radiology, operating rooms and equipment and critical care beds are limited and must be carefully managed. The hospital is in a damage-control mode where the minimum resources are utilized for each patient to maximize surge capability.[3] Management is directed at saving life and limb while keeping the hospital functioning effectively. Phase 2 lasts for a few hours only.

Phase 3: Consolidation. All casualties have been received and the casualty receiving area is stood down. Most critically injured patients have had limited diagnostic work-up and damage-control procedures. Some are still in operating rooms and some walking wounded are still being assessed.

During this phase there is consolidation both of the clinical status of the patients and a restocking of the hospital's depleted resources. All patients are tallied with a full list of injuries identified so far. Full tertiary surveys document investigations to date, outstanding diagnostic work-up and likely subsequent operating room requirements. Once all diagnostics have been completed, planning can begin for definitive care (Phase 4). The emergency department, operating rooms, critical care areas and blood bank are re-stocked and staff rotated out for rest and recuperation. Phase 3 usually lasts ~24 h.

Phase 4: Definitive Care. This phase may last several weeks. These severely injured patients have large operating-room and critical-care needs which require extra resources for effective management. Patients have multiple trips to the operating rooms for fracture stabilization, wound debridement and reconstructive procedures. Extra operating time and medical and nursing staff reinforcement are required. Frequent multidisciplinary meetings for status updates and effective planning are required.

Phase 5: Rehabilitation. This phase may last several months. Survivors have intensive and specialist acute rehabilitation needs which need to be resourced effectively. Some patients continue to require further reconstructive surgery. Mental and physical rehabilitation teams work within the acute care setting to optimize patient outcomes.

The first two phases have been discussed elsewhere in this book. This chapter concentrates on the final three phases of consolidation, definitive care and rehabilitation. These important periods are rarely incorporated into major incident planning for hospitals. There is an expectation that these patients will simply be absorbed into routine activity. However these multi-dimensional, multi-system injured patients[3] are resource-intensive and exert significant ongoing demands on a system that must also recover from what has gone before. Additional resources are consumed managing families, police and media. Casualties of a terrorist event acquire a special status, but they must be managed within, and not compromise the care of, the existing patient population. Thus a smaller but significant amount of additional capacity sufficient for both groups must persist over the medium term.

Failure to understand and plan for the demands and complexities of these phases will result in additional strain on an already stressed system. It must also be recognized that the efficiency and quality of care in these later phases is very dependent on the effectiveness and attention to detail of the initial response.

After the terrorist bomb attacks in London on 7 July 2005, 197 patients were admitted to the Royal London Hospital, of which 27 patients arrived with a priority triage status and 10 patients were critically injured. Seventeen patients required surgery on the day of the incident and seven patients were admitted to the intensive care unit (ICU). This moderate casualty load placed a significant burden on the hospital over the next weeks and months. The 27 patients required 183 hours of theatre time over the next 14 days. Median stay in ICU for the seven patients admitted there was 12 days, with a maximum of 22. Maximum hospital stay was 64 days.[1] There was no provision for this ongoing workload in the hospital's Major Incident Plan.

Maintaining capability to optimally manage casualties requires rapid assessment of numbers and severity of injuries; a systematic stock-taking of depleted resources and an effective system for their replenishment. Resources at a premium can be summarized as space, staff and equipment.

Space: In the casualty receiving phase, space is generated throughout the hospital by rapid movement of patients or by temporarily upgrading or re-designating existing areas. While appropriate for the initial response, these areas need to be returned to routine use to allow normal hospital functions to resume.

For example, converting a post-operative recovery area into a satellite ICU is a simple and effective capacity-building measure. However, if the need for this space persists, lack of recovery facilities will slow the throughput of surgical cases. Conversion of other facilities, such as an endoscopy suite, will have similar implications. Maintaining capacity in these temporary spaces is difficult, more expensive and may have knock-on resource implications: for example, if piped oxygen is not available, there will be a steep increase in the requirement for bottled oxygen.

Operating room space also needs to be assessed. Extra operating room time is required along with associated staff and equipment costs. A temporary reduction in the routine workload may have to be accepted, for example, by the cancellation of more elective work.

Incident victims may be scattered throughout the hospital, wherever space could be generated at the time of the incident. There are several advantages to bringing them together in one ward. It aids the coordination of specialist care, simplifies security and allows the patients to group together for mutual support. A disadvantage is the concentration of large numbers of high-acuity trauma patients as well as the combined psychological and emotional impact on the staff of that ward.

Staff: In the initial phases of the incident, the dedication and enthusiasm of staff will ensure that staff numbers are adequate to manage the casualty influx, although the demand for some key specialists may be excessive. Some departments may find that they actually have too many staff—for example, the cancellation of elective radiography could lead to an abundance of radiographers. These staff will be required in the days and weeks to come and excess staff should be identified and sent home to rest as soon as possible. An estimate of current and future needs can be made relatively early after an incident begins—certainly after all scenes have been cleared and casualties triaged. Extra duty shifts should be arranged as necessary. Major incident plans should contain clear authority for department heads to fund extra shifts as they see fit.

During the incident, staff will grow tired. The acuity of the casualties and the external pressures of these unusual events may impair the performance of some. Senior clinicians must assess at an early stage how best to husband the potentially scarce resource of personnel through enforcing rest, rotating staff through different roles and controlling when to call in off-duty workers. The needs of staff for food, rest, accommodation and other services must be met. Some situations may require provision to be made for staff to leave to care for their homes or families which have themselves been involved in the event.

Care should be taken to identify and manage burn-out and compassion fatigue. Rest should be enforced and duties shared appropriately. De-briefing is important but the benefit of formal counselling is unclear, especially in the early days and weeks following an event.

Equipment: Successful planning for likely major incident scenarios should prevent hospitals from exhausting stocks of important consumables, including blood and drugs. However, critical shortages will occur if resupply is not effective. Pre-defined agreements should be in place with outside agencies. Policies with suppliers should include provision for mass casualty events. This is especially true of contracts with outside agencies providing vital services such as sterile supplies, orthopaedic fixation devices and specialist ventilators or beds. Suppliers should be queried as to their capacity to meet obligations made to nearby hospitals as well as your own.

Clinical care of the casualties during the consolidation and definitive care phases of the incident response also requires a coordinated, anticipatory strategy. This has four key elements:

- *Reassessment.* All severely injured patients must be continually reassessed, often several times a day. Tertiary surveys[4] should be carried out on all patients admitted to identify missed injuries and outstanding diagnostic imaging requirements.[3] These may need to be repeated as blast injuries evolve and diagnostic information becomes available.
- *Restructuring.* During the casualty receiving phase of the major incident many patients are managed simultaneously. Many of the clinicians involved during the initial response may not routinely treat trauma patients. A restructuring of care needs to take place to allocate patients to trauma specialties appropriate to their clinical requirements. In addition, concentrating responsibility in the hands of a few prevents dilution of experience and aids coordination. Responsible clinicians in other specialties, such as radiology and anaesthesia, should be appointed for the same reasons. Care must be taken not to allow the full workload and emotional burden to fall on a single clinician in any specialty.
- *Coordination.* The responsible clinicians should meet to discuss the patients' care at least daily. All departments caring for the patients or providing services for them should be included. These meetings are aimed at resolving confusion

generated during the chaos of the initial phases of the incident. The key outputs from these meetings are the management plans for individuals and the estimate of resources that this requires. Clinical information is shared, operating room time apportioned and prioritized. Thus managers should be represented alongside clinicians.

• *Quality* is ensured by examining care already given and jointly planning further treatment across specialty boundaries. Lessons should be identified, to be raised during debriefing. These meetings should continue for as long as they remain useful; they may last just a few days or may evolve, with changing attendance, to plan the late care and rehabilitation of victims.

These processes continue throughout the definitive care and rehabilitation phases. Gradually they become less frequent and less intensive. As patients move into the rehabilitation phase, new specialist staff are rotated in and some are no longer required. However multidisciplinary coordination and integration of care are vital at all stages, and become even more important as patients are readied for transfer to community care.

Security During a Major Incident

The security of the hospital site is of paramount importance—failure to ensure this can lead to threats to the hospital's ability to function from many sources:

• Uncontrolled movement of patients, especially the walking wounded
• Friends and relatives, or people searching for unidentified victims
• The media
• Curious members of the public
• Impostors posing as staff
• Terrorists

Hospitals are difficult places to secure. They are usually built to be welcoming and aesthetically pleasing. Many hospitals expand and modernize by the serial building of large extensions, often in a haphazard fashion. They may have multiple entrances and access through these may be necessary for patient care during a major incident. In general, hospital staff have a poor sense of ownership of security—wearing of ID badges is a chore and staff seldom challenge strangers moving about the hospital. The number of security personnel available may be small, particularly at night. Thus securing the hospital site during a major incident presents a considerable challenge.

Security departments must have their own major incident plans. During the major incident security staff will be stretched and call-out arrangements should include the ability to call on additional staff from private agencies. During the 7 July 2005 London bombings, security staff at the Royal London Hospital had to be diverted from the outer cordon to marshal two busloads of walking wounded who arrived unexpectedly. Aggressive members of the media, mostly freelance photographers, then invaded the ambulance area outside the emergency department, making ambulance movement extremely difficult.

The basic principle of hospital site security is the 'rings of protection',[5] a commonplace security concept. The outer ring is the boundary of the hospital site, next is the hospital buildings themselves and last is the inner ring surrounding critical areas and personnel. Each ring has associated physical, procedural and staffing measures to keep it secure—examples of these are, respectively, gates and doors, card readers and security patrols. Minimizing the number of points of access at each ring is crucial.

The security department must understand which parts of the hospital will be most important to the major incident response so that they may be protected, access to them controlled and movement between them facilitated. Coordination with the needs of other departments is the key. There is little point securing the Emergency Department (ED) by blocking the passage to the radiology department.

Most major incident plans will call for all staff to wear their ID badges and for these to be checked regularly. It is pointless to attempt this if staff do not routinely wear them. Effective major incident security therefore begins with effective routine security. Where ID cards include digital photographs, copies of these can be held centrally and new or temporary cards issued to staff whose identity can be verified.

A clear policy for dealing with 'good Samaritans' must be set out—these may be healthcare professionals from other institutions, concerned but unskilled members of the public, and charlatans or miscreants. No one should be employed in patient care who cannot establish their identity and qualifications. In general, utilization of people who do not routinely work in the hospital is counter-productive. There is almost always an initial surfeit of staff, and outsiders are not familiar with personnel, physical locations and local practices. The process of verifying identities and qualifications and of providing appropriate security badges diverts stretched resources from other vital functions.

After the immediate response to a terrorist incident has subsided there will still be considerable demands on the security department. In particular, victims admitted to the hospital must be secured from the unwanted attentions of the press and public. This is facilitated by concentrating the patients in one place. However, constant identity checks can be burdensome to patients, staff and relatives: clear explanations must be given as to why they remain necessary. The security department will also be expected to cooperate with the police in the gathering of evidence. Hospitals are also likely to enjoy visits from VIPs, who will have exacting security requirements at such times of enhanced threat.

Media Relations

Proper handling of media relations during a hospital's response to a terrorist incident is vital. Good use of the media can prevent the spread of disinformation, reduce (or increase) the influx of relatives and good Samaritans, reassure the public or educate them as to the symptoms of chemical or biological attack. How the media are handled during a major incident can have a lasting impact on the image and status of a hospital.

The crucial point to understand in interacting with the media is that journalists have to acquire a story (and pictures or film to go with it). This Darwinian imperative drives all news reporting. The vast majority of journalists are responsible and seek the truth through legitimate means. A hospital's response to a terrorist incident *is* a story. The job of a hospital's media relations staff is to ensure that the media have access to this story without the need to resort to unregulated means of acquiring it. Thus the hospital's story can be told while patients remain protected from intrusion.

Hospital media relations staff must have their own major incident plan, including many of the elements common to other plans such as divisions of responsibility, call-out plans and guides to available resources. Facilities must be set aside for the media. A room that might be appropriate for the use of the media in normal times may be useless during the initial response phase: journalists and, still more, photographers will wish to be near the Emergency Department (ED) entrance watching the arrival of ambulances.

Media relations staff should give the media regular, factual updates on the hospital's response. The earlier an initial statement can be made the better. The media services will quickly understand that information will be forthcoming and that they will have the opportunity to interact with senior staff and ask pertinent questions. This will reduce attempts to secure stories by other means. Journalists understand that confidential information cannot be disclosed but will expect to be given an idea of numbers and severity of injury. Statements to the press should therefore be drafted in consultation with senior managers and clinicians. It is vital that only verified facts are promulgated—journalists will be unforgiving if misled.

As the situation matures the media will wish to conduct interviews with members of staff. It is important that this happens under the supervision of media relations personnel. Staff should all be instructed to direct requests for interviews to them. Ideally, staff members who are to be interviewed should be relatively senior and have undergone media training.

Ultimately the media will also want to interview victims. This represents a legitimate public interest. Access to patients can only be allowed with their consent. However, it must be explained to patients that they are likely to single themselves out for sustained media attention in the weeks and months ahead. Great caution must be exercised by hospital staff and the patients themselves.

Handling of Relatives

Four types of relatives may be encountered following a terrorist incident:

- Relatives of identified in-patients
- Relatives of identified walking wounded (not admitted)
- Relatives of the missing
- Relatives of the dead

These four groups have very different needs. Relatives of identified in-patients require space to wait, refreshments, information about their relatives and, eventually, access to them. Relatives of the walking wounded have similar needs but also require advice on how to care for their relatives at home, including advice on specific symptoms to be alert for and contact details for follow-up and management of later emotional or psychological sequelae.

Relatives of the missing should ideally be directed to facilities such as phone lines administered by the civil authorities. However, in practice these can take some time to set up. Hospitals must make provision to accommodate these people, who may be highly distressed, until systems to find their relatives are available. These relatives may well arrive at a hospital other than that to which their relatives have been taken. A coordinated system agreed in advance between the hospitals and civil authorities would be of benefit but is rarely available.

The hospital also has a responsibility to work with the police and other agencies to identify casualties as quickly as possible. Documentation is often poor during the initial phases, but initial attention to detail has major benefits in the long term. The simple act of asking victims their names before intubation can save days of police work and relatives' anguish.

Relatives of the missing and of the deceased should ideally be accommodated separately from each other and from the first two groups. Hospital bereavement services will also be stretched by a terrorist incident—even if the total number of dead only equals that which the hospital normally has to deal with over a few days, they will all have been unexpected deaths in the most traumatic circumstances for the families. This will be compounded by the forensic requirement to delay disposal of the bodies. In addition, staff in many departments must be assigned to deal with victims' property. These may be contaminated, possibly even with the body parts of others. Staff must be prepared for this and understand the need to handle victims' effects without destroying evidence. Carefully ensuring that patients' effects are kept separate from others can aid the identification of the multiply injured.

Debriefing

Debriefing is a fundamental part of successful management of a hospital's response to a major incident. The debrief has many purposes, including much needed catharsis for hard-working staff and an opportunity for good work to be acknowledged. However the chief goal must be to identify lessons from this incident so that a better response may be mounted in future. No exercise can fully simulate a real incident; indeed a hospital's response to a small incident may well prove the most realistic and informative exercise in preparation for a big event.

It is important to begin the process while memories are still fresh. However, it must be remembered that different departments are involved in the response at different times. Hence a 'hot debrief' of emergency department staff will likely occur at a time when intensive care staff are busy admitting patients from the operating rooms.[1] This must be clearly acknowledged if large, open debrief sessions are conducted, to avoid the impression that continuing work is being ignored and some departments are excluded from the process. Such sessions, particularly when held soon after the incident, are perhaps most likely to be used to let staff get issues off their chests and for senior staff to thank their colleagues. Cold debriefs, some weeks after the incident when data has been collected and analysed, may be more effective in the long term for future planning.

Debriefing is not the only process that is required after a terrorist incident. Equipment usage should be inventoried. All patients should be added to a trauma database. Care of severely injured patients should be subjected to morbidity and mortality peer-review. Where the exigencies of the circumstances meant that sub-optimal or non-standard care was delivered this should be acknowledged and the cause found. The database should include information on patient movements so that a picture of the usage of the hospital facilities can be built up and bottlenecks identified.

All this activity will produce a wealth of information about the nature of the incident and the hospital's strengths and weaknesses in response. This must be put to good use. Internally, a designated officer should ensure that identified lessons are acted on. Major incident plans should be altered and the effect of changes audited after subsequent exercises and live incidents. Data gathered from the incident response should be used to inform future planning and exercises. Data on patient flow can be used to make exercises more realistic and validate computer models of major incident response.[6] These in turn can lead to realistic planning. Clinicians who have responded to significant terrorist attacks should publish the data they collect; few hospitals will encounter these events with sufficient frequency to be able to rely on their own experience.

Impact on Primary Care

Members of the primary care community may be affected in several ways by terrorist incidents. Primary care facilities are effective early triage and treatment posts of the walking wounded. If used effectively they can significantly reduce the burden of walking wounded on hospitals and allow concentration of resources on the critically injured.

As hospitals generate capacity, patients will be discharged. Enhanced primary care involvement in the early care of this group may help to identify those who need additional support and ongoing care. It has been suggested that primary care practitioners may identify patients who were discharged early and may allow minor problems to be treated early, preventing readmission.[7] Equally, a willingness by family practitioners to provide an enhanced level of care in the community could help to relieve pressure on hospital resources by reducing admissions of routine (i.e. not related to the terrorist incident) patients. However, family practitioners cannot be expected to provide in-patient care and, in particular, do not have the qualifications or resources to care for the acutely injured.

Primary care has an important role in the rehabilitation phase, as victims return to the community where their rehabilitation will be overseen and family doctors will be best placed to identify the signs of emotional and psychological consequences of the attacks. Liaison between hospital staff and primary care is important at this stage. There will be a large amount of information on each of the critically injured patients that needs to be transferred to community healthcare providers to ensure continuity of care. Health authorities should ensure that information and education is made available to support primary care in this role.

Healthcare as the Victim of Terrorism

The 9/11 Commission reported that the attacks were able to occur because there was a 'failure of imagination' among those responsible for anticipating this. Regrettably, there is no need for imagination when considering the possibility of terrorist attack on healthcare facilities. Such attacks are a common feature of insurgent activity in Iraq; at least 10 such incidents occurred in 2005.[8] In the same period attacks on hospitals were reported in India, Gaza and Jordan. Attacks on healthcare facilities in Western countries have not been a feature of the current terrorist threat, but they are by no means unheard of. The Provisional Irish Republican Army (IRA) exploded a bomb at Musgrave Park Hospital, Belfast, in November 1991, killing 2 and injuring 11 including a 5-year-old girl and a 4-month-old baby.[9] And in July 2006, Hezbollah fired a missile from Lebanon into the Western Galilee Hospital in northern Israel. Although the ophthalmology wing was destroyed, there were no casualties because patients and personnel had been moved to a protective area.[10]

Healthcare is integrated into the community and location it serves. It uses the same infrastructure, trades in the same currency and recruits from the same population. Thus as the community suffers from terrorism, healthcare suffers with it. Apart from the broader injury to society caused by terrorism, healthcare can suffer material losses, whether by being directly targeted or as collateral damage.

It is instructive to consider the causes of the failure of healthcare systems (particularly hospitals) in regions of larger scale conflict.[11] These give a guide to the means by which terrorism could impair the functioning of a healthcare system (Table 4.1).

Healthcare facilities and healthcare systems that may face these threats need to be able to maintain or restore their capabilities in the face of such events. This ability is known as resilience.[12] Resilience to terrorist threats will also increase resilience to other dangers such as natural disasters and industrial accidents and these should be considered as part of the same process. UK law (the Civil Contingencies Act 2004) requires 'Category 1 Responders', including emergency services, to have plans to maintain their services in the event of an emergency. This includes normal functioning of all their services, not just those needed to respond to the emergency.

Healthcare organizations should employ the principles of business continuity management (BCM) to attenuate the effect of terrorist incidents (and other events that might threaten their function). BCM requires the identification of the key activities and resources an organization requires in order to maintain its outputs (business impact analysis). A risk analysis then allows a measure to be taken of the threat to these factors. BCM strategies are then adopted to overcome these where feasible. These include plans for dealing with incidents such as real or threatened bombings,

TABLE 4.1. Failures and Impairments related to Conflicts and Terrorism

Causes of failure in areas of conflict	Causes of impairment due to terrorist action
Loss of physical infrastructure	Damage by direct attack
Loss of utilities	Direct attack on utilities and public infrastructure such as transport
Loss of skilled staff	Injury or death due to terrorist attack
Failure of routine services followed by loss of emergency care	Saturation of hospital facilities, for example, ICU beds. Loss of treatment opportunities for and revenue from elective care
Loss of emergency medical services and referral system, so patients cannot reach those facilities still functioning	Ambulance service may be overwhelmed during incident, to the detriment of other patients
	CBRN contamination of ambulances may render them useless
Loss of consumables, drugs and related items	Extraordinary consumption of particular drugs or other items, for example, atropine after chemical agent usage; ciprofloxacin after biological attack.
Breakdown in morale and motivation	Damage to community cohesion
	Fear of CBRN contamination
Forced closure	Secondary CBRN contamination due to arrival of victims
	Hospital usage restricted because of status as a crime scene
	Bomb threats

plans for restoring disrupted services and provision of additional resources to replace those that may be lost. The BCM strategy of a wealthy commercial bank may extend to a full alternative business site with a complete IT system shadowing that at the bank's normal premises. Duplication of a complex facility like a hospital is clearly impractical. However, duplication of a hospital's computerized patient records on another site would be a sensible defence against many threats, including fire. Finally BCM strategies should be exercised and BCM embedded in the culture of an organization. International standards in BCM have been promulgated.[13]

Hospitals must acknowledge the possibility of direct attack. As before, ownership of the issue of security by staff in normal times is needed. Routine checks of identity and restriction of access to sensitive areas are fundamental to making hospitals secure from terrorism and other, commoner threats, such as child abduction. Major incident plans for response to terrorist incidents elsewhere must include searches of the hospital site for secondary devices. Basic coordination of attacks in this manner is a common characteristic of the current terrorist threat. Security departments must have plans for use in the event of bomb threats or suspicious devices.

In the event of an actual attack on a hospital it will be necessary to evacuate parts of the hospital. Standard procedures are based on responding to small, isolated fires and use the principle of horizontal evacuation. Attacks using a small degree of coordination such that damage and fire occurs in more than one part of a hospital with rapid spread can make this inappropriate.[14] Low staff:patient ratios, particularly at night and compounded by the use of temporary staff unfamiliar with procedures, could lead to slow, ineffective evacuation and consequently increased loss of life.

A successful direct attack on a hospital is likely to impair its function, or force it to close. Reduced capacity may follow other events outlined above. In these cases healthcare systems at a regional or national level must have made provision for moving patients to other facilities. This will require adequate transport, involving ambulances being drawn in from elsewhere, and the production of additional capacity at receiving hospitals. Thus a cascade of further major incidents and disruption to hospital services will ensue. In metropolitan areas it will not be difficult to divert patients from a closed or impaired facility. However, in a rural context the loss of the only accessible hospital could have serious consequences—in this situation the identification of a suitable temporary facility for use after a terrorist incident or natural disaster may be appropriate.

Much more likely than direct attack on a hospital is damage to important local resources and infrastructure. Attacks on public transport systems are common. Particularly in urban areas, hospitals may depend on these to transport their staff to work. Public transport, particularly the London Underground, was severely disrupted following the 7 July 2007 bombings. The Royal London Hospital has now implemented a system of pre-designated collection points around London where staff can be asked to gather for transport by chartered coaches in the event of similar problems in future. Public utilities may also be targeted by terrorists; water supplies are particularly likely to be used to disseminate chemical, biological, radiological, nuclear (CBRN) hazards. Most hospitals have electrical generators and water tanks sufficient to cope with short-term losses of utilities but provision must be made for reinforcing these measures where terrorist attacks cause longer-lasting problems.

Whether by displacing patients from the hospital, blocking treatment facilities such as the operating rooms (OR), recovery suite and ICU or by preventing patients attending hospital, terrorist incidents can produce considerable lost revenue for hospitals. At the same time, multiply-injured patients require complex and expensive care and there are additional costs to cover staff overtime and other extraordinary activity. Effective hospital response to terrorist incidents is a vital part of national resilience. Thus, whether in a state or privately financed system, it is vital that mechanisms exist to adequately recompense hospitals and other providers for the expense of managing these complex incidents.

Consequences of Terrorism on Healthcare Policy

The purpose of terrorist actions is to bring about political change. It is rare for terrorists to directly succeed in altering the political make-up or foreign policy of a nation. However, even quite small terrorist incidents can lead to enormous political activity and indeed changes in policy. These changes are chiefly in the areas of civil rights, policing, homeland security and intelligence. Alterations in governmental funding priorities follow. Responding to a terrorist threat represents both an opportunity and a trap for healthcare organizations and systems. There is an opportunity to gain political leverage with which to argue for resources. But there is a trap of funding being distorted by political assessments of public health priorities.

There are grounds to believe that the attacks of 11 September 2001 and the subsequent anthrax attacks led to a distortion of US government funding for public health.[15] Initial proposals included a $1Bn smallpox vaccination program, later shelved after questions were raised as to its necessity and scientific basis. Subsequently billions of dollars of bioterrorism preparedness funding have been announced by the US Department of Health and Human Services (HHS). Proposed HHS spending on terrorism preparedness for FY 2008 is $4.3Bn.[16] This compares with proposed National Institutes of Health research spending of $2.3Bn on cardiovascular disease.[17] The terrorism preparedness funding is almost entirely directed towards biological threats, to the exclusion of other terrorist weapons, particularly the far more common conventional bomb and the trauma care needed to deal with it. Two people were killed as a result of inhalation of *Bacillus anthracis* at postal facilities in October 2001[18]; 3,400 died in the (non-CBRN) 9/11 attacks; 700,142 Americans died of heart disease in 2001.[19]

It should be noted of course that government will always be the sole or primary funder of terrorism preparedness whereas there are other sources of spending on cardiovascular disease research, prevention and treatment. In addition, terrorism preparedness is not only a health activity but also part of government's primary duty of defending the nation and maintaining peace and security. Nevertheless, a disconnection between funding levels and the actual risk to health that different types of terrorism present must be avoided.

References

1. Aylwin CJ, Konig TC, Brennan NW et al. Reduction in critical mortality in urban mass casualty incidents: analysis of triage, surge, and resource use after the London bombings on July 7, 2005. *Lancet* 2006;368(9554):2219–25.
2. Stein M, Hirshberg A. Medical consequences of terrorism. The conventional weapon threat. *Surg Clin North Am* 1999;79(6):1537–52.
3. Kluger Y, Mayo A, Soffer D, Aladgem D, Halperin P. Functions and principles in the management of bombing mass casualty incidents: lessons learned at the Tel-Aviv Souraski Medical Center. *Eur J Emerg Med* 2004;11(6):329–34.
4. Enderson BL, Reath DB, Meadors J, et al. The tertiary trauma survey: a prospective study of missed injury. *J Trauma* 1990;30(6):666–9.
5. Current Healthcare Security Issues and Countermeasures. http://www.ihf-fih.org/pdf/2roll.pdf. Accessed December 2, 2007.
6. Hirshberg A, Scott BG, Granchi T, Wall MJ, Jr., Mattox KL, Stein M. How does casualty load affect trauma care in urban bombing incidents? A quantitative analysis. *J Trauma* 2005;58(4):686–93; discussion 694–5.
7. Beyond a Major Incident. http://www.dh.gov.uk/prod_consum_dh/idcplg?IdcService = GET_FILE&dID = 14238&Rendition = Web. Accessed December 2, 2007.
8. Blackwell JK. Hospital Security and Force Protection: A Guide to Ensuring Patient and Employee Safety. http://www.tvfr.com/Dept/em/dnld/Blackwell_thesis-SECURITY_FP_GMP_0406.pdf. Accessed December 2, 2007.

9. Hodgetts TJ. Lessons from the Musgrave Park Hospital bombing. *Injury* 1993;24:219–21.

10. Gannon K. Hezbollah Rocket Hits Israel Hospital (Associated Press). http://www.breitbart.com/article.php?id = D8J53MH01&show_article = 1. Accessed February 29, 2008.

11. Ryan JM, Mahoney PF, Macnab C. Conflict recovery and intervening in hospitals. *BMJ* 2005;331:278–280.

12. UK Resilience. http://www.ukresilience.info/. Accessed December 2, 2007.

13. ISO/PAS 22399:2007. Societal Security—Guideline for Incident Preparedness and Operational Continuity Management. Geneva, Switzerland: International Organisation for Standards; 2007.

14. Hancock C, Johnson CW. Thinking the Unthinkable: Exposing the Vulnerabilities in the NHS Response to Co-ordinated Terrorist Actions. http://www.dcs.gla.ac.uk/~johnson/papers/NHS_terrorism.pdf. Accessed December 2, 2007.

15. Frank E. Funding the public health response to terrorism. *BMJ* 2005;331:378–379.

16. Advancing the Health, Safety, and Well-Being of Our People. FY 2008 President's Budget for HHS. http://www.hhs.gov/budget/08budget/2008BudgetInBrief.pdf. Accessed December 2, 2007.

17. Estimates of Funding for Various Diseases, Conditions, Research Areas. http://www.nih.gov/news/fundingresearchareas.htm. Accessed December 2, 2007.

18. Follow-Up of Deaths Among U.S. Postal Service Workers Potentially Exposed to *Bacillus anthracis*—District of Columbia, 2001–2002. *MMWR Weekly* 2003;52(39):937–938.

19. Anderson RN, Smith BL. Deaths: Leading causes for 2001. *Natl Vital Stat Reports* 2003;52(9):59–78

5
Terror Medicine: Education and Training

Yuri Millo

If a mass casualty incident (MCI) occurs on American territory, the main difficulty with disaster response is not from a lack of resources or volunteers but from a lack of a properly managed disaster plan. In fact, first responders and local healthcare practitioners, and even non-clinical locals rush to the scene and to local healthcare facilities to offer their services or make donations. The presence of so many volunteers and donations can be of great help during a disaster if properly managed. Even before 9/11, hospitals were required to have a disaster plan and ensure that their employees were familiar with it. Very few hospitals, however, actually worked on coordinating their disaster response plans with other hospital facilities, Emergency Medical Services (EMS), or local governmental facilities to offer a united response in case of a disaster.[1] Healthcare institutions therefore had difficulties not only working with other institutions preparing for a disaster but also were often unprepared for managing unexpected resources from the community.

Institutional readiness for disasters has improved somewhat since 9/11, with the new government-mandated National Incident Management System (NIMS) compliant Hospital Incident Command System (HICS)[2] and increased clinician familiarity with disaster protocol. Commonly cited references for medical practitioners such as Up-To-Date.com now describe how to manage disaster victims and describe the different signs and symptoms of major biological and chemical weapons of mass destruction.[3] Disaster drill frequency has increased across the country. However, even now, post-9/11, disaster preparedness is in its infancy. A 2007 Centers for Disease Control and Prevention (CDC) study on terrorism preparedness for office-based medical practitioners from 2003 to 2004 showed that less than 50% of physicians received some kind of training on at least one terrorism-related disease.[4] An even smaller percentage of allied health professionals received this training. The debacle of coordinating an efficient response to the flood victims in Louisiana also indicates that more training and education in the field of disaster medicine is needed. Training for the specialized field of terror medicine is also necessary as long as governments are an active target of terrorists.

S.C. Shapira et al. (eds.), *Essentials of Terror Medicine*,
DOI: 10.1007/978-0-387-09412-0_5, Springer Science+Business Media, LLC 2009

The specific challenges that any education and training for terror medicine must face in order to be effective, efficient, and customizable for specific kinds of MCI include the problems of engagement, finances, and the need to retrain. First, how should an institution respond to a terrorist attack? The details of a particular hospital's response plan are not obvious and require thoughtful development by administrators, clinicians, and other hospital staff who are well versed in NIMS protocols. As well, the plan needs to be rolled out to staff in a timely and efficacious manner. Second, financial planning for an MCI is essential: technologically advanced, sturdy, or space-saving medical equipment designed for MCI and often applicable for patient care during normal operations is available. Financial managers should be trained in how to incorporate MCI equipment purchases into their budgetary outlays in order to save expenses later during a real MCI. Third, terror medicine addresses incidents that – by definition – occur infrequently and unpredictably, but have high casualty rates when they do happen. Hospital staff may be trained once in the proper management protocols for MCI, but since they do not practice using these guidelines frequently, they will not be able to recall them quickly during an MCI. In a MCI, losing minutes of time can equate to losing patients. Basic education and training for terror medicine is similar to other situations like fencing: the fencer practices parries and reposts for hours until they are a part of his unconscious muscle memory and he can focus on his overall strategy. In a similar fashion, a doctor should not have to be struggling with putting on the right kind of boots and helmet while a patient lies dying at his feet. Much time can be wasted searching for the location of Personal Protective Equiment (PPE), the right persons to contact for interfacility risk communication, or the right way to request consults during an MCI. Proper education and training before MCI is essential.

The targets of terror medicine education and training are not only physicians and allied health professionals but also administrators, protective service personnel, lab technicians, and other hospital staff.

Physicians need to be ready for two kinds of training. First, they must learn how to recognize the signs and symptoms specific to particular kinds of terrorist weapons. An educational system should be available so that they can be trained on basic clinical guidelines at minutes' notice, since the specific kind of weapon (e.g., anthrax or nuclear) employed by a terrorist is difficult to predict beforehand and victims usually start arriving at local hospitals within minutes of an attack. A low-frequency/high-casualty MCI can have devastating effects if clinicians in the casualty receiving areas are not ready to apply the appropriate prophylactics, or use current treatment protocols.

Second, clinicians must be ready to adopt management principles that are the same for all MCI but differ from typical medical training, which focuses on managing a single patient well. Since these principles do not vary much for different MCI, they can be rolled out to clinicians well in advance of an MCI. The main management principles are how to manage multiple patients simultaneously, focus on the emergent patients that cannot be shunted aside, and manage time, departmental personnel, and resources (such as Personal Protective Equipment) effectively.

Hospital administrators must be trained in how to support the clinical teams during the stress and time constraints of an MCI. During an MCI, chief administrators in areas away from direct patient care need to be available to manage resources essential for patient care like clinical supplies, transport, and the personnel pool. Administrators must also be prepared to liaise with local government and EMS agencies, and to engage in astute risk communication with the local populace and media. They also need to prepare their facility according to federally mandated and researched management guidelines for the onslaught of an MCI – before it occurs.

Protective service personnel have a key role in MCI management. They serve to protect the hospital environment from hostile attack and maintain order in a chaotic MCI situation. They need to achieve competency in an "all-hazards" approach to handle threats, including MCI and terrorist attacks against their facility. They must be trained to analyze and plan for future threats to hospital security. In order to protect the innocent patients and hospital staff, they also need to analyze the mindset and motives of those who would inflict harm on the hospital. They should be ready to implement the tools available in their institutions to detect potential threats in the hospital.

Clinicians can flood the labs with certain types of lab requests during an MCI. To prevent backup in returning results, lab technologists should be prepared to "surge." They should also be trained to prioritize between the lab tests that need to be done immediately, and others that are less urgent. Other hospital staff should be given guidance about what procedures to follow if an MCI occurs; for instance, that they must absolutely show their ID badge in order to enter the facility. They should also be trained in general knowledge about the different kinds of disaster codes that are called at their facility and how they affect the day-to-day operations of the hospital at large.

When it comes to understanding how their role as physicians (or as other hospital staff) change in the event of an MCI, a systematic education and training program is useful. For convenience, terror management learning can be classified into three categories: education, training, and exercises and drills.

Education

The goal of terror medicine education is to improve patient care in both predicted and unpredicted situations. Educating for terror medicine encounters the challenge of all new disciplines in that it has had no systematic foundational treatises until now. Terrorists by definition try to shock and surprise their victims, so specialists in terror medicine must also constantly evolve to adapt to new psychological techniques and technological advances, while at the same time searching for underlying emergency management principles that are useful for predicting and responding to most terrorist incidents. In addition, authoring educational material for the field is difficult because terror medicine is based upon low-frequency/high-consequence events, which consequently have few subject matter experts.

The types of weapons used as instruments of terror are now classified as chemical, biological, radiological, nuclear, and explosive (CBRNE), but that division is a recent one and explosive) in the history of MCIs. Early uses of terror weapons do not usually show a systematic application; usually the technology was developed carefully but not applied in the most strategic manner. Conventional weapons were the first to be used in mass casualty events. A very early example of a conventional attack resulting in mass casualties was Archimedes's burning mirrors used against Roman soldiers.[†]

The pioneer of chemical weaponry was Thomas Cochrane. In the Napoleonic Wars, he proposed that the British navy use sulfur dioxide, which had a poisonous smoke. In the right wind conditions, it "would drift onto the object of attack with the dual purpose of providing a dense smokescreen and asphyxiating or driving off the defenders."[5] While this use of toxins is a creative approach to chemical weaponry, it is clear that the tactic could easily turn on those who used it. Later, in World War I, chemical weapons were used more frequently. Chlorine gas was used experimentally by the Germans at Ypres in 1915 but the commanders were unprepared for its deadly success in collapsing the Allied line. The great advantage of surprise was thereby lost for an unsystematic attack with limited goals, as Heller points out.[6] If the Germans had been educated in the likely outcome of the attack, that is, the routing of thousands of Allied soldiers from their front, they would have more likely employed the new weapon more strategically. As it happened, the Allies had time to develop and roll out gas masks (primitive personal protective equipment) to their soldiers (Fig. 5.1).

No one recognized the true advantages that mass casualty weapons have until World War II. During that period, the effort was made to develop CBRNE weapons as true mass casualty weapons. Discoveries in atomic physics, for instance, led to the development of fusion and fission bombs by the Allies. The bombing of Hiroshima and Nagasaki in 1945 are the first clear examples of deliberate, systematic MCI weapons deployment in human history: a mass casualty weapon was deployed and the ensuing casualty levels and threat of future incidents were key factors in the surrender of Japan shortly thereafter.[‡] The Japanese government and healthcare

---

[†] When Marcellus [the Roman commander attacking Syracuse, Archimedes' city] withdrew them [his ships] a bow-shot, the old man [Archimedes] constructed a kind of hexagonal mirror, and at an interval proportionate to the size of the mirror he set similar small mirrors with four edges, moved by links and by a form of hinge, and made it the centre of the sun's beams – its noon-tide beam, whether in summer or in mid-winter. Afterwards, when the beams were reflected in the mirror, a fearful kindling of fire was raised in the ships, and at the distance of a bow-shot he turned them into ashes. In this way did the old man prevail over Marcellus with his weapons.
John Tzetzes, Chiliades, Book II, Lines 118–128.
[‡] Moreover, the enemy has begun to employ a new and most cruel bomb, the power of which to do damage is, indeed, incalculable, taking the toll of many innocent lives. Should we continue to fight, not only would it result in an ultimate collapse and obliteration of the Japanese nation, but also it would lead to the total extinction of human civilization. Such being the case, how are We to save the millions of Our subjects, or to atone Ourselves before the hallowed spirits of Our Imperial Ancestors? This is the reason why We have ordered the acceptance of the provisions of the Joint Declaration of the Powers.
Hirohito, August 14, 1945, capitulation announcement.

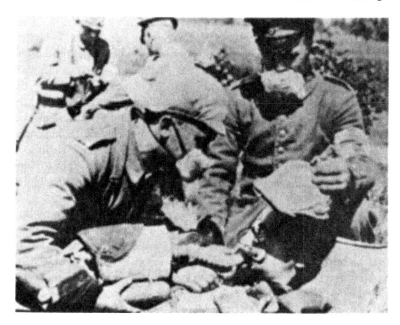

FIG. 5.1. German medics, wearing an early mask, giving oxygen to gas victim, 1915. British, French, and Russian prototype masks were similar in design. Gas masks being used by World War I medics is evidence of terror medicine educational preparedness. From Heller Combat Studies Institute (Public domain).

personnel were completely unprepared to handle such a disaster. They had no reliable method of communication in a disaster and at first officials refused to believe that an MCI of such a great extent could occur. Their response to the disaster exacerbated the resulting medical problems faced by the victims. Biological and radiological weapons and education have proceeded apace.

While terror medicine tends to focus upon MCIs, individual persons – such as Alexander Litvinenko, victim of radiation poisoning – can also be victims of terror attacks, and clinical physicians need to be educated to face these threats as well so that they can not only treat the patient rightly but also know when it is necessary, and how to protect other patients from contamination. Medical practitioners also need to be trained to quickly recognize a victim of a biological attack, so that the appropriate antidote can be applied.

Terror medicine education has a clear goal: to impart information on how to manage patients and communications during a disaster to minimize patient suffering and maximize the use of institutional resources. As shown historically, with the rise of MCI attacks, having greater disaster education can help mitigate the severity and duration of victim injuries should an MCI occur. Because much of the field is in constant flux, however, pedagogical material must often be modified and revised, and should require a low level of investment to create. The earliest educators for MCI were in the military, since historically military personnel have borne the brunt of mass casualties. Military healthcare educational research facilities shared a background with military medicine during the cold war, and were the first to approach the challenge of educating on terror medicine. The U.S. Army Medical Research Institute of Infectious Diseases (USAMRIID, http://www.usamriid.army. mil/index.htm), the center of excellence for the Department of Defense medical biological defense research, was founded in 1969. The education section of the Institute focuses on instructing military personnel on defending against biological weapons but recently has branched out to include civilian clinicians in biological terror medicine education.[§]

Several major civilian research facilities exist in America that provide education for MCI. In the civil healthcare environment only a few academic and hospital based institutes took the initiative and developed content for healthcare providers. Most of the work on terror was developed by grants provided by the CDC and tailored for public health with the assumption that terrorism is a public health domain. A full list of courses and publications is available. The Center for Public Health Preparedness at Harvard has developed partnerships with local, regional, and statewide organizations to promote emergency preparedness educational opportunities (homepage: http://www.hsph.harvard.edu/hcphp/products/ webcasts/index.html). The Integrative Center for Homeland Security at Texas A&M University (homepage: http://homelandsecurity.tamu.edu/) has begun to collaborate with Texas A&M faculty to offer courses for degree credit in the field of emergency preparedness and related areas. The Johns Hopkins Bloomberg School of Public Health offers a wide variety of educational material for terror medicine through its Public Health Preparedness division (homepage: http://www.jhsph.edu/ preparedness/).

Most of these opportunities, however, focus upon how a system – such as a hospital, clinic, or EMS division – should respond to a terror incident. They do not, however, offer assistance on how to medically manage patients who are victims of an MCI. Several institutions are beginning to respond to this need. The George Washington University School of Medicine, partly because of its location in central Washington, DC, offers an interdisciplinary Disaster Preparedness track program lasting throughout medical school (curriculum: http://www.gwumc. edu/smhs/students/opportunities/ep_curriculum.htm). In Israel, a relatively large number of healthcare providers and researchers have had firsthand experience of

---

[§] The USAMRIID offers several satellite-recorded civilian clinician courses such as "Medical Defense Against Biological Agents Botulinum Toxin," http://www.usamriid.army. mil/education/satellite.htm.

MCI. At Hadassah University Hospital in Israel, various training and educational materials are offered on terror medicine management (http://www.hadassah.org.il/English). The ER *One* Institute at the Washington Hospital Center Department of Emergency Medicine, located close to the heart of Washington, DC, offers a variety of educational material specific for clinicians managing patients in the wake of a terror incident (homepage: http://EROneInstitute.org). In particular, the Simulation and Training Environment Lab Learning Management System is an eLearning platform that provides sophisticated and continuously updated education for healthcare providers based upon Israeli and American terror medicine expertise (www.sitel.org, www.web.sitelms.org). The Institute for Bioterrorism and Emerging Disease (BEPAST, homepage www.bepast.org) researches, collects, and shares information, and is chartered to facilitate up-to-date resource planning and the dissemination of knowledge on emerging diseases related to terrorism or natural disease outbreaks.

Educational deliverable options vary, and deciding which one is most suitable depends on several variables. First to be considered is the educational time frame. That is, the educational coordinator must consider if the occasion is emergency preparedness education, but without an impending MCI occurring or, on the contrary, if a Code Orange for anthrax contamination was just called overhead. Second, the number of students must be considered; if large, an institutionalized, easily accessible course would be appropriate, but if small, a department-specific inservice might be better. Third is the educational budget. Finally, the preferences of the clinical personnel should be considered. Some have familiarity with web-based training and are more likely to enjoy being educated online, but others are more comfortable with printed material, and will absorb the information more easily that way.

Educational material can be accessed in hardcopy mainly through journals, since few books in English have yet been specifically aimed at terror medicine education. Both disaster-specific journals and terror-medicine articles in emergency medicine serials are now easily available to most medical education facilities, and since 9/11 the number of articles pertaining to terror medicine has "increased tremendously," according to G Kelen and L Sauer (Acad Emerg Med Volume 14, 5 Supplement 1, 189–190).[¶] In fact, we are on the cusp of an upsurge in terror medicine educational material in all media, not simply through the printed word. Online terror medicine education is available through satellite lectures,[∥] online recorded lectures and/or

---

[¶] Cf. for instance *Disaster Medicine and Emergency Health Preparedness*, started in 2007. ISSN: 1935-7893, The Official Medical Journal of the World Association for Disaster and Emergency Medicine and the Nordic Society for Disaster Medicine, and the *American Journal of Disaster Medicine*.

[∥] The CDC and the Johns Hopkins School of Public Health also offer education via satellite links. See also http://www.usamriid.army.mil/education/satellite.htm

PowerPoint presentations,** question-and-answer scenarios†† and online printed material‡‡ workshops, and seminars.

At this point, terror medicine is yet to be academically recognized in its own right, although the closely related fields of Disaster Medicine and Homeland Security are disciplines at accredited American institutions. We expect that this book will be the cornerstone for establishing the field of terror medicine as a global discipline. In order to progress in the field, researchers should gather experts from around the world in order to compile evidence-based learning into one standardized manual. Educational experts should consult those medical professionals in China who have experienced SARS, garner the expertise of African physicians who have seen Hemorrhagic Fever Virus firsthand, confer with Israeli security experts on Conventional MCI, and learn from Russian physicians who experienced treating patients from radiation incidents. Terrorists do not restrict their attacks to one nation or one type of weapon. Likewise, terror medicine experts should gather educational material to rollout for every current feasible terror weapon to assist their clinicians in the front lines of attack, whether be it on a battlefield or at Ground Zero.

Training

Training involves teaching students to practically apply cognitive knowledge about a field so they can reach a competency level in it. The most effective training has been found to be systematic, which uses structured tools and has relatively stand-ardized measurements of success. While education for terror medicine is based upon different kinds of lectures and is largely theoretical, the demands of an actual MCI require that students learn pragmatic MCI management skills by hands-on courses. The goal of a systematic terror medicine training program, then, is to teach students how to practically apply the appropriate knowledge both as an individual and as an integral member of a team.

Throughout history, many types of training for events with large numbers of casualties have been developed. Most of the preparations were for bringing about MCI rather than for responding to it. Even so, it is useful to review historical types of training because the principle of preparedness remains the same: regularized training is remarkably effective. Students who were trained in these systems were often demonstrably more successful during combat than their counterparts, who

---

** For instance, see The Yale New Haven Center for Emergency Preparedness and Disaster Response at http://ynhhs.emergencyeducation.org/ and the Simulation and Training Environment Lab Learning Management System (LMS) at www.web.sitelms.org.

†† The Question and Answer format for diagnosing different types of biological MCI victims at http://www.bioterrorism.uab.edu/home.html through the University of Alabama School of Medicine.

‡‡ See the Johns Hopkins Bloomberg School of Public Health for examples of online printed material.

had little or no standardized training. The Spartans, for instance, were famous for the harsh training and indoctrination of their citizen-soldiers.[§§] Because of this training, they were the most feared soldiers in ancient Greece due to their immaculate discipline and valor.[¶¶]

Early on, the Romans had professionalized gladiator training; later, they realized that this training could carry over into other areas and applied it to their soldiers so that they were well versed in sophisticated weapons tactics.[‖‖] Later, starting in 1493 A.D., the Ottoman Empire systematically trained thousands of enslaved children of Christian subjects to be Janizaries, elite guards, and soldiers.[***] Ever since the Renaissance, most military and paramilitary institutions have employed

---

[§§] Plutarch, Lives of the Noble Greeks and Romans: Lycurgus.
At the age of seven, Spartan boys left home and went to live under military discipline. Those who showed the most skill and courage were appointed by the old men to be leaders, with the authority to order the other boys and the power to punish disobedience. The main subject they studied was command and obedience. Spartan boys learned enough reading and writing to be literate, but learning how to endure pain and conquer in battle was considered even more important.

[¶¶] See Thucydides describing the surrender of the Spartans at Pylos (Tr. Hobbes: Thucydides, The English Works, vol. VIII (The Peloponnesian War Part I, IV:40) [1839]).
Of all the accidents of this war, this same fell out the most contrary to the opinion of the Grecians. For they expected that the Lacedæmonians [Spartans] should never, neither by famine nor whatsoever other necessity, have been constrained to deliver up their arms, but have died with them in their hands, fighting as long as they had been able: and would not believe that those that yielded, were like to those that were slain.

[‖‖] As Valerius Maximus (ca. 20 ad) wrote in Factorum et dictorum memorabilium libri ix (Nine Books of Memorable Actions and Speeches) 2.3.2,
The practice of weapons training was given to soldiers by P. Rutilius, consul with C. Mallis. For he, following the example of no previous general, with teachers summoned from the gladiatorial training school of C. Aurelus Scaurus, implanted in the legions a more sophisticated method of avoiding and dealing a blow and mixed bravery with skill and skill back again with virtue so that skill became stronger by bravery's passion and passion became more wary with the knowledge of this art.
(Tr.: The Latin Library at Ad Fontes Academy.)

[***] See Islamic History Sourcebook: James M. Ludlow: The Tribute of Children, 1493. From: Eva March Tappan, ed., The World's Story: A History of the World in Story, Song and Art, (Boston: Houghton Mifflin, 1914), Vol. VI: Russia, Austria-Hungary, The Balkan States, and Turkey, pp. 491–494.
… [M]any thousands of the European captives were educated in the Mohammedan religion and arms, and the new militia was consecrated and named by a celebrated dervish. Standing in the front of their ranks, he stretched the sleeve of his gown over the head of the foremost soldier, and his blessing was delivered in the following words "Let them be called Janizaries [yingi-cheri–or 'new soldiers']; may their counternaces be ever bright; their hand victorious; their swords keen; may their spear always hang over the heads of their enemies; and, wheresoever they go, may they return with a white face." …. Such was the origin of these haughty troops, the terror of the nations.… Both classes [of Janizaries] are kept under a strict discipline. The former especially are accustomed to privation of food, drink, and comfortable clothing and to hard labor. They are exercised in shooting with the bow and arquebuse by day,

systematic training. The more rigorous the training, in general the more successful were the students.

Until the past half-century, systematic training regimens were largely used for military training and readiness and no programs for training clinicians to *respond* appropriately to a mass casualty event were implemented significantly. In the present day, educators and trainers have realized that training military members for war is similar in principle to training responders for MCI preparedness. Both involve readiness for low-frequency/high-casualty events: even though a battle may not loom in the near future, still, military personnel must be ready for it when it occurs. Likewise, physicians should be ready to lead their teams in the event of an MCI, and systematic training should give them the skills necessary to respond effectively. Training clinicians for terror medicine is thus a new and – given the worldwide terrorist threat levels – vitally important field. Training now involves two steps. The student must reach a competency level in a particular subject, and then undergo exercises to maintain the ability to perform that procedure. The frequency of exercises for the second step varies inversely to how often a procedure is performed in medical practice. Some procedures are crucial and have a high level of complexity, so require ongoing training. For example, C-sections are complex procedures, yet are central to obstetrics/gynecology practice, so a resident in the field must frequently be tested on the ability to perform the procedure. Other protocols are straightforward and may only be necessary if an MCI were to occur. Thus, training for these procedures can be rolled out on an ad hoc basis and is called "Just In Time Training." For instance, clinicians do not need to know how to use a cyanide antidote kit in nearly every medical situation, so it would not normally be worthwhile for them to memorize the proper steps in the application of the antidote. However, if patients could have been poisoned by a cyanide agent, then they would need to be trained speedily in the proper application of the antidote.

Several different types of medical training vehicles are useful in terror medicine procedures. Training on real, living patients is the traditional way that clinical personnel have learned how to perform procedures. The advantage of training on live patients is clear: since the patients have complete fidelity to actual victims, then the physician learns exactly how to do a procedure correctly. Since terror medicine focuses upon low-frequency events, it is not ideal to rely upon live patient training to teach physicians the proper MCI response: most clinical personnel would not encounter a terror victim until an actual MCI, when large numbers of patients would threaten to overwhelm his or her ability to treat them. Other methods of training

---

and spend the night in a long, lighted hall, with an overseer, who walks up and down, and permits no one to stir. When they are received into the corps of the Janizaries, they are placed in cloister-like barracks, in which the different odas or ortas live so entirely in common that the military dignitaries are called from their soups and kitchens. Here not only the younger continue to obey the elders in silence and submission, but all are governed with such strictness that no one is permitted to spend the night abroad, and whoever is punished is compelled to kiss the hand of him who inflicts the punishment.

have recently been developed in response to the problem of training for MCI and use simulation, "the artificial representation of a situation, environment, or event that provides an experience for the purposes of learning, evaluation, or research."[7] High-fidelity patient simulators are "[c]omputer-controlled, full-body mannequins ..." They serve many purposes, such as "imitate[ing] cardiovascular and pulmonary physiology well and allow[ing] verbal interactions with a patient," and can also specialize in "simulating regional anatomy." Twenty patient simulators are being rolled out at different facilities across the country for various purposes. At the National Capital Area Medical Simulation Center at Walter Reed Army Hospital, Washington, DC, a number of advanced patient simulators for MCI are used in courses for MCI preparedness as well as for clinical training (http://simcen.usuhs.mil/). The National Capital Area (NCA). Simulation Center has several training departments, including Clinical Skills Teaching and Assessment Laboratory, the Virtual Training Center (VTC), Room and Computer Laboratory, and the Surgical Simulation Laboratory. The SiTEL Clinical Simulation Centers at the Washington Hospital Center in Washington, DC, and the Union Memorial Hospital in Baltimore, MD, partner with the leading manufacturers of clinical simulators to develop, research, and evaluate new products and technologies to fit the next generation of Clinical Simulation Centers (www.csc.sitelms.org and www.sitel.org) (Fig. 5.2).

A number of medical schools now incorporate training on high-fidelity simulators into their core curriculum, although most use them for conventional medical

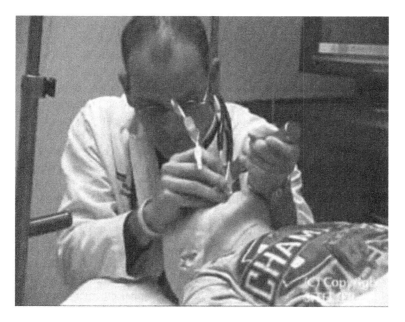

FIG. 5.2. A resident physician being trained to perform intubations on a high-fidelity patient mannequin (Courtesy of Dr. Cory Wittrock and the Washington Hospital Center Department of Emergency Medicine)

training rather than for MCI training. In Israel, the Medical Simulation Center (MSR) trains clinicians on the appropriate responses to an MCI patient with a high-fidelity patient simulator (http://www.msr.org.il/Courses_Medical_Simulation_Center/166.htm).

Using standardized patients – who are actors or volunteers simulating an illness or disorder – are another excellent way that institutions provide training to clinicians for MCI responses. To increase realism, a standardized patient can even be moulaged in imitation of a real patient. The Federal Emergency Management Agency (FEMA) uses the Nobel Training Center for courses on emergency preparedness. The Military USMARIID offers courses for bioterrorism preparedness with standardized patients. The National Disaster Life Support Foundation offers standardized patients in their Basic Disaster Life Support and Advanced Disaster Life Support courses (http://66.160.8.45/index.asp). The American Burn Association provides the American Burn Life Support hands-on course that utilizes standardized patients to train clinicians and first responders on how to treat burn patients (http://www.ameriburn.org/). The ER *One* Institute at the Washington Hospital Center offers the Hospital Disaster Life Support (HDLS: www.HDLS.SiTELMS.org) and Hospital Disaster Life Support II (HDLS II: www.HDLS2.SiTELMS.org) courses. The Armed Forces Radiobiology Research Institute (AFRRI) also utilizes standardized patients during training (http://www.afrri.usuhs.mil/www/news/previousheadlines/terror_disaster_drill.htm). Finally, standardized patients are commonly used by medical schools to teach students the appropriate ways to respond to a patient situation without compromising quality of care for any real patient.

In the constantly evolving field of terror medicine training, the most recently developed training method is by a virtual simulator. Instructional designers and multimedia programmers develop and deploy online educational training games which offer a powerful way to educate and train on competencies-based content for healthcare providers. The teaching method employed is often a first-person interactive simulation training whereby the user will be placed in a virtual Emergency Room, Emergency Operation Center, or other key emergency preparedness position (Fig. 5.3).

The user will be required to perform various tasks that will reinforce the best practice procedures for MCI, and his adherence to these protocols is scored (Fig. 5.4).

Sometimes the virtual simulator will include a pre and post test to test the user's acquisition of knowledge. The participant will have learned the correct disaster responses so that when a real MCI occurs, he will know how to respond calmly and efficiently. One virtual simulator available publicly, "Emergency Room: Code Red," trains the participant in clinical management of cases typical during an MCI.[8] "Code Orange," developed by SiTEL at the ER *One* Institute, is a serious game which uses the techniques of the commercial strategic games (such as "Civilization"[†††]) and applies it to the field of hospital emergency management where it trains the participant in managing communication, personnel, supplies,

---

[†††] Created by Sid Meier for MicroProse in 1991.

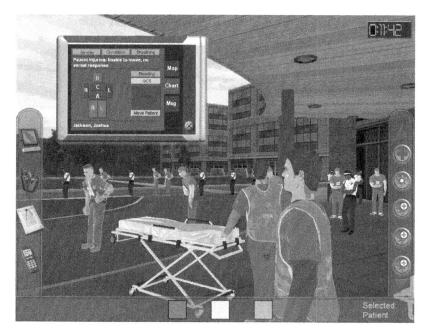

Fig. 5.3. An overview of a virtual, interactive Emergency Department that locates patients, other player movements, and supplies along with a map of the scenario. (Courtesy of the Code Orange Simulation by SiTEL© and the ER One Institute)

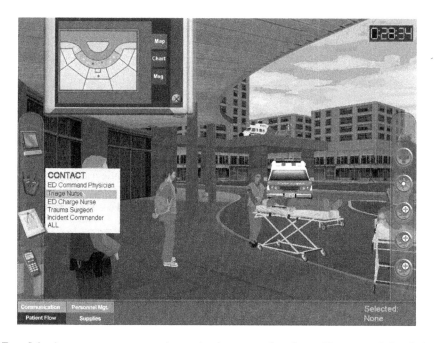

Fig. 5.4. An emergency preparedness simulator user interface. (Courtesy of the Code Orange Simulation by SiTEL© and the ER One Institute)

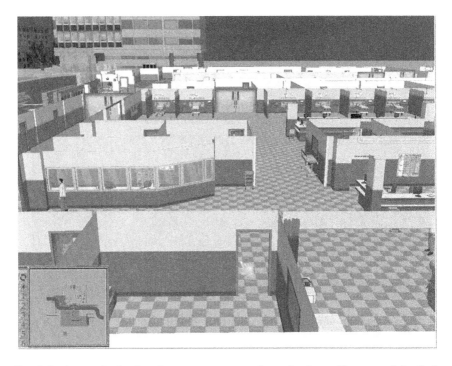

Fig. 5.5. A recently developed emergency preparedness simulator. (Courtesy of the Code Orange Simulation by SiTEL© and the ER One Institute)

and patient flow effectively according to government-mandated incident command standards (NIMS and HICS) (Fig. 5.5).

Training for an MCI has evolved a long time from the days of the Spartans, and the field is still constantly changing. In the future, training can be expected to involve more technological developments and will become integral to core medical training. The challenge will be to make sure that clinical students do not lose sight of the patient, the individual person who is suffering the effects of an MCI, behind all of the exciting technological enhancements.

Exercises and Drills

Once a student completes the initial training for a high-casualty/low-frequency event, then the student's competency needs to be maintained by exercises and drills. Logistically, exercises and drills are the same, and so can be considered together, but their purposes are different. An exercise is when a student gives a hands-on demonstration of what he has been trained to do. The purpose of an exercise is to allow the student to maintain his competency. Unlike exercises, which test students in an expected way, drills test student(s) in unforeseen scenarios. The reason a drill is conducted is to find a gap in preparedness: the drill administrators want to see where the system lacks resources or where competencies are not fulfilled. Based upon the results, a drill may also provide a way for an institution to improve future training.

Historically, training, exercises, and drills were considered under the same rubric. For instance, in ancient Greece, training for Olympic events was combined with exercise and drills, as Epictetus writes.[‡‡‡] Men who wanted to be Olympic victors had to swear that they had been in training (which implies exercises and drills to test the contestant's body) for at least ten months prior to the contest.[9]

In modern days, hospital planners realized the potential usefulness of drills and exercises for emergency preparedness. They can be designed based upon the identified stresses specific for the institution's locations. For instance, on the West coast a drill scenario might involve a nuclear accident if the facility is near a nuclear plant, a tsunami, or an earthquake, while elsewhere in the country a flood or hurricane might be the tested scenario.

Hospitals must incorporate drills and exercises into their facility planning, per the Joint Commission (TJC), which mandates as a minimum two exercises per year. One involves the community and the other must be a full hospital-scale exercise. According to TJC, exercises have a cycle: planning, exercising, and a post-action report. Most of the drills and exercises promoted by TJC are intended to test the integrity of the system and the effectiveness of an institution's teamwork during a simulated MCI, and assess the competencies of individual practitioners only secondarily. They occur across the country, since they must be done at every institution that can be considered a casualty receiver from an MCI. Several planned exercises, however, are noteworthy for their complexity and fidelity to a real MCI. Operation Kerkesner, a first-year medical student exercise, and Operation Bushmaster, are an exercise and drill for the Uniformed Services University of the Health Sciences and involve medevac as well as regular first responders and hospital facilities (http://www.usuhs.mil/mem/operationinformation.html) (Fig. 5.6).

In the north/central Washington, DC, area, the multi-campus Collaborative Multi-Agency Exercise (CMAX) drill is held and involves Georgetown University Hospital, the National Institutes of Health, Sibley Hospital, Suburban Hospital, the Walter Reed VA Hospital, and the Washington Hospital Center.

[‡‡‡] You say, "I want to win at Olympia." … If you do, you will have to obey instructions, eat according to regulations, keep away from desserts, exercise on a fixed schedule at definite hours, in both heat and cold; you must not drink cold water nor can you have a drink of wine whenever you want. You must hand yourself over to your coach exactly as you would to a doctor. Then in the contest itself you must gouge and be gouged, there will be times when you will sprain a wrist, turn your ankle, swallow mouthfuls of sand, and be flogged. And after all that there are times when you lose.
Epictetus, Discourses 15.2-5, trans. W.E. Sweet cit. ap.

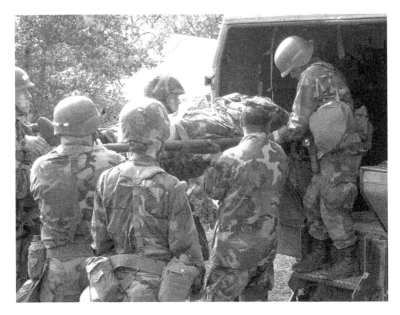

Fig. 5.6. An exercise at the Uniformed Services University of the Health Sciences. Photo from: http://www.usuhs.mil/images/jpg/operations4.jpg. (Courtesy of Uniformed Services University of the Health Sciences)

Recently, emergency preparedness experts have developed a range of types of exercises and drills. The first is a Tabletop and requires the least manpower to implement but likewise has the least fidelity to a real scenario. Tabletops are most effective if coupled with a walk-through. The other options fall under the category of a live scenario. Some exercises and drills use live actors or volunteers from the community, who simulate injuries. Other exercises and drills can utilize moulaged actors. The make-up adds to the reality of the drill.

While the drill becomes more realistic when volunteer "victims" flood the Emergency Department (ED) and other key areas, they use space that could be used for patient care and require dedicated manpower. High-fidelity manniquins can also be used and allow for testing of invasive, realistic treatment of injuries (Fig. 5.7).

The most cost-effective and convenient way to implement drills and exercises is through web-based virtual multi-player simulations, which are available 24/7/365 and are not restricted to one location.

Through these simulations different skills such as resource, personnel, and time management can be tested. No real patient care is affected since personnel are managing patients in cyberspace, and virtual simulation uses the least amount of hospital resources. The disadvantages are that – even with workarounds – the scenario is not being played in realtime, and even if the graphics are excellent, the virtual patients lack fidelity to real persons.

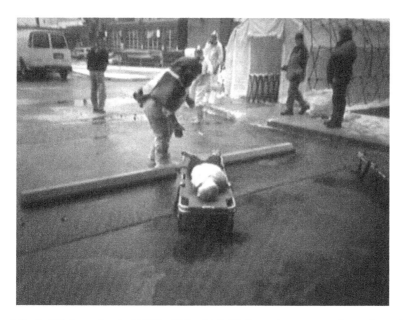

FIG. 5.7. A drill for a chemical MCI utilizing high-fidelity patient mannequins and attendees wearing personal protective equipment. (Courtesy of SiTEL© and the ER One Institute)

While teamwork and system integrity are essential during a real MCI, hospital planners should consider going beyond the minimum requirements of TJC emergency preparedness. The competency of individual practitioners to respond effectively and efficiently to an MCI should also be tested, and can often be done most easily by using an innovative format for the drill or exercise.

Conclusions

Terror medicine education and training offer diverse options customizable for institutions' or individual physicians' needs. Before implementing any learning program, however, it is necessary to consider what constitutes a successful curriculum.

Since terror medicine learning is a field in its earliest stages, it is relevant to consider historical antecedents for successful systematic education and training. All military and Greco-Roman athletic training had one simple, common factor so far as success was concerned: a successful student was a victorious one. Coming in second place militarily was certainly not an option, and likewise only Olympic victors were remembered. No second place prizes were awarded.

For modernity, defining what constitutes successful education and training can vbe more complex and controversial, especially when it comes to terror medivcine, as Asher Hirshberg pointed out.[10] Disasters will always occur, hospitals will continue to receive large numbers of victims, and not all of them can be treated optimally within a short span of time. In a real MCI, the percentage of patients with critical injuries demanding immediate attention is small, and although they are most in need of care, they are often the patients who are less likely to demand attention in the turmoil of a casualty receiving area. Physicians and other clinicians should therefore be trained to recognize and focus upon the few critically injured patients, and firmly transfer resources from less critically injured patients to rescue the ones severely injured. It may seem callous, but there can be no simple triumph in MCI management, and emergency preparedness planners should recognize that fact.

Finding real, solid data about a particular institution's response to an MCI in order to analyze its effectiveness – and, implicitly, the efficacy of its education and training programs – is difficult, however. The crux of education and training for terror medicine thus lies at the borders of an institution's surge capacity. When an institution's surge capacity is approached, the larger the number of critically injured patients, the lower the level of care.[11] No hospital, however, has ever reported a gradually failing trauma line,[12] and few agencies admit to mismanagement during an MCI.§§§ Criteria for successful training and education can sometimes be obvious, for example, showing that concretely measurable protocols such as the JCAHO Standardized Stroke Measure Set (Harmonized Measures) were implemented.¶¶¶ The standard for successful education and training for terror medicine, however, can vary depending on institutional capabilities. A Level One Trauma Center with a certified Burn Center should be held to a different standard than a small, community hospital. The measurement for a successful response to an MCI should be that, without exaggerating real hospital and first responder capabilities, if physicians and other staff are trained well, they should let as few truly emergent patients die as possible.‖‖‖ (Also see chapter 11 for more on these concepts.)

Most facilities do not have the opportunity to learn from a real MCI to plan a better curriculum for the future. Several types of metrics used by the education and

---

§§§ Cf., for instance, the response to the London bombing in July 2005: "The Metropolitan Police said it and the British Transport Police felt their radio systems worked well and they were able to work around the difficulties communicating underground. 'We didn't feel that was detrimental to our response,' said Asst Comm Alan Brown." Yet a London Assembly report found that "[p]oor communication and a lack of basic medical supplies hampered the 7 July bombings rescue operation," BBC online International Version, "7 July report highlights failings," June 5, 2006:

http://news.bbc.co.uk/2/hi/uk_news/england/london/5046346.stm.

¶¶¶ See the Joint Commission Primary Stroke Centers Standardized Stroke Measure Set (Harmonized Measures) available at: http://www.jointcommission.org/CertificationPrograms/PrimaryStrokeCenters/standardized_stroke_measure_set.htm.

‖‖‖ An MCI is an incident that does not overwhelm all medical facilities' surge capacities: that is a catastrophe. Training and education for terror medicine as proposed in this chapter does not look at catastrophes, because in that event, no strategic planning can prevent the deaths of many critically injured patients.

training programs described above have been developed by leading subject matter experts and can provide simulated ways to track the successfulness of terror medicine education and training. For education, post-quiz results can be compared with pre-quizzes, and the successful completion of a course can be determined if the student demonstrates a better grasp of the material after completing the educational module than before he learned it. For training and exercises for terror medicine, a student can show competency in a certain procedure by demonstrating it (with a live, standardized, or virtual patient). Successfully completing exams that propose scenarios similar to the ones the student encountered in training are also possible. An individual clinician or a team (such as the Triage Area) can be considered successfully prepared for an MCI if he or the team shows resiliency during a drill.

Overall, education and training for terror medicine is critically important. Many areas of cross-disciplinary research and development are available in this new area. For instance, emergency planners are working on developing reliable metrics for education and training in book, journal, and web-based formats, MCI subject matter experts are beginning to work hand-in-hand with clinical educators and internet gamers to develop multi-player virtual simulators, while computer programmers work to develop internet-based platforms to support these projects.

References

1. Auf der Heide E. Disaster planning, Part II. Disaster problems, issues, and challenges Identified in the research literature. Emergency Med Clin North Am. 1996 May; 14(2): 453–455, 469.
2. Information about NIMS: http://www.fema.gov/emergency/nims/whats_new.shtm. Direct link to the relationship between ICS and NIMS: http://www.fema.gov/txt/emergency/nims/nims_ics_position_paper.txt.
3. See UpToDate ® articles: Christopher W Woods, MD, MPH and David Ashford, DVM, MPH, DSc: "Identifying and managing casualties of biological terrorism," John F Beary, III, MD, William S Aronstein, MD, PhD, and Arkadi A Chines, MD: "Chemical terrorism: Diagnosis and treatment of exposure to chemical weapons," Joseph Y Allen, MD, and Erin E Endom, MD: "Clinical features of radiation injury in children" and "Management of radiation injury in children," Jamie K Waselenko, MD, FACP, James O Armitage, MD, Nicholas Dainiak, MD, John R Wingard, MD, "Treatment of radiation injury in the adult," Debra L Weiner, MD, PhD: "Emergent evaluation of acute respiratory distress in children," Rose H Goldman, MD, MPH: "Information and educational resources for occupational and environmental health" and "Overview of occupational and environmental health," Baruch Krauss, MD, Salvatore Silvestri, MD, and Jay L Falk, MD: "Carbon dioxide monitoring (capnography)," Thomas J Marrie, MD: "Epidemiology, pathogenesis, and microbiology of community-acquired pneumonia in adults," Steven Bird, MD: "Organophosphate and carbamate toxicity," Nicholas Dainiak, MD, and Jamie K Waselenko, MD, FACP: "Biology and clinical features of radiation injury in adults."
4. Niska RW, Burt CW. National Ambulatory Medical Care Survey: terrorism preparedness among office-based physicians, United States, 2003–2004. Adv Data. 2007 July 24; (390):1–16.

5. Stephenson C. Stink vessels. History Today. 2006 Nov; 56(11): 2–3. Available online at http://www.historytoday.com/MainArticle.aspx?m=318848amid=30234971.

6. Chemical Warfare in World War I: The American Experience, 1917–1918. MAJ(P) Charles E. Heller, USAR. Combat Studies Institute, Leavenworth Papers US ISSN 0195 3451.

7. Lammers RL. Simulation: the new teaching tool. Ann Emerg Med. 2007 Apr; 49(4): 505–507. Epub 2006 Dec 18.

8. "Emergency Room: Code Red" developer and publisher: Legacy Interactive, Inc., release date: 10/2001.

9. Kyle DG. Winning at olympia: Ancient olympics guide. Archaeology. 2004 Apr 6. Available at: http://www.archaeology.org/online/features/olympics/olympia.html. Accessed October 10, 2008.

10. Asher Hirshberg, MD, FACS. "Issues with Hospital Training & Drills: A Trauma Care Perspective," 3rd Annual Conference, ER One Institute, January 19–20, 2006, Washington, DC (unpub PowerPoint Presentation).

11. Asher Hirshberg, MD, FACS. "Issues with Hospital Training & Drills: A Trauma Care Perspective," p. 22, 3rd Annual Conference, ER One Institute, January 19–20, 2006, Washington, DC (unpub PowerPoint Presentation).

12. Asher Hirshberg, MD, FACS. "Issues with Hospital Training & Drills: A Trauma Care Perspective," p. 21, 3rd Annual Conference, ER One Institute, January 19–20, 2006, Washington, DC (unpub PowerPoint Presentation).

6
Modeling and Simulation in Terror Medicine

Asher Hirshberg and Kenneth L. Mattox

Amid the wailing sirens of approaching ambulances, the screams of wounded patients, the hectic activity of trauma teams, and the emotional outrage of the public, it is often easy to forget that at the heart of the medical response to urban terrorism is an organizational challenge known as resource allocation problem.[1] As trauma care providers or administrators, we know that the success of our institution's response to a mass casualty incident (MCI) hinges not on the management of individual patients, but rather on the ability of our system to rapidly accommodate a sudden large influx of casualties on very short notice.[2] However, when trying to think quantitatively about these abstract concepts, we encounter significant difficulties.

While terrorism-related MCIs have become a ubiquitous global threat, they remain very rare events for any single institution or emergency system. When such incidents do occur, they are typically brie, though they carry a high public profile as well as a substantial emotional impact. All these factors stand in the way of researchers wishing to apply evidence-based approaches to disaster research and emergency planning.

Prospective studies are obviously not an option, but even retrospective analysis is problematic because there is no standard methodology to study the administrative and logistic aspects of the medical response to terrorism. Not surprisingly, attempts to examine past incidents from the organizational perspective (as opposed to the clinical one) have had mixed results.[3,4] Furthermore, it is often unclear whether lessons learned from a past event are institution-specific or exportable to other systems.[5]

Complex resource allocation problems inaccessible to traditional analytic methods are amenable to computer modeling. The modeling approach is widely used in operations research, engineering, and industry.[6] In the past decade, there has been a growing interest in the use of computer modeling and simulation methods in disaster planning.

This chapter is an accessible nontechnical overview of computer modeling and simulation as a research tool in terror medicine. Our aim is to introduce the reader to the fundamentals of disaster modeling, explain how models are developed and used, and review the published literature in this rapidly evolving field.

S.C. Shapira et al. (eds.), *Essentials of Terror Medicine*, 79
DOI: 10.1007/978-0-387-09412-0_6, Springer Science+Business Media, LLC 2009

Some Principles of Modeling and Simulation

What Is a Computer Model?

A model is a simplified representation of a system, developed to help answer a specific question about the behavior of that system. Model building must be a goal-oriented activity with specific aims in mind. One cannot undertake to build a "general purpose" model without a clear and carefully formulated specific question that the model will help to answer.[7]

A computer model is a program with which we try to simulate (or mimic) the behavior of the real system. *Modeling* is the process of writing the program, which typically consists of a set of mathematical equations or logical statements. *Simulation* is the process of running the program (i.e. solving the equations numerically) to produce results.[8] The term "disaster simulation" is sometimes used to refer to the immersion of medical care providers in a physical or virtual environment of a disaster scenario for training purposes. Use of such "simulations" as educational tools is addressed in another chapter of this book.

Before the early 1990s, computer modeling was the province of the select few who mastered the relevant mathematics and programming skills in addition to their specific domain of expertise. This changed dramatically with the introduction of personal computers and especially the graphical user interface in the early 1990s. Personal computing brought with it a host of user-friendly yet powerful software packages that greatly simplified the modeling process. Using these new software tools, one can draw a diagram of the system on the computer screen using simple graphical building blocks, while the software handles the underlying mathematics in the background.[6] This quiet revolution has made computer modeling eminently accessible to researchers and disaster planners who wish to incorporate quantitative thinking into their professional toolkits.

Why Model Disasters?

Computer models offer a useful means of exploring our assumptions about the behavior of a system, and confront us with the consequences of these assumptions. They allow us to test our intuitive impressions within a "virtual laboratory," a strictly controlled experimental environment. At the same time, modeling also provides a quick and easy way to manipulate and modify this environment. The modeling approach is especially useful when test-driving the real system would be very difficult or prohibitively expensive.

In planning the medical response to terror-related MCIs, computer models offer three unique advantages:

1. They enable us to create a virtual MCI on our desktop, play out various "what if" scenarios and explore the effects of alternative plans – all without moving a single patient or opening a single facility.

2. Hospital disaster planning relies heavily on intuitive impressions and static metrics. For example, in trying to assess how many casualties can be treated in a medical facility, planners typically consider numbers of beds and available staff. However, the ability to accommodate a large number of casualties, the so-called surge capacity, is a dynamic concept related to casualty processing rates (i.e. casualties processed per unit of time) rather than storage capacity. Modeling allows us to capture, analyze, and manipulate these dynamic variables.

3. Full-scale disaster drills are expensive productions conducted in unrealistic time frames.[1] A drill may be useful as a training tool, but is an extremely poor data source for planning the medical response. In contrast, a computer simulation evolves within a realistic time frame and utilizes surgical resources and assets as they would be used in a real-time event. A trauma laparotomy takes the same time within a simulation as it would in real life, and a trauma team will be composed of the same staff members that would manage a real casualty.

The Modeling Cycle (Fig. 6.1)

Every modeling project evolves through a well-defined sequence of steps.[8] The crucial first step is formulating a good *question* that the model will attempt to answer. The chosen question has to be important enough to warrant the effort and specific enough to have a reasonable chance of reaching a meaningful answer. For instance, the question "what is the impact of triage on the hospital disaster response?", though important, is much too general and fuzzy. A related question that is more specific and therefore amenable to modeling would be "How does over-triage affect the flow of critical casualties through the trauma resuscitation area of the Emergency Department (ED)?"

The next step is developing a *conceptual model*, typically a simple schematic drawing or diagram that captures the essential features of the system. A simple block diagram of the movement of casualties between hospital facilities can be the beginning of a conceptual model of the hospital disaster response. This step requires original thinking and may be the most creatively challenging step of the entire project. *Model construction* is the labor-intensive technical process of translating the conceptual model into a set of mathematical equations and an executable computer program.

Solving the equations (or running the program) cannot be done until the model is *calibrated* by inserting parameters from the real world into the equations. To calibrate a model, it is necessary to obtain data from the real system by performing an audit. In modeling the hospital response to an MCI, the most important data set is an inventory of casualties, their injuries, treatment, and outcomes. Additional required data include the amount of time each casualty spends at each service point, transport times, and capacities (i.e. how many patients can be treated simultaneously). Since it is obviously impossible to perform such an audit in the midst of a real-life MCI, disaster modeling must rely on data obtained from normal daily activities. Thus we assume that the duration of the initial assessment

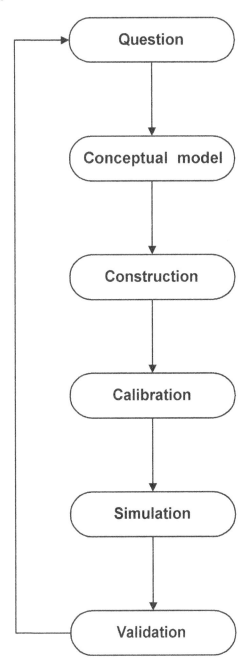

FIG. 6.1. The typical steps in a modeling cycle. Modeling is a dynamic iterative process and the cycle leads to sequential and progressive refinement of the computer model.

of injured patients in the trauma resuscitation bay or the length of surgical procedures in an MCI would be roughly similar to their duration in patients with comparable injuries treated on a normal working day.

The next step in the modeling process is *simulation*, when the computer program is run and the model equations are solved numerically. During a simulation run, the model "comes alive" and produces results that mimic the behavior of the real system. Results are then collected and analyzed, providing new insights into the behavior of the system. Comparing the simulation results to data obtained from the real system is *model validation*, which allows assessment of the usefulness of the model and the soundness of the underlying assumptions.

At the end of the modeling sequence we may have answered our original question, but this is not the end of the process. Almost invariably, these answers lead to new questions which take us back to the beginning of another modeling cycle. The entire process is therefore a dynamic iterative process of ongoing refinement, improvement, and intellectual exploration.

Two Types of Models

It is important to understand the fundamental difference between two types of models: deterministic and stochastic.[6,7] In a deterministic model, each input parameter is a specific number, so that every simulation run always produces the same result. In a stochastic (Monte Carlo) model, the input parameters are randomly sampled numbers from a statistical distribution, and therefore each simulation run produces a different result. For example, in a deterministic model the arrival rate of casualties in the ED may be set at 20 casualties per hour (i.e. an interval of 3 min between arrivals). In a stochastic model, casualties would arrive randomly with inter-arrival intervals that correspond to a probability distribution around a mean of 3 min.

Stochastic models are more complex, but have the advantage of better resembling the random nature of real-life processes. A stochastic model typically requires a large number of simulation runs to produce meaningful results, which are also given as statistical distributions. The great majority of computer models of disasters are stochastic.

Limitations of Modeling

A computer model is a cartoon; it is not a photograph of reality. The question is not whether the model faithfully reflects the real system (which it never does), but whether it captures some key features of the system and is useful in answering important questions about the behavior of the system.

The perpetual challenge of modeling is striking the fine balance between the desire to capture details of the clinical situation and the need to simplify the model to reach a workable set of equations. Occam's razor, a fundamental principle of modeling, states that a model should not be more complicated than is absolutely necessary.[7] More realism in modeling inevitably means higher complexity and, hence, more opportunity for errors.

A model is only as good as the assumptions built into it. This elicits obvious concerns about the exportability of results from a model to the real world. In many fields we can validate a model by comparing the results of simulation runs to data obtained from the real system. However, in modeling the medical response to an MCI, such validation is virtually impossible because real-life data often do not exist. Reports of the medical response to MCIs focus on clinical problems and outcomes,[3,5] rarely addressing organizational issues.[4] Furthermore, clinical outcomes are typically reported as global statistics (e.g. mortality rate for the entire group of severe casualties), not individual outcomes.[9] No report has ever been published on delays or preventable deaths and complications in an MCI, and no hospital has ever reported being overwhelmed by a terror-related incident. This inability to validate the results of disaster models means that special caution must be taken in drawing conclusions from them.

The Medical Response from a Systems Perspective

Every modeling project hinges, first and foremost, on a thorough understanding of the system being modeled. We cannot develop models of the medical aspects of terror-related MCIs without a clear view of how the system works.

Using the vocabulary of systems thinking and operations research, medical care in an MCI is a multistep serial workflow process.[10] Much like a car-wash operation or a fast food restaurant, it is based on moving products (casualties) through a series of service points (hospital facilities) where the products are processed (given medical care) in a stepwise fashion. Each service point requires staff and resources, has throughput (processing capacity) and turnover times between casualties. However, the hospital disaster response has several unique features that set it apart from other serial workflow processes.

Hospital administrators often fail to recognize that in an MCI, the hospital operates not one, but two service lines working in parallel to treat critical and noncritical casualties, respectively. The service line for critical casualties is the hospital trauma system: the staff and resources that treat severely injured patients during normal daily operations. This line consists of trauma resuscitation bays, CT scanners (and other imaging modalities), operating rooms, and surgical ICU beds. It is staffed by trained trauma care providers. The second service line is designed for noncritical casualties and typically consists of other areas of the ED and related facilities (such as radiology), where noncritical patients are evaluated and treated by ED staff reinforced by medical and nursing staff from the hospital floors.

From a system perspective, there are crucial differences between these two service lines. The trauma service line for critical casualties is a tightly coupled serial workflow process,[10] meaning there are no "storage areas" between service points where critical casualties could wait for the next step in their management plan. Hence, a casualty cannot be moved from a resuscitation bay to the CT scanner until the latter becomes available. This stands in sharp contrast to the other service line for noncritical casualties, a loosely coupled process in which the ED serves as a "storage area" where casualties can wait for the next steps in their medical care.

Regardless of the mechanism or specific circumstances of an MCI, only about 10% of casualties arriving in an ED are critically injured and require urgent trauma care. Most others sustain only minor or nonurgent injuries and can tolerate significant delays and suboptimal care.[2,11] This universal severity distribution forms the foundation of both hospital disaster plans and computer models. It means that coping with a large casualty load entails diverting assets and resources from mildly injured to severely wounded casualties. While the mildly injured majority may be the focus of attention from the customer service perspective, the critically wounded few are much more important from the clinical perspective. Providing optimal care to this small group of severely injured casualties is the crux of the entire medical response.[1,2]

Another salient characteristic of the hospital response to an MCI is its mode of failure. A serial workflow process typically fails abruptly, thereby creating long delays in service and resulting in long queues of objects waiting to be processed. In a hospital trauma service line, long delays are uncommon and occur very late when the number of casualties is truly overwhelming. Failure occurs gradually, with progressive degradation of the level of care as casualties are treated by less-experienced providers in suboptimal (or improvized) facilities. Thus, the first severe casualty will be greeted in a fully stocked shock room by the best trauma team that the hospital can provide. The 20th severe casualty will be lucky to be treated by an ATLS Advanced Trauma Life Support trained physician in an improvized trauma resuscitation bay.[2]

Each arriving casualty must be routed (or directed) to the appropriate service line. This routing function is called triage and is typically begun at the ED door.[12] The accuracy of the triage process is a major consideration in every disaster plan. Overtriage refers to routing noncritical casualties into the critical trauma service line, while under-triage is the erroneous direction of critical casualties into the non-critical service line.[12] Since critical casualties compete for limited trauma assets and resources (such as the attention of a trauma surgeon or an available CT scanner), over-triage sharpens the competition and hampers the ability of the trauma service line to cope effectively with a large number of critical casualties.[9,12] Under-triage, on the other hand, puts the individual mistriaged critical casualty in jeopardy but has much less impact on the system. Effective hospital disaster planning sees both types of triage errors as inevitable and employs mechanisms to identify them and mitigate their adverse consequences, a planning principle known as "error-tolerant design." For example, repeating triage at multiple service points enables quick identification and correction of initial routing errors.[12]

Another unique system characteristic of the hospital disaster response that is a key to effective model building is that patient flow is driven entirely by clinical decisions. In other serial workflow processes, the product moves to the next service point when it is ready. The process is automatic and typically does not require individual decisions at every step. In a hospital coping with an MCI, no casualty will be moved to the next service point unless someone has made a clinical decision. Therefore, the real engine behind the hospital response, the driving force that keeps casualties moving through the system, is a limited number of trauma professionals who can make clinical decisions on complex, severely injured patients.[1,2]

Tools for Modeling the Disaster Response

To build and implement computer models, we need a computing environment that can perform a long series of sequential stepwise calculations. While any programming language and many applications (such as spreadsheets) can be used for this purpose, it is much easier to employ a dedicated modeling software package. These software tools provide a user-friendly interface, facilitate simulation and enhance collection and analysis of results. Each software package is based on a specific modeling paradigm, the theoretical or mathematical basis upon which the software is designed. In this section, we discuss modeling tools that are particularly suitable for modeling medical systems and their response to disasters.

Discrete-Event Simulation (Fig. 6.2)

By far the most useful environment for modeling the medical aspects of a disaster is discrete-event simulation (DES). DES is based on queuing theory, a branch of operations research that is concerned with mathematical analysis of waiting lines.

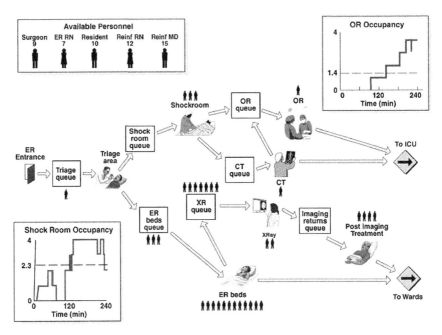

FIG. 6.2.   An artist's depiction of the key elements of a discrete event simulation model. The computer screen shows the dynamic flow of casualties between service points in and around the Emergency Department. The software keeps track of available personnel (upper left corner) and moves patients between service points. During each simulation run, the software also collects metrics (such as shock room occupancy or wait times) and displays them as numbers or graphs.

DES is a methodology for the study of objects (e.g. casualties, surgeons, or units of blood) as they move through a system (e.g. an Emergency Medical Services [EMS] system or hospital facilities).[8] The model is constructed by defining a set of computable logical statements that describe how objects change from state to state (from a waiting patient to a treated patient), or interact with other objects (patient with nurse). The time at which an object changes from state to state is defined as an "event," hence the term DES. Each model is an executable computer program that moves the objects through the system and monitors interactions with other objects. DES is used extensively in operations research and engineering to address such diverse problems as facility design, traffic management, or complex scheduling issues.[8]

A DES model is constructed by creating a graphical representation (flow diagram) of the system on the computer screen. Icons are used to represent entrance, sequential service points, and exit (Fig. 6.3). Connecting arrows are used to model the direction of flow between facilities. The model is stochastic, so that key parameters such as arrival rates or service times are randomly sampled from probability distributions derived from data obtained from the real system. The software allows rapid multiple simulation runs and collects the results. It also provides statistical analysis of key performance variables such as waiting times, delays, throughput, and percent of time that a specific service point was busy during the simulation run.

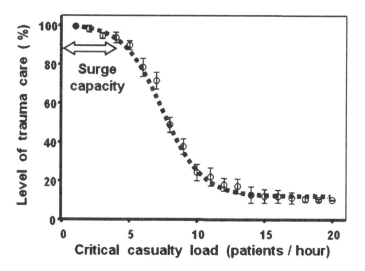

FIG. 6.3. Model prediction of the effect of critical casualty load on level of trauma care. Each data point represents the mean ± 95% confidence interval obtained from 100 simulation runs of the model. The level of trauma care is expressed as percentage of the optimal level of care, which is defined as care given to a single trauma patient on a normal working day. A sigmoid function was fitted through the data. The surge capacity of the hospital trauma service line is the casualty load corresponding to a 90% level of care on the fitted curve[37].

System Dynamics

This popular and versatile modeling platform is based on an approach to understanding the behavior of complex systems developed by Jay W. Forrester of MIT.[13] Forrester showed that the dynamic behavior of complex systems can be modeled using a few simple building blocks. Software tools based on this paradigm were originally designed for deterministic modeling of continuous processes, particularly feedback loops.[13,14] However, the modeling paradigm was later expanded to include stochastic workflow models.[10] The system dynamics approach is especially useful for models that combine both discrete events (such as patients moving between facilities) and continuous variables (such as cost or quality of care) in the same model.

Agent-Based Modeling

In this more recent modeling approach, a system is represented as a group of autonomous decision-making entities ("agents").[15] During a simulation run, each agent repeatedly assesses its situation in relation to other agents or to the environment and executes actions based on predefined rules. The interactions of a group of agents, each following the same simple rules, can lead to unanticipated dynamics and new behavior patterns, a phenomenon known as emergence. Agent-based modeling differs from other modeling paradigms because it looks at the system from the bottom up rather than from the top down. It is especially useful in studying processes where the behavior of any single object is unpredictable, such as during emergency evacuation of a facility, crowd behavior during a stampede, the spread of epidemics in an urban population or the creation of traffic jams.

Review of Published Models

Beginnings

Published reports on computer modeling of the medical response to MCIs represent only a small fraction of the work done in this field. Many disaster models remain unpublished, either because they are classified (like models used by the military or by government agencies to predict the consequences of unconventional terrorism) or because they are considered institution-specific and therefore of limited interest to the general public.

The quantitative approach to medical disaster planning was pioneered by De Boer.[16-19] He showed that the medical severity of an MCI and the capability of medical systems to cope with it can be predicted using simple empirical calculations. De Boer was the first to express the hospital treatment capacity as a rate (casualties treated per hour) rather than a number of hospital beds.[19] He estimated this capacity at roughly one critical casualty per hour per 100 hospital beds during normal daily operations, with an increase to two to three casualties when the hospital disaster response is fully deployed. This is surprisingly close to more recent estimates of hospital surge capacity derived from much more complex dynamic modeling. De Boer's major contribution was moving disaster planning from the traditional qualitative and vague frame of reference based on intuitive impressions and "guesstimates" to a firm quantitative data-based footing.

Modeling the Pre-Hospital Phase

An excellent example of the use of DES to help analyze the performance of an EMS system and suggest ways to improve it was published by Su and Shih,[20,21] who developed a computer model of the EMS system of Taipei, Taiwan. While their model addresses normal daily operations, the methodology applies equally well to unusually large casualty loads in large-scale events. A similar clinically oriented approach was used by Stevenson et al.,[22] who studied field triage strategies for trauma patients with severe head injuries in Wales. They asked themselves whether outcome could be improved by bypassing hospitals without neurosurgical facilities, and used their analysis to identify triage and transfer strategies that may offer a significant outcome advantage over existing policies. Again, while this study addressed normal daily operations within a specific EMS system, the methodology is eminently applicable to modeling MCIs in any emergency medical system.

Christie and Levary[23] developed a DES of the pre-hospital response to airplane crash scenarios in the St. Louis metropolitan area. They focused on the effectiveness of casualty evacuation by ambulance, but did not proceed to draw operational conclusions that could have been applied to the real system. More recently, Inoue et al.[24] demonstrated the importance of pre-hospital triage during an MCI in an airport. They showed how casualty survival can be improved by employing pre-hospital triage as compared to a "first come first served" approach, and proposed practical ways to redesign casualty evacuation to improve outcome. Ohboshi et al.[25] modeled on-scene triage during a major disaster using a workflow modeling tool. Calibrating the model to data from the Great Hashin-Awaji earthquake in 1995, they showed the importance of triage duration (the time it takes to reach a triage decision) on the flow of casualties in large-scale disasters.

There are currently no published models of pre-hospital medical care during terror-related conventional MCIs, such as urban bombings. This is not surprising since in these incidents evacuation from the scene is typically very swift[26] and is only partially controlled by pre-hospital care providers. Many mildly injured or noninjured casualties arrive in hospital independent of the EMS system. Since the general pre-hospital philosophy in an urban MCI is "scoop and run" field treatment stations are rarely (if ever) deployed, and the pre-hospital phase is almost never a significant bottleneck. All these factors combine to make modeling of medical care at the scene more complex and of less practical value than modeling the hospital phase.

There is, however, a plethora of published models on the medical response to unconventional terrorism, especially large-scale biological events.[27-33] Since the medical response to a large-scale biological event relies primarily on a robust public health system and since there is virtually no experience with such events, many organizations rely on computer modeling to help design and test their response plans. One such example is InfluSim,[27] a modeling tool that is freely available online. InfluSim helps planners predict the time-course and healthcare impact of a pandemic influenza outbreak and develop an effective response.

In the wake of the mail anthrax attacks in the USA in the fall of 2001, Hupert et al.[29] used DES modeling to analyze staffing arrangements and patient flow rates for antibiotic distribution centers in a large-scale bioterrorism attack. Their study is another demonstration of the usefulness of computer modeling in planning and preparing for terror-related incidents.

Modeling the Hospital Response

Levi and Bregman [34,35] pioneered the use of DES to study the surgical capabilities of Israeli trauma centers during prolonged periods of high casualty load. From their experience in the use computer simulation as a training tool, Levi and Bregman realized that DES can also be useful in emergency planning. Their landmark study compared OR utilization in a wartime scenario in six Israeli hospitals.[34] The model was based on clinical data from 900 real war casualties and the simulation time was 10 days, a time frame that is more representative of a large-scale military conflict rather than a terror-related MCI. The simulation revealed wide variability in the operative surge capacity of the modeled trauma centers and showed that the number of hospital beds is a poor predictor of that capacity. More importantly, the study illustrated how a computer model can be used to study institutional capabilities under emergency conditions and to "test drive" various approaches to offloading surgical facilities during MCIs.

The first wave of suicide bombings in Israel (1994–1998) led to re-examination of hospital disaster plans across the nation and to intense discussions of casualty flow patterns and institutional capabilities. The Israeli Ministry of Health arbitrarily directed hospitals to achieve and maintain a target surge capacity of 20% of the total number of hospital beds. This arbitrary determination seemed unrealistically high to Israeli trauma surgeons, and led to a project that critically analyzed the disaster plan of the Sheba Medical Center, a 1,400-bed university hospital and trauma center, using a computer modeling approach.[36]

The Sheba disaster plan was translated into a DES model using casualty profiles and severity distributions obtained from a registry of 771 casualties from 12 urban terrorist bombings across Israel maintained by the Trauma Division of the IDF Israel Defense Force Medical Corps. By running each simulation for four virtual hours, the simulated casualty load exceeded that of any single urban terrorism event in the Israeli experience. The study allowed an evidence-based determination of staffing needs for large casualty loads and, more importantly, identified bottlenecks to patient flow in the trauma resuscitation bays and the CT scanners. Based on these findings, the hospital disaster plan was revised by adding improvized resuscitation bays and restricting access to the CT scanners. This study underscores the practical usefulness of modeling as an adjunct to hospital disaster planning,[37] and provided a realistic data-driven estimation of the surgical resources and assets required to deal with a terror-related MCI.

One crucial aspect of trauma care in MCIs is the relationship between casualty load and the level of trauma care. The prevailing view is that a heavy casualty load adversely affects the quality of care for critically injured patients, because a large number of critical casualties is competing for limited hospital resources.[1,2] However, this relationship has never been defined nor formally studied using quantitative tools. Furthermore, despite fears of additional large-scale terrorist attacks in the wake of 9/11, the surge capacity of US trauma centers remains largely unknown. More importantly, there is no standard accepted definition of surge capacity and no agreement on how it should be measured.

In 2003, the authors of this chapter, in collaboration with Dr. Michael Stein in Israel, addressed this conundrum of unresolved issues through what can only be described as a substantial leap of the imagination. We developed a model that simulates how a US Level 1 trauma center is coping with a stream urban bombing casualties from Israel.[37] We began by constructing a system dynamics model of the disaster plan of the Ben Taub General Hospital in Houston.[38] We then generated a virtual stream of patients based on the clinical profiles of 223 urban bombing casualties treated at the Rabin Medical Center in Petah Tikva, Israel.

The heart of the model (and the reason for choosing a system dynamics platform) was a set of equations that calculated the level of trauma care for each new arriving casualty based on the availability of trauma staff and facilities. This level of care was graded on a numerical scale where the highest grade (i.e. optimal care) is the care given to a single critically injured patient on a normal working day. The model demonstrated a clear sigmoid-shaped relationship between the casualty load (number of casualties arriving per hour) and the level of trauma care that each critical casualty received (Fig. 6.3). The upper flat portion of the curve corresponds to a multiple casualty incident, a situation in which the trauma service line of the hospital is strained but not overwhelmed. The steep portion represents mass casualty, with gradual degradation of the trauma care capabilities as more and more casualties arrive. The lower flat portion of the curve corresponds to a major disaster, where the casualty load is so large that most critically injured patients cannot even gain access to the trauma facilities and staff of the hospital.

This quantitative analysis led to a quantitative definition of the hospital surge capacity as the maximal critical casualty load that can be managed without a precipitous drop in the level of care. Obviously, this surge capacity is not a finite number of casualties (or beds) but rather a casualty arrival rate.

The study demonstrates how computer modeling and simulation can help us not only to analyze the details of specific disaster plans but also to resolve conceptual questions at a higher level. Thus while the specific numbers in Fig. 6.3 may vary between institutions, the sigmoid shape of the curve is an inherent characteristic of any hospital dealing with an MCI, and the degradation of the hospital trauma assets and resources is a gradual process that can be mitigated by effective planning and preparation.[37]

Conclusion

The evolution of computer modeling and simulation and the availability of powerful modeling software packages have transformed disaster research from intuition-based qualitative "guesstimates" into an evidence-based quantitative activity. Computer models helps us not only to gain a better understanding of the complex dynamic processes involved in the medical response to terrorism but also serve as a useful adjunct to practical contingency planning within institutions and systems.

Computer modeling, once the province of the select few, is now within easy reach of any of us who wish to use this modality to study and improve the response of our systems to terrorism-related MCIs using modern quantitative tools. Models capture and analyze critical variables of the disaster response as though multiple data collectors, statisticians, and system analyzers were auditing the hospital response on a real-time basis. Modeling and simulation, when applied correctly, allows clinical decision-makers and managers to test their assumptions about the resource allocation, asset use and casualty flow dimensions of a terror-related MCI. The methodology also promises to provide trauma systems and centers with variable resources with a common language to realistically and effectively prepare for the future challenges of terror medicine.

Acknowledgments: The authors gratefully acknowledge the outstanding editorial assistance of Mary K. Allen, Administrative Coordinator at the Michael E. DeBakey Department of Surgery, Baylor College of Medicine, Houston, TX, USA.

References

1. Hirshberg A. Multiple casualty incidents: lessons from the front line. Ann Surg 2004; 239:322–324.
2. Hirshberg A, Holcomb JB, Mattox KL. Hospital trauma care in multiple-casualty incidents: a critical view. Ann Emerg Med 2001; 37:647–652.
3. Aylwin CJ, Konig TC, Brennan NW, Shirley PJ, Davies G, Walsh MS, Brohi K. Reduction in critical mortality in urban mass casualty incidents: analysis of triage, surge, and resource use after the London bombings on July 7, 2005. Lancet 2006; 368:2219–2225.
4. Aschkenasy-Steuer G, Shamir M, Rivkind A, Mosheiff R, Shushan Y, Rosenthal G, Mintz Y, Weissman C, Sprung CL, Weiss YG. Clinical review: the Israeli experience: conventional terrorism and critical care. Crit Care 2005; 9:490–499.
5. Almogy G, Belzberg H, Mintz Y, Pikarsky AK, Zamir G, Rivkind AI. Suicide bombing attacks: update and modifications to the protocol. Ann Surg 2004; 239:295–303.
6. Hannon B, Ruth M. Dynamic modeling. New York: Springer; 2001.
7. Starfield A, Smith KA, Bleloch AL. Introducing models. In How to model it: Problem solving for the computer age. Edina, MN: Burgess International Group; 94 A.D.:1–14.
8. Pidd M. Tools for thinking: Modelling in management science. Chichester: John Wiley & Sons, Ltd.; 2003.
9. Frykberg ER. Medical management of disasters and mass casualties from terrorist bombings: how can we cope? J Trauma 2002; 53:201–212.

10. McGarvey B, Hannon B (eds). Dynamic modeling for business management. New York: Springer; 2003:106–139.

11. Stein M, Hirshberg A. Medical consequences of terrorism. The conventional weapon threat. Surg Clin North Am 1999; 79:1537–1552.

12. Frykberg ER. Triage: principles and practice. Scand J Surg 2005; 94:272–278.

13. Taylor RA. US Department of Energy's introduction to system dynamics. http://www.albany.edu/cpr/sds/DL-IntroSysDyn/inside.htm. 1997.

14. Richmond B. An introduction to systems thinking. Hanover, NH: High Performance Systems; 2001.

15. Resnick M. Turtles, termites, and traffic jams: Explorations in massively parallel microworlds. Camridge, MA: MIT Press; 1997.

16. de Boer J. Tools for evaluating disasters: preliminary results of some hundreds of disasters. Eur J Emerg Med 1997; 4:107–110.

17. de Boer J. Criteria for the assessment of disaster preparedness – II. Prehosp Disaster Med 1997; 12:13–16.

18. de Boer J. An attempt at more accurate estimation of the number of ambulances needed at disasters in the Netherlands. Prehosp Disaster Med 1996; 11:125–128.

19. De Boer J. Order in chaos: modelling medical management in disasters. Eur J Emerg Med 1999; 6:141–148.

20. Su S, Shih CL. Resource reallocation in an emergency medical service system using computer simulation. Am J Emerg Med 2002; 20:627–634.

21. Su S, Shih CL. Modeling an emergency medical services system using computer simulation. Int J Med Inform 2003; 72:57–72.

22. Stevenson MD, Oakley PA, Beard SM, Brennan A, Cook AL. Triaging patients with serious head injury: results of a simulation evaluating strategies to bypass hospitals without neurosurgical facilities. Injury 2001; 32:267–274.

23. Christie PM, Levary RR. The use of simulation in planning the transportation of patients to hospitals following a disaster. J Med Syst 1998; 22:289–300.

24. Inoue H, Yanagisawa S, Kamae I. Computer-simulated assessment of methods of transporting severely injured individuals in disaster – case study of an airport accident. Comput Methods Programs Biomed 2006; 81:256–265.

25. Ohboshi N, Masui H, Kambayashi Y, Takahashi T. A study of medical emergency workflow. Comput Methods Programs Biomed 1998; 55:177–190.

26. Einav S, Feigenberg Z, Weissman C, Zaichik D, Caspi G, Kotler D, Freund HR. Evacuation priorities in mass casualty terror-related events: implications for contingency planning. Ann Surg 2004; 239:304–310.

27. Eichner M, Schwehm M, Duerr HP, Brockmann SO. The influenza pandemic preparedness planning tool InfluSim. BMC Infect Dis 2007; 7:17.

28. Aaby K, Abbey RL, Herrmann JW, Treadwell M, Jordan CS, Wood K. Embracing computer modeling to address pandemic influenza in the 21st century. J Public Health Manag Pract 2006; 12:365–372.

29. Hupert N, Mushlin AI, Callahan MA. Modeling the public health response to bioterrorism: using discrete event simulation to design antibiotic distribution centers. Med Decis Making 2002; 22:S17–S25.

30. Giovachino M, Carey N. Modeling the consequences of bioterrorism response. Mil Med 2001; 166:925–930.

31. Kleinman KP, Abrams A, Mandl K, Platt R. Simulation for assessing statistical methods of biologic terrorism surveillance. MMWR Morb Mortal Wkly Rep 2005; 54 Suppl:101–108.

32. Medema JK, Zoellner YF, Ryan J, Palache AM. Modeling pandemic preparedness scenarios: health economic implications of enhanced pandemic vaccine supply. Virus Res 2004; 103:9–15.
33. Riley S, Ferguson NM. Smallpox transmission and control: spatial dynamics in Great Britain. Proc Natl Acad Sci USA 2006; 103:12637–12642.
34. Levi L, Bregman D, Geva H, Revah M. Does number of beds reflect the surgical capability of hospitals in wartime and disaster? The use of a simulation technique at a national level. Prehosp Disaster Med 1997; 12:300–304.
35. Levi L, Bregman D, Geva H, Revach M. Hospital disaster management simulation system. Prehosp Disaster Med 1998; 13:29–34.
36. Hirshberg A, Stein M, Walden R. Surgical resource utilization in urban terrorist bombing: a computer simulation. J Trauma 1999; 47:545–550.
37. Hirshberg A, Scott BG, Granchi T, Wall MJ, Jr., Mattox KL, Stein M. How does casualty load affect trauma care in urban bombing incidents? A quantitative analysis. J Trauma 2005; 58:686–693.

7
National Coordination and Integration

Shlomo Mor-Yosef and Shmuel C. Shapira

Every terror incident, no matter its size, location, or nature, is a national event. National efforts before, during, and afterwards include introduction of preventive measures, preparedness, event management, and dealing with the after-effects on individuals and communities.

Attacks launched with conventional weapons or with biological, chemical, or radiological agents will have a direct impact on the health system. Because of the medical implications of such events, healthcare workers will be involved no matter the number of casualties.[1] Cyber-terrorism could also profoundly affect the coordination and integration of the medical system. Although this form of terrorism is the focus of another chapter, it is worth underscoring its potentially devastating effects on traffic control and healthcare networks, which have become dependent on computers and computer-associated equipment.[2]

Although the responsibilities of a national health system are many and varied, effective communication and cooperation are vital to proper performance under dire circumstances.

Intelligence Information

Evaluation and Forwarding of Processed Data to Hospitals and Pre-Hospital Systems

The intelligence information cycle is composed of collection, analysis, production of reports, identification of gaps, and dissemination.[3] This information is divided into two categories: long range and short range. Long-range information relates to strategic and extended threats that could affect the nation. Although terrorism has become a worldwide phenomenon, the probability of an attack differs from one country to another, and may change over time for a particular country. Long-range information serves as the basis for ongoing national preparedness of emergency systems for an extended period into the future. Short-range intelligence relates to threats that may be realized in the coming hours, days, or weeks. Such information demands urgent attention and readiness in the face of a likely imminent assault.

S.C. Shapira et al. (eds.), *Essentials of Terror Medicine*,
DOI: 10.1007/978-0-387-09412-0_7, Springer Science+Business Media, LLC 2009

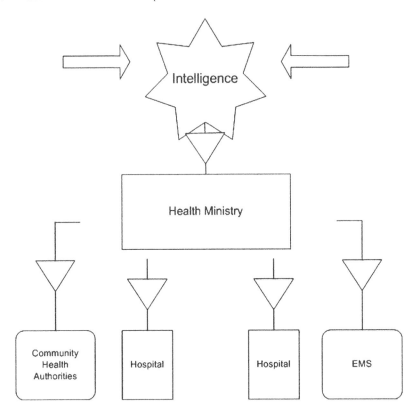

Fɪɢ. 7.1. Flow of intelligence data.

Following receipt of intelligence information, data must be evaluated, processed, and transferred from the Ministry of Defense to the Ministry of Health. A particular threat for which procedures are to be defined is characterized as a "reference threat." A reference threat comprises a working hypothesis for all those who need to prepare. The flow of intelligence data is described in Fig. 7.1. The level of the reference threat can be the same for the entire country or vary from one region to another. The differences among regions may be attributable to varied population densities, demographics, locations that encompass strategic facilities, regions that have symbolic significance to the country or to the terror organization, soft targets that are easy to access, and regions that are within geographic proximity to exit points for terror organizations.

Strategic intelligence preparedness and reference threats are developed at a national level by political, security, and military authorities. From the moment the reference threat has been established it is the responsibility of various national systems to prepare for it. It is beyond the scope of this text to relate to political and military systems, and here we will deal with civilian emergency preparedness and in particular preparedness of medical systems.

Partners: Integration and Cooperation

One must first define the various authorities that deal with terror events and then the nature of their interaction[3]:

- Essential civilian industries and services
- Fire Department
- Health System
- Home Front Command
- Intelligence and Counter-Intelligence Agencies
- Media
- Municipal Authorities
- Police

These systems are coordinated on national and regional levels via a special National Emergency Coordination Committee (NECC), representing all of the relevant authorities. This committee must make decisions with regard to reference threats and actual terror events – how to deal with them and their consequences.

It is not necessary for the entire committee to meet each time there is a new threat. Rather, the declared level of the threat should determine the extent of involvement of the various authorities. Meetings should be routinely convened for the purposes of policy making and defining Standard Operating Procedures (SOP). During elevated alerts or an actual attack, meetings should be held more frequently in order to make real-time decisions. These meetings can be face-to-face round table discussions or conducted by video conferencing.

The extent of the NECC involvement is determined by the nature and magnitude of the attack, that is, conventional, mass-conventional (e.g., September 11), use of weapons of mass destruction (WMD). An assault on a nuclear reactor, for example, would warrant an approach far different from an attack with biological weapons, though either would draw more multi-agency involvement than, say, an explosives attack in an urban shopping mall.

The NECC needs to establish guidelines as to how each participating emergency agency deals with terror preparedness, which includes providing for physical infrastructure, acquisition of emergency equipment, responsibilities of senior personnel, development of SOP, and training and exercises.

Despite overlapping paths of action, preparedness for a conventional terror attack is different from preparedness for a WMD threat.[4] Additionally, the nature and urgency of the threat will require distinctive protocols, methods of preparedness, and responses. An attack with a toxic material that affects a vast area would be handled differently from one that is limited to a train station or an entertainment hall. While no single SOP could apply to such disparate events, neither can distinctive procedures be written for all possible scenarios. The challenge is to prepare for as many reference threats as can be reasonably anticipated, and also to allow for flexibility so that protocols can be adjusted to unanticipated needs.

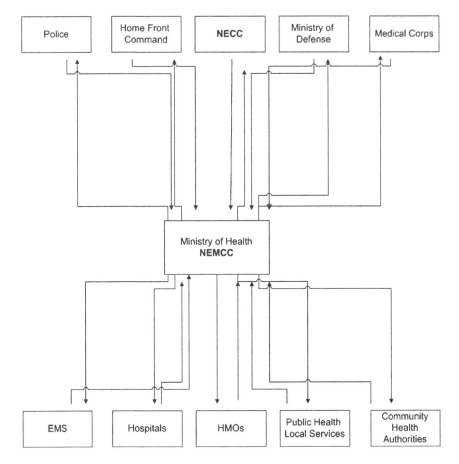

FIG. 7.2. Coordination with the Ministry of Health throughout the terror attack (EMS –Emergency Medical Services, HMOs – Health Management Organizations, NEMCC – National Emergency Medical Coordinating Committee, NECC – National Emergency Coordinating Committee).

Within the health system there must be coordination among the participants from every sector (Fig. 7.2):

- Primary and community medical care
- Emergency Medical Services (EMS), which provides pre-hospital triage, emergency treatment, and evacuation to hospitals
- General hospitals of varying levels
- Rehabilitation facilities
- Outpatient treatment and care
- Organizations that provide support and follow-up for individuals who were exposed to the attack but not physically injured or in need of acute care

At the time of an attack, the most challenging location to manage is the immediate attack zone, which is often chaotic and subject to the danger of repeated follow-up attacks. In contrast to permanent facilities, such as hospitals that are in regular service, the zone cannot be prepared in advance. First responders at the site of an attack include medical teams, fire and rescue personnel, hazard materials (HAZMAT) teams, police, home front command, and local municipal teams. Ongoing communications and reporting must be maintained among the different authorities. The police are usually in command and for complex events an incident command post is often established on the scene.

The Israeli Model

In order to maintain coordination among these various authorities, which normally operate independently, the National Emergency Medical Coordinating Committee (NEMCC), a division of the National Emergency Coordinating Committee, was established in Israel.[5] Managed by the Director General of the Ministry of Health, the NEMCC deals with the reference threats to the health system, establishes the responsibilities and tasks of the member authorities in the health system, and coordinates emergency response during large-scale attacks. All the health system authorities that participate in emergency preparedness are represented on the NEMCC, including the Medical Corps of Israeli Defense Forces, the Ministry of Health, and the Health Management Organizations.

Preparation of SOP

SOP preparation for each authority in the system is vital to effective outcomes. The NEMCC is responsible for establishing the subjects that should be included in the SOP for different scenarios and reference threats. It then becomes the responsibility of each authority to develop its own protocols subject to review and approval by the NEMCC. The process relies heavily on cooperation among the various authorities, especially in the case of complex mass terror events. For example, when victim extrication is required, coordinated action by relevant divisions in the Ministry of Health and Home Front Command is essential.

Israel's EMS' SOP includes the following topics:

- Operation of the regional dispatch center
- Communications
- Coordination with other onsite rescue teams
- Coordination with EMS headquarters and neighboring EMS regions
- Onsite command and operations
- Guidelines on extent of treatment, such as triage and "scoop and run" (quick removal of victims from attack site)
- Managing WMD events, including identification of nature of attack, hot zone, self protection, antidotes, and extent of pre-hospital decontamination

A key responsibility of the NEMCC is to delineate the roles of the various authorities during emergency situations. For example, the role of an individual hospital is determined by two principal criteria: first, its size and extent of medical capabilities such as trauma and other specialty departments; and second, its location – a small facility in an isolated area has greater responsibility than one with other hospitals nearby that could offer back-up.

In order to make optimal decisions a national database should include detailed capabilities of every hospital in the country. This registry is regularly updated to reflect even slight changes in infrastructure, such as the purchase of an additional bed or imaging device, or the addition of an operating theater.

Every hospital staff member must undergo instruction in SOP and participate in periodic drills. Moreover, each hospital must be able to quickly expand bed capacity and patient services by at least 20% beyond its usual capacity. The expansion must take into consideration not only the numbers of patients that might arrive at the institution but also the rate of influx. A hospital that is prepared to receive 50 emergency victims during a 2-hour period could be overwhelmed if they arrived in half that time. Thus, a hospital's SOP must allow for a combination of issues that includes the volume of victims that can be received, the number expected to arrive in a given time period, and the nature and severity of the injuries.

As part of the triage, which occurs at the event site, the standard procedures delineate hospital evacuation and destination plans. This includes advance understanding about protocols for patient distribution to various hospitals. Transference of patients will depend in part on the classification of injury (Fig. 7.3). In an attempt to achieve

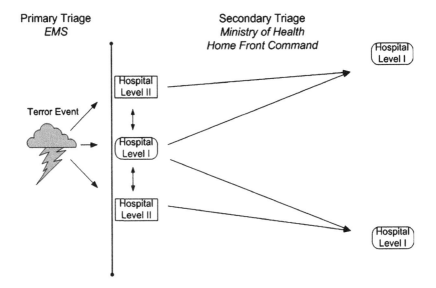

FIG. 7.3. Patient flow during primary and secondary triage (EMS – Emergency Medical Services)

optimal outcomes – reduced mortality, morbidity, and disability – NEMCC also oversees plans to distribute patients so that no hospital is overloaded.

The location of the event often determines the role of a particular hospital following an attack. During a mega terror event there might be a need to define a "triaging hospital" which functions as one big Emergency Department (ED) and transfers all victims who are stable and therefore transportable, to other hospitals. The concept of a triaging hospital is a key element of response procedures in a mass terror event. Another task of the NEMCC is to make decisions regarding classifying hospitals as triaging facilities. Only the national coordinating system, which sees the larger picture, can make timely and informed decisions that specify a particular hospital as a triaging facility. The decision is made well in advance of a hospital's reaching maximum capacity, when pressures on the institution and staff are still less intense. It is at this point that the many and varied capabilities of the health system come into play.[6]

In general, hospital SOP should include the following topics[7]:

- Introduction: detailing the relevant scenarios with general guidelines depending on the magnitude of the attack
- Triage
- Additional admission sites: options and modes of operation
- Managing WMD events: identification of nature of attack and agent; hot zone, decontamination, self protection, and antidotes
- Checklist for hospital management
- Operations as a triaging hospital
- Manpower management
- ED
- Operating theaters
- Intensive care
- Relevant department activities
- Blood bank
- Security
- Public Information Center
- Spokesperson

Exercises and Rehearsals

The NEMCC oversees drills conducted by health and hospital personnel within the medical system, and also multidisciplinary drills with role players from outside the system. The NEMCC, in conjunction with its constituent agencies, establishes the type and frequency of drills to be conducted. Some hospitals rehearse disproportionately for specific scenarios and others hold more drills for many possible scenarios. Thus, certain hospitals may be especially proficient in dealing with particular types of attack. But all facilities are to some degree multidisciplinary and conduct drills with various parties including EMS, fire, police, and HAZMAT personnel. Exercises may also include mock victims whose numbers and rate of arrival at the hospital help frame the nature of the drill.[8]

Elective hospital activity is commonly reduced to a minimum during an exercise. Thus, increased frequency of drills affects the availability of the staff for normal hospital routines. Enhanced preparedness, therefore, comes at both an economic cost and a temporary reduction of elective services. But this tradeoff is understood to be indispensable by most members of a society that has endured repeated terrorist attacks.

Another vital part of the drill is the summation held immediately afterwards, which includes lessons learned from the exercise. Remedies for deficiencies discovered in the course of a drill are rapidly incorporated into standard procedures. No less important than the implementation of corrections locally is the distribution of the findings to parties outside the area. Thus, the benefits of a local drill redound throughout the national system.

Emergency Stockpiling

The NEMCC is responsible for the provision of equipment, disposable materials, and drugs that might be needed for a range of possible assaults, including from terrorists using biological, chemical, radiological, or conventional weapons. Each scenario generates particular requirements and calls for distinctive supplies. The NEMCC determines the type of equipment and drugs required for each reference threat, and it also defines the scope of activity for each medical authority. In conjunction with these understandings, hospitals are guided in their own acquisition of equipment and supplies. While scenario-specific supplies are stored in each hospital, backup quantities are also held in dedicated national stockpiles.[9]

Following the determination of the type and quantity of equipment required, sources of funding need to be assigned. Israel's emergency preparedness model provides that funding comes from the government and not the individual medical authorities. The principal responsibility of a local medical authority in this regard is to locate storage space for the equipment and oversee its maintenance.

The precise location and time of a terror attack is rarely known in advance, which limits preparatory time for a hospital to change from routine operations to emergency functioning. Thus, storage locations for equipment should be in close proximity to where it will be used.

In areas where terror attacks have been rare, much of the stored equipment and supplies may go unused for long periods. But it remains important that all such equipment be maintained in working order, that it be refurbished as needed, and that the staff continues to rehearse operational procedures. Finally, medications and other materials with limited shelf life must be periodically checked and replaced in advance of their expiration dates.

In Israel, the NEMCC plays the additional role of training medical, paramedical, and administrative teams. Training includes instruction about the stages of preparedness and the manner of coping with emergency operations. Distinctions are carefully drawn between various scenarios based on the types of weapons that may be used. For conventional weapons attacks, training focuses on treating trauma with reference to some aspects specific to terror.[10] Emphasis is also placed on organizational preparedness related to the admission of a large number of patients within a short period of time, as in a mass casualty event (MCE). Optional patterns of the flow of victims between the various medical authorities should also be part of the curriculum.[11]

Biological, chemical, and radiological attacks are rare, so medical teams have had little experience with them. In fact, these threats are associated with a unique pathophysiology that is unfamiliar to most clinicians. Thus, training to deal with unconventional terrorism should include essentials about the relevant pathophysiology as well as diagnosis, treatment, and organizational aspects such as protection, containment measures, and decontamination.[12] For example, it should be understood by healthcare providers that a covert biological attack could go unrecognized until patients become ill, which might not happen until days or weeks after the microbe was released. In the case of an attack with chemical weapons, the effects are likely to be more immediate and identification would come much sooner.[13]

The NEMCC is responsible to ascertain that each authority's SOP not only contains relevant information but that it is updated regularly according to changes in reference threats, clinical practices, recommended treatments, personnel, and physical matrix. Updated protocols also reflect organizational changes within the authority itself and lessons learned during previous drills and actual terror events.

The NEMCC contains a unit that determines that each authority implements all the guidelines in preparation for the various scenarios. The determination is made by audit, which includes review of hospital protocols, site visits to the hospital and to the emergency equipment storage facilities, participation, and oversight during drills, checking of the paging system that reaches employees during emergencies, and surprise inspections of both the logistical and emergency medical systems.

The NEMCC must be the ultimate repository of all medical information concerning preparedness and emergency operations. Gathered in a centralized repository, this information can then be disseminated to all medical authorities within the system.

Alert Levels

Another area requiring national coordination is the defining of medical alert levels. In Israel, five levels have been designated, each with distinctive SOP[14]:

1. Routine
2. Nonfocused threat
3. Focused attack that is, the existence of an estimated location and time of attack
4. A violent attack without victims, but which may turn into an MCE
5. MCE

For application of these different levels to recommended operations, see Table 7.1.

Table 7.1. Preparedness procedures by level of alert

Level of alert	Preparedness procedures
Routine	Preparations, instructions, drills
Nonfocused threat	1. Review of all hospital systems to ensure proper functioning and preparedness: inventory levels; equipment and necessary elements; senior personnel paging system; ensuring availability of senior personnel; briefing and training of key personnel and reinforcements for trauma and emergency units, operating rooms and recovery.
	2. Ensuring the activation, within 20 min, of the core emergency team which shall include a medical manager, a nursing manager, and an administrator.
	3. Ensuring the ability of the surgery/trauma, anesthesiology, and emergency on-call physicians to arrive at the hospital within 20 min of being paged.
	4. Ensuring the arrival of reinforcements for the nursing team in the emergency department (ED) and operating rooms within 30 min of the page. During regular hours – 50% reinforcements and after hours – 100%.
Focused threat	1. Activating the core emergency team (as described above) with the addition of a nurse.
	2. Ensuring the ability of the surgery/trauma, anesthesiology, emergency, orthopedics, neurosurgery, vascular surgery, cardiac-thoracic surgery, intensive care, pediatric surgery, pediatric intensive care, and imaging services on-call physicians to arrive at the hospital within 20 min of being paged (according to the specific departments existing in the hospital).
	3. Ensuring the arrival of reinforcements for the nursing team in the ED and operating rooms within 20 min of the page. During regular hours – 50% reinforcements and after hours – 100%.
	4. Ensuring the arrival to the hospital of key personnel from maintenance, supply, sterile supply, pharmacy, patient admission, and computer services within 20 min of the page.
A violent attack without victims which may turn into a mass casualty event (MCE)	1. Activating the core emergency team which shall include a medical manager, a nursing manager, and an administrator.
	2. Activating on-call physicians from the hospital's surgery/trauma, anesthesiology, and EDs.
	3. Activating nursing reinforcements in the ED, operating rooms, and recovery suites. During regular hours – 50% reinforcements and after hours – 100%.
	4. Ensuring the ability of the orthopedics, neurosurgery, vascular surgery, cardiac-thoracic surgery, intensive care, pediatric surgery, pediatric intensive care, and imaging services on-call physicians to arrive at the hospital within 20 min of being paged (according to the specific departments existing in the hospital).
	5. Ensuring the arrival to the hospital of key personnel from maintenance, supply, sterile supply, pharmacy, patient admission, and computer services within 20 min of the page.
MCE	Activities according to MCE Standard Operating Procedures.

The NEMCC is responsible for declaring an alert level based on intelligence and developments in the field. That decision is immediately forwarded to all medical authorities. With the exception of the MCE level, where there is no time to convene the authority, authorized officials are appointed by the NEMCC to engage the hospitals in preparedness.

Physical Structure

The ability of a hospital to admit numerous victims within a short period of time requires special physical preparedness. Additional admitting areas may be needed, as well as extra decontamination capabilities. Hospitals should have the ability to convert pre-designated areas to emergency admission areas. Under normal circumstances these spaces serve other purposes, that is, entryways, lobbies, hallways, ambulatory care areas.[15]

During construction of new hospital buildings or additions to existing buildings, the issue of emergency preparedness should be taken into account. For example, oxygen and vacuum lines may be placed in ceilings and walls of public areas so they can be easily exposed and put into use during emergencies. At the entrance to EDs, an infrastructure could be installed that would serve the staff during a chemical, biological, radiological, or nuclear attack. This area includes multiple water outlets that could be quickly hooked up to provide decontamination showers, and airlocks and filtered vents that could recirculate uncontaminated air.[16]

All admission areas should be directed and coordinated via a central hospital command station. Besides emergency admitting and treatment areas, other sites in the hospital would also require special consideration in the event of a chemical, biological, or radiological attack. Operating theaters and intensive care units in particular would need to be sealed and isolated from the infected air outside.

Because these structural accommodations are expensive, not every hospital is in a position to implement them. Moreover, since the degree of threat may vary according to location, not every hospital needs the same level of preparedness. But advanced structural preparedness should be required in at least one or two hospitals in every region of the country. This is especially true in high-risk metropolitan areas.

Identification of Unknown Victims

Casualties from terror attacks may vary markedly in number and type of injury, often depending on the weapons used. Conventional explosives detonated at close range may mutilate victims, making their identification difficult.[17] This problem can be addressed in part by recording descriptive information and taking digital photographs soon after hospital admission. The earlier the better since facial features may become distorted by edema or masked by tubing and other medical equipment.

When terror victims are admitted, a hospital should also set up a Public Information Center to respond to inquiries from family, friends, and the media.[18] (Fig. 7.4) In the interest of privacy rights, information exchange with other hospitals and the forensic institute can be conducted via a secured network.

The process of scientific identification of the deceased can be complex and should take place in state-of-the-art forensic institutes. There is a need for clear guidelines requiring all unidentified deceased persons to be transferred to the forensic institute accompanied by all items found within their proximity. Scientific identification of bodies is dependent on fingerprints, odontology, and DNA comparisons.[19]

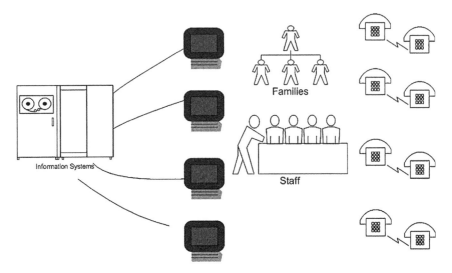

FIG. 7.4. Public Information Center. Receiving phone calls, arriving relatives, and sharing information with other centers through a centralized computer system.

Following an event with an unconventional weapon, it might be necessary to perform an autopsy to confirm the nature of injury or disease, and to help identify the causative agent. Following an attack with biological or chemical weapons, it is also necessary to protect all of the individuals who handle the human remains. There is a need for clear guidelines about how to deal with the bodies and, if necessary, special burial procedures.

Helping the Public

Terror attacks may affect individuals who were not physically injured, but who were in the vicinity of an event. Many will need psychological assessment, and sometimes treatment.[20] Dealing with family members of a severely wounded victim can be especially challenging. Multi-disciplinary teams of psychologists, social workers, and administrative personnel should be made available by local authorities to help with temporary housing, damage repair, and other immediate needs. Special efforts should be directed to underprivileged and otherwise needy individuals.

Emotional coping both in the long and short terms requires addressing post-traumatic stress disorders (PTSD): identifying such patients, convincing them they need help, and guiding them to a treatment facility.[21] Special attention should also be given to rescue workers, who may be suffering emotional trauma from attending to numerous terror events.

The Role of the Media

Terror attacks are often intended by the perpetrators to be media events or to otherwise gain public attention. But such displays also can be detrimental to a terrorist's intentions by antagonizing viewers and by preserving on film actions that could be used as evidence against the perpetrators.

In fact, the media can provide the public with a range of important information about an event including its scope, rationale, characteristics of the perpetrators, and the number and identity of victims. It can also be a pivotal transmitter of public announcements, such as providing phone numbers of helplines or conveying calls for blood donors.

Ideally, media contacts with hospital and other authorities should be centrally managed, focused, and scheduled. The aim is to provide the press with the most accurate and up-to-date information in real time from one central source that represents the principal participants – from the EMS and hospitals to police and fire officials. Conflicting information from different bodies can only lead to confusion, false rumors, and lack of confidence on the part of the public.

Closing the Circle: Debriefing

An after-action debriefing should follow every terror attack, MCE, or drill. Participants should include all interested parties – from the treating teams in the field and emergency room personnel to hospital administrators. Principles must be established as to the type of debriefing required for different scenarios. Debriefings are basic to risk management and essential to identifying areas in need of improvement. They are at the core of information management within the organization, allowing it to become a "learning institution" that quickly implements adjustments to performance.

The debriefing is not designed to dwell on operational failures or to investigate those at fault. But all relevant information should be transparent and available to anyone involved with preparedness, rescue, treatment, or oversight. All such reviews should lead to improved efficiency of operations and enhanced patient care. While lessons learned should be implemented locally, they should also be disseminated at the national level to be used as learning tools. Thus, these lessons may contribute to improving the preparedness and functioning of hospitals throughout the country.

The absence of a common template for hospital debriefings can impair consistency in evaluation of performance. Without uniform debriefing procedures there is a risk that successes and failures could either be overlooked or exaggerated. To help avoid this pitfall, a singular debriefing form that is neither complicated nor long should be used by all relevant institutions.

The Israeli Debriefing Method

In Israel, debriefing meetings are held as soon as possible after an event. The aim is to avoid the unintentional cognitive process of mixing facts with desired outcomes, which becomes more likely with the passage of time.

Israeli guidelines for the process include

1. Debriefings by individual units that participated in particular aspects of the event, such as ambulance teams, ED units, and other relevant hospital teams.

The smaller the team, the more efficient the process. Debriefings of individual units take place simultaneously, not in sequence.

2. Similarly, debriefings by higher-level units also are conducted simultaneously, including by regional EMS management, hospital administration, etc. and at the coordinating level by the Division of Emergencies in the Ministry of Health. The debriefings should relate to the specific activities of the division and not to the attack as a whole. At this stage, representatives of other relevant responder units such as the police, fire department, Home Front Command, and the municipality should participate. The debriefing of individual units takes place as soon after the attack as possible in accordance with the debriefing protocol below.

3. Summaries of the debriefings and recommendations are forwarded to the NEMCC and to the directors of the EMS and hospitals.

4. Debriefing procedures for management-level units should be the same for all such groups and should take place after the summary reports are received from the individual units. Management unit debriefings are then held in the presence of senior representatives from all of the authorities that have already conducted their internal debriefings.

5. Finally, at a later time, an overview of those findings is conducted under the initiative of the NEMCC.

Managing the Debriefing

1. A debriefing protocol includes the following: location, timetable, relevant participants, presentation aids, and other accessories such as lists of victims, maps, media, or amateur video clips.

2. A chairperson is appointed and all participants are asked to review their roles in accordance with the chronological order of events. Remarks and discussion follow the individual presentations.

3. During the debriefing, notes are taken which will be used as the basis of a summary protocol. A final draft of the protocol is reviewed and authorized by the chairperson.

Debriefings shall take place on two levels:

1. Organizational operational debriefings (Table 7.2): An organizational terror MCE debriefing shall relate to the following four stages: preparatory phase, admittance phase, treatment phase, and return to routine operations.

2. Professional medical debriefing and discussion to include modes of injury, evacuation, triage, flaws in diagnosis and treatment, and availability of resources directly needed for patient care.

The conclusions of the debriefing need to be distributed on a national level to all parties that were involved, and to those who are apt to be involved in similar events in the future.

TABLE 7.2. Organizational operational debriefing

Stage		Definition
1	Preparations	From receipt of initial call until the patient admission begins
2	Admittance phase	From admission of the first victim at the hospital until the last victim is admitted and registered in the admittance area
3	Treatment phase	From admission of the first victim until the last victim from any site is discharged
4	Return to routine operations	From the discharge of the last victim from any site until the facility is ready to absorb victims of the next attack

Conclusion

Terror attacks produce major challenges for the medical system. Some events, especially those that produce mass casualties, can place extremely heavy demands on scarce resources. A goal of medical management is to oversee rapid and appropriate care for victims and a return to routine order as quickly as possible. Healthcare providers are often unfamiliar with certain terror scenarios, such as those associated with unconventional weapons, and they require special instruction in those areas.

Terrorism can induce anxiety, depression, and other negative emotions in victims, families, emergency responders, and caregivers including medical teams. All need observation and perhaps counseling to help assuage their emotional stress.

The location and time of a particular attack may not be known in advance, but in view of repeated occurrences throughout the world, more assaults can be expected. Medical managers have an obligation to prepare their facilities and teams for the worst. Preparedness should include familiarity with plausible threats, written SOP, acquisition of equipment and drugs, periodic drills and exercises, and maintenance of decontamination apparatus, isolation areas, and other such essential facilities. Proper preparedness will decrease mortality, morbidity, and disability while strengthening a society's resilience in the face of further terrorist threats.

References

1. Peleg K, Aharonson-Daniel L, Stein M, Shapira SC. Patterns of injury in hospitalized terrorist victims. Am J Emerg Med. 2006;21:258–262.
2. Federal guidelines for protecting information. In: Federal information management act of 2002 (FISMA): http://csrc.nist.gov/policies/FISMA–final.pdf. Accessed September 1, 2007.
3. Shapira SC, Mor-Yosef S. Terror politics and medicine – The role of leadership. Studies in Conflicts and Terrorism. 2004;27:65–71.
4. Shapira SC, Mor-Yosef S. Applying lessons from medical management of conventional terror to responding to Weapons of Mass Destruction terror: The experience of a tertiary university hospital. Studies in Conflicts and Terrorism. 2003;26:379–385.
5. Ministry of Health Emergency Division. National Standard Operating Procedures. http://www.health.gov.il/emergency/mamarim/mishpatiim_8.htm. Accessed August 8, 2007.

6. Leibovici D, Gofrit ON, Heruti RJ, Shapira SC, Shemer J, Stein M. Interhospital patient transfer – A quality improvement indicator for prehospital triage. Am J Emerg Med. 1997;15:341–344.

7. Tadmor B, Poles L, Shapira SC. In: Kamien DG, ed. *The McGraw-Hill Homeland Security Handbook*. 1st ed. New York, NY: McGraw-Hill; 2006:721–737.

8. Gofrit ON, Leibovici D, Shemer J, Henig A, Shapira SC. The efficacy of integrating "smart simulated casualties" in hospital disaster drills. Prehosp Disas Med. 1997;12:26–30.

9. Shapira SC, Shemer J. Medical management of terrorist attacks. IMAJ. 2002;4:489–492.

10. Sheffy N, Mintz Y, Rivkind AI, Shapira SC. Terror related Injuries: A comparison of gunshot wounds versus explosives' secondary fragments induced injuries. J Amer Col Surg. 2006;203:297–303.

11. Avitzour M, Liebergall M, Assaf J, et al. A multicasualty event: Out-of-hospital and in-hospital organizational aspects. Acad Emerg Med. 2004;11:1102–1104.

12. Lawrence DT, Kirk MA. Chemical terrorism attacks: Update on antidotes. Emerg Med Clin N Am. 2007;25:567–595.

13. Macintyre AG, Christopher GW, Eitzen E, et al. Weapons of mass destruction events with contaminated casualties. JAMA. 2000;283:242–249.

14. Israel Ministry of Health Levels of Hospital Alerts. Committee chaired by Shmuel C. Shapira, 2001.

15. Shapira SC, Shemer J, Oren M. Hospital management of a bioterror event. IMAJ. 2002;4:493–494.

16. Shapira SC, Cole LA. Terror medicine: birth of a discipline. J Homeland Security Emerg Manag 2006; 3: www.bepress.com/jhsem/vol3/1ss2/9. Accessed September 1, 2007.

17. Shapira SC, Adatto-Levi R, Avitzour M, Rivkind AI, Gertsenshtein I and Mintz Y. Mortality in terrorist attacks: A unique modal of temporal death distribution. World J Surg. 2006;30:1–8.

18. Liebergall MH, Braverman N, Shapira SC, Picker Rotem O, Soudry I, Mor-Yosef S. Role of nurses in a university hospital during mass casualty events. Am J Critical Care. 2007;16:480–484.

19. Hiss J, Kahana T. Suicide bomber in Israel. Am J Forens Med Path. 1998;19:63–66.

20. Tuval-Mashiach R, Freedman S, Bargai N, et al. Coping with trauma: Narrative and cognitive perspectives. Psychiatry. 2004;67:280–293.

21. Shalev AY, Freedman S. PTSD following terrorist attacks: A prospective evaluation. Am J Psych. 2005;162:1188–1191.

8
Response Planning

Jorie D. Klein

The World Trade Center, September 11, 2001, terrorist attacks and Hurricanes Katrina and Rita, in the Gulf in 2005, have produced significant changes in emergency response planning and potential funding opportunities in the United States. Hospitals, healthcare organizations, and acute care providers are now active in community disaster response preparation, planning, and mitigation strategies. Isolated-silo, preparation, and planning is now considered unacceptable. Local and county emergency operations centers, emergency medical services (EMS), hospitals, acute care providers, community agencies, and volunteer agencies now work in collaboration to develop community and regional response plans. Laws and regulatory requirements for preparedness and planning have gone through several revisions and amendments at the Federal and State level. Accreditation organizations such as the Joint Commission have revised their emergency management standards to reflect a stronger emphasis on system integration and sustainability. This chapter will focus on the hospital planning phases of emergency response. Planning is considered the most important aspect of the emergency response process. The planning process brings together multiagencies and multidisciplines to review the response history of the community, define threats, define gaps in hospital response, and develop strategies to improve the overall response plans.

Preparation

Preparation begins with a framework that is in compliance with the Stafford Act, National Response Framework, and Homeland Security Presidential Directive #5. In addition to these Federal mandates, the hospital planners should review the published disaster management mass casualty principles and the critiques of past disasters. The local Office of Emergency Management typically defines the preparation and planning for the local community response which includes EMS and field triage response capabilities. Hospital Environment of Care Committees typically have the responsibility and oversight of the hospital's disaster response planning. Many hospitals create a subcommittee specifically to address their disaster or emergency management activities. The Joint Commission uses the term "emergency operations"

S.C. Shapira et al. (eds.), *Essentials of Terror Medicine*,
DOI: 10.1007/978-0-387-09412-0_8, Springer Science+Business Media, LLC 2009

plan and "emergency response" in their standards rather than "disaster." Both terms are used in this chapter.

The Robert T. Stafford Disaster Relief and Emergency Assistance Act (Stafford Act 1988) is the legislation governing the federal response to disasters in the United States.[1] The Stafford Act defines the chain of command for declaration of an emergency, types of assistance that are available, and cost sharing agreements between the State, Federal, and local communities. It created the system by which the Presidential Disaster Declaration of an emergency triggers financial and physical assistance through the Federal Emergency Management Agency (FEMA). The chain of command for activation of this response moves from the local office of emergency management, to the county judge, to the regional district, to the Governor's office, and then to the President of the United States. FEMA serves as the overall executive branch coordination agency for a Presidential Disaster Declaration. FEMA has the responsibility and authority for coordinating all government relief efforts.[2] All 50 states and the 6 territories have emergency management agencies that fall under this executive branch of the State government.

The Homeland Security Act of 2002 established the Department of Homeland Security as a cabinet-level executive agency. Department of Homeland Security consolidated 22 agencies and unified many federal functions into a single agency dedicated to protecting America.[3] FEMA is now an agency within the Department of Homeland Security. FEMA continues to be the lead coordinating agency for all disaster response in the United States, under the oversight of the Department of Homeland Security. The Secretary of Homeland Security has the authority to initiate a Federal response under the Stafford Act without prior consultation with the President under certain emergencies. In 2003, the President issued Homeland Security Presidential Directive #5 to enhance the ability of the United States to manage domestic emergency.[4]

The Secretary of Homeland Security directed the development of a single, integrated Federal Emergency Operations Plan. The National Response Plan was the outcome of this directive. The National Response Plan has 15 Emergency Support Functions. These typically exist within multiple Federal agencies and are coordinated by a single emergency support function coordinator.[5] Emergency Support Function #8 is the Public Health and Medical Service. Acute medical care and mass casualty care are included in this emergency support function. The Emergency Response Plan, now the Emergency Response Framework, provides guidance on Federal, State, and local emergency response systems. The Homeland Security Act defines the term "emergency response provider" to include Federal, State, and local emergency public safety, law enforcement, emergency response, emergency medical (including hospital emergency facilities), and related personnel, agencies, and authorities.

Homeland Security Presidential Directive #5 also called for the development of a standardized incident management system to facilitate interoperability and integration of the many Federal, State, and local response organizations. The National Incident Management System (NIMS) provides this standardization.[6] It is a nationwide framework in which the local, State, and Federal government and private sector can work effectively and efficiently to prepare, plan, mitigate, respond, and recover from incidents regardless of their cause, size, or complexity. The NIMS is mandated for all agencies in the federal government. Federal funding for disaster and homeland security initiatives is directly tied to the use of NIMS in preparation, planning, and response. Hospitals have defined NIMS elements of performance that are mandated to be inline with Federal funding initiatives, grants, and response reimbursement.

The Joint Commission has historically been the leader in developing accreditation standards for healthcare agencies in the United States. Joint Commission accreditation is required for reimbursement of services under Medicare and Medicaid. The Environment of Care Standards and the Emergency Management Standards define the standard requirements for accreditation. The proposed 2009 Joint Commission Standards recommend that emergency management planning be separated from the typical Environment of Care Committee and become a stand alone committee dedicated to preparation and planning for the hospital emergency operations plan and system integration.

Preparation for hospital disaster management begins with a full review of these regulatory mandates that govern the hospital's emergency response performance. These include the NIMS elements of performance, Joint Commission standards, and the Federal, State regulations. Information regarding NIMS is available at http:// fema.gov/emergecy/nims/. Joint Commission standards specific to disaster planning can be accessed on their website[7]: www.jcrinc.com/perspectivesspecialissue -26K or www.hcma;larketplace.com/prod-3803.htm-25K.

Commitment

Hospital Board of Managers and Administration must commit resources for a successful emergency response plan. Hospitals may develop Medical Staff and Hospital Board Resolutions that define the adoption and integration of the NIMS and defined Joint Commission regulatory guidelines by the hospital system. Defining a specific emergency management cost center will assist in defining the actual employee salary dollars, operational budget dollars, and expenditures to sustain the emergency operations plan. This will also facilitate tracking the available grant dollars dedicated to emergency management. Hospitals may choose to appoint a Disaster Medical Director(s) who has the authority and oversight to lead the emergency response acute care medical response. This individual is responsible for medical staff leadership in an emergency response, defining minimal care standards, triage systems, overall care coordination, and patient flow from the emergency triage/receiving area to the operating room, intensive care units (ICUs), general care units, and the clinical resources to support mass casualty care. This individual must have taken the required courses mandated by NIMS. All individuals who have the job titles and responsibility for emergency operations planning should have the mandated course requirements and credentials (NRP-800, NIMS 700, ICS 100, and ICS 200). The NIMS elements of performance for 2008 require specific individuals to complete defined courses. The course certificates of completion should be kept on file and tracked to ensure compliance.

The final phase of preparation defines the community response plan, community capabilities, capacity, and the hospital's role in the community response. A comparison of the hospital's current response plans to the defined regulatory and compliance standards defines a performance gap analysis. The gap analysis defines the planning priorities for the next 12 months. The core elements of preparation are related to understanding the rules, regulations, and standards for disaster response and the hospital's ability, capacity, and capabilities to meet these expectations.

Planning

The hospital emergency operations planning committee members must understand all required standards and elements of performance mandated for emergency management to be an effective committee member. In addition, they need to understand all rules and regulations regarding reimbursement for a disaster response. NIMS elements of performance define that the leaders of the hospital have training in the NIMS to apply for federal grants or response reimbursement. These leaders are defined by the planning committee. These individuals must attend training courses or complete the online training course http://training.fema.gov/EMIWEB/IS/is700. asp. Completed course certificates must be on file for record keeping and available during all regulatory reviews.

The Emergency Management Committee should include emergency medicine physicians, trauma surgeons or general surgeons, anesthesiologists, orthopedists, neurosurgeons, intensive care medical directors, infectious disease physicians, and behavioral medicine physicians. Hospital administrators, nursing directors/managers, clinical support departments, human resources, educational services, public relations, safety, hazmat, and security personnel should be represented on this planning committee. The teamwork and relationships that develop from this planning activity is a significant benefit to the hospital during crisis. The process outcomes of this effort are often considered more important than the written completed plan, due to the team building, system knowledge that is gained, and opened communication lines across all disciplines.

The planning committee (subcommittee) is typically led by the individual responsible for the overall hospital disaster preparedness. The committee reviews the hospital's disaster response history. This includes reviewing critiques and after-action reports from past drills and actual events. These reports establish the hospital's actual performance capabilities. Records in the local Office of Emergency Management are reviewed to define historical data in the community. These records identify past events and current threats such as flood plains, pipeline locations, geographic and natural threats. This review will assist in defining the community's resources and expectations of the hospital during a disaster, and also may define the resources and capabilities of a regional response to a disaster.

Hazard Vulnerability Analysis

Completion of a hospital hazard vulnerability risk assessment is the second deliverable of the planning committee. The hazard vulnerability assessment (HVA) must be reviewed and updated annually.[8] Hospitals utilize the completed community risk assessment information to begin their HVA. This assessment will define all possible threats to the hospital. These threats or hazards can be categorized into natural and manmade.

Each defined hazard is reviewed to define the probability of risk for the hazard occurring. The probability of the hazard occurring is categorized into high, medium, low, and not likely. Scores are assigned to each category. The probability of occurrence is derived from the defined community assessment, information gained from the Local Emergency Management Office, and the hospital's past experience.

The hazard's potential severity of impact on the community and hospital is defined. This phase of assessment defines if the hazard has the potential to produce life-threatening events, health and safety risk for citizens/staff, and whether it poses a high, moderate, or low risk of disruption of community social structure.

The hospital response plans, and the community's level of preparedness for each identified hazard are assessed in the last phase of the HVA. This assessment focuses on the documented response plan, and staff's knowledge and competency associated with each response plan. Assessment includes the training program, insurance coverage, volume of supplies on hand, staff's availability to respond, and available backup utility systems. The signed mutual assistance agreements with community agencies, coordination with local and state agencies, coordination with local healthcare facilities, and coordination with community special treatment facilities are included in the risk assessment. The planning committee and hospital leaders may chose to have the HVA findings reviewed by legal counsel to determine if the assessment has potential legal risk. The HVA is a tool to systematically assess the hospital's risk. Failure to exercise due diligence when conducting and HVA may have adverse consequences ranging from loss of life, business interruption, damage to reputation and litigation from inadequate emergency planning.

Communications Systems

The Dallas aircraft crash in 1985 defined significant communication failures between the scene, local agencies, and the hospitals.[9] The Katrina events in New Orleans in 2005 demonstrated the impact of communication failures between the site, planning agencies, State and Federal agencies. Communication continues to be listed as a failure or weakness in most disaster drill evaluations.[10,11] Communication is used to mobilize the hospital emergency responses procedures, notify essential staff, notify community agencies, and coordinate the overall integrated response. Hospitals must plan for redundant communication systems and backup communication resources. All communication capabilities available in the hospital and in the community are assessed to define communication strengths, weaknesses, and opportunities. There are many forms of communication used in a disaster response. Telephones, fax capabilities, portable radios, ham radios, satellite phones, cellular phones, computer soft phones, Internet/Intranet systems, and private networks are examples of communication options. The critical issue regarding communication is sustainability during a disaster response, and redundant backup systems to maintain the core function. These are critical elements that must be addressed by the planning committee. Equipment and reserve power sources must be available during all hazards. Communities and regions that invest in developing regional communications systems, backup systems, and backup power sources are likely to be more successful, because information assists in the response coordination. The use of common terminology, definitions, and resource typing (NIMS) enhances information sharing, communication, and coordination.

Patient tracking systems and hospital capacity systems are essential for an effective and efficient emergency response. These systems are components of communication and facilitate integration with the community response. The planning committee must define how these systems are to be activated, who has access to this information and who is responsible for the oversight of these systems. Equipment and training to support and sustain these tracking systems must be outlined in the response plan.

Communication systems to provide situational or status reports for all employees are required for regulatory requirements. The frequency of these updates are specific to the type of event. Procedures define who is responsible for these updates, the type of information to be communicated, and how the information will be disseminated. Communication systems to support this function must be in place. This can be addressed through websites, Intranet, Internet, or written document disseminated to all areas.

System response planning must include media communication and prepared crisis communication plans. The location for media coordination and tools to facilitate media communication need to be in place with backup systems and redundancy. Mass casualty events will create a mass media response. Communication capabilities must address this predicted need. Updates and news conferences are scheduled at frequent and regular intervals to provide the information media timelines. The media receiving area needs to be away from the EMS receiving area, medical decontamination, triage, emergency department, incident command centers, and the casualty's family center. The Public Information Officer (PIO) is the individual responsible for all hospital media requests. The best hospital and community disaster plans involve the media in this planning process. This promotes teamwork, collaboration, and relationship development, as well as provides the media an opportunity to have input on plans that directly impact their performance.

Safety and Security

Securing the facility, EMS access, and traffic routes around the hospital are essential components of the hospital response. The planning committee defines the areas that need additional security during response. These areas are typically the areas that individuals migrate to for information, casualty receiving areas, or identified risk areas, such as utility or physical plant resources. Security must participate in a leadership capacity for effective and efficient response planning. Activation of the emergency response plan requires implementation of a lock-down procedure that restricts hospital access. The severity and degree of the lock-down procedure and access restrictions is defined by the event. Emergency response activation to assist with medical decontamination, escalated threats from the community, quarantine events, mass prophylaxis, and VIP situations require specific security plans. The mass shootings occurring throughout the nation, in all types of environments require hospitals to do due diligence in developing security plans to prevent and respond to mass shooting in the health-care environment. In addition, security measures to prevent acts of terrorism must be addressed. These issues and their priority in response planning are defined through the HVA.

The planning committee defines a central location for community donations, and who is responsible for the acceptance of these donations. Security must be available to screen donations to protect the patients, staff, and visitors. Community volunteer access and identification procedures must be in place. Security must be present or immediately available to these screening locations. The planning committee defines the locations where the community volunteers are staged as they wait for an assignment. The hospital plan may require security to use the community volunteer's driver's license to complete a background check. Security procedures and capabilities must be defined in advance for this level of response.

Hospital Police/Security departments across the nation are typically understaffed, and have limited resources. The planning committee defines the expectations of security and the resources required to address the functions of security. If these expectations are not attainable with the current resources, the planning committee must make the hospital leaders aware of the critical issues and assist in developing budget request, or alternate plan such as outsourcing and contract services. Other departments, such as engineering, and other facilities, may be targeted to assist with security functions. Signed, "Memorandum of Sharing" agreements with other law enforcement agencies and hospital security departments in the community are encouraged. Hospitals that are in close proximity may choose to develop a collaborative, integrated security management plan to conserve resources.

Emergency Operations Plan

The hospital's *emergency operations plan,* or disaster plan, serves as the hospital's business response plan to incidents that partially or completely disrupt normal hospital operations. The four key components of an emergency operations plan are *mitigation*, *preparedness*, *response*, and *recovery*. Joint Commission and NIMS compliance require an *all-hazards* approach to emergency response planning. An all-hazard response allows hospitals to be prepared to respond to events of all types, while maintaining the necessary flexibility to adapt to the specific circumstances of an event. The emergency operations plan defines the framework and hospital's organizational structure for managing the impact of all disaster scenarios realistically. The goal is minimum disruption of services, while still meeting the needs of the event. Efficient, effective, and coordinated disaster planning is an investment for the hospital and community. It should be addressed in the strategic initiatives and viewed as a component of the hospital's long-range business plan.

Common Terminology

The planning committee must adopt and define common terminology (NIMS) that is utilized in developing and responding to disasters. Common terminology and definitions facilitate communication and *interoperability*, as previously reviewed. Terms that are common in disaster and emergency response may not be common to the physicians, nurses, engineers, and other hospital personnel. A list of definitions should be readily available during a response, and should be included in the employee's educational overview of the disaster plan.

Mitigation

Completion of the hospital HVA defines the priorities of emergency response planning. Activities initiated based on the HVA in advance to lessen the severity and/or impact of a potential hazard is mitigation. Mitigation may reduce or eliminate the possibility of the disaster occurring altogether. This is considered a primary prevention, or it may reduce the adverse consequences of an event or secondary prevention.

Preparedness

Preparedness includes the activities that address and coordinate capacity expansion and increase capability. These aspects of the disaster planning address the additional resources and consumption of resources during an emergency response. Inventory management systems, defined capabilities, and procedures to expand the capabilities to meet the projected response needs through prearranged agreements are examples of preparedness. Preparedness activities are ongoing processes that require re-evaluation of resources to define changes in equipment needs, changes in procedures, or standards of care. NIMS and Joint Commission require an inventory management system, planning to address surge needs, alternate case sites, and a plan for hospital 96h of sustainability. Preparedness activities will address measures to support each of these standards.

Response

Response procedures define the guidelines, steps, and protocols for the all-hazard response to an event. Response plans include the processes to mobilize the disaster response, notify essential staff, and measures to establish the incident command system. Procedures for casualty management, patient flow, documentation, and demobilizaton are components of the response plan. This part of the plan involves the procedures for *crisis management*. It will provide details for staff to follow when activated; what they are expected to do, where to report, whom to report to, and the chain of command.

Recovery

Recovery is the consequence management of the disaster response. Recovery defines how the hospital will demobilize their disaster response. Business recovery and the processes to return to normal operation are the priorities. The activation of insurance coverage policies, review of the inventory available, and steps to define procurement needs for full hospital services are addressed during the recovery phase. Outsourcing and contract management are addressed in the recovery section of the disaster plan. Staff scheduling, staff availability, building recovery, and psycho-emotional management for all providers are standard priorities during recovery. This is the *consequence management* phase of a disaster response.

Essential Elements of the Disaster Plan

The completion of the written plan is the beginning of the *process* of preparedness. The infrastructure, provider training and education to support and sustain the response plan must be completed. Staff education is an ongoing evolution. Emergency response plans are integrated into the hospital orientation and annual mandatory education. The response plan must be flexible, adaptable, and include the NIMS elements of performance and the Joint Commission Emergency Management standards compliance to ensure potential Federal grant funding or Federal reimbursement for an emergency response.

Incident Command System

NIMS elements of performance require adoption of the Incident Command System (ICS). Hospitals must integrate the NIMS concepts and principles of flexibility and standardizations into their emergency operations plan. The ICS is modular and scalable. ICS develops in a top-down modular fashion that meets the size and complexity of the event. ICS incorporates measurable objectives which ensure completion of incident management goals. ICS develops and issues assignments, plans, procedures, and protocols to meet the management objectives. The Incident Action Plan provides a method of communicating the overall incident objectives for operational and support activities. The span of control of any individual with incident management supervisory responsibility ranges from three to seven subordinates. The type of event, nature of tasks, and defined hazards influence span-of-control considerations. The hospital planning committee integrates the NIMS elements of performance and the Hospital Incident Command Structure (HICS IV) into their response plans.[12] HICS IV is a *crisis management* tool for hospitals to use to facilitate and coordinate their emergency response procedures. There are five functions in HICS IV comparable to the functions of the pre-hospital ICS: Command, Logistics, Operations, Planning, and Finance/Administration. The goal of the ICS is to create a system that improves effectiveness, accountability, communications, and interoperability during a disaster response. The incident command system uses an incident action planning process that is comprehensive and has the ability to link multiple agencies and emergency response disciplines. The unified command concept used in the ICS provides processes for coordinating and directing multiple disciplines during a disaster.

The goals of HICS IV are to define function, create effective *span-of control*, and provide a "modular" organizational response to ensure that critical role job functions are completed. Each section of the incident command system is designed to promote the responder's concentration on their primary assignment. HICS IV allows the incident commander to escalate response or to decrease the modular response based on need.

The Command Center, or *Incident Command*, is designed to provide the authority and leadership for the hospital's response. The command staff includes the Incident Commander, PIO, Safety Officer, and the Liaison Officer. The ICS roles are assumed by those individuals most qualified for the position.

The Incident Commander has overall incident management responsibilities delegated by the hospital executive officers. The Incident Commander develops the incident objectives that guide incident response and recovery efforts. The commander approves the incident action plan and all requests pertaining to the ordering and releasing of incident resources. The Incident Commander performs all major incident command system functions, operations, logistics, planning, and finance/administration until one or more of these functions are delegated, based on the event. The Incident Commander's role is to establish general policy and decision-making for the organization's overall response efforts. The Incident Commander approves public information release, and coordinates the hospital's response with the other public officials and agencies.

The PIO is responsible for the interfacing with the public, media, and other organizations with incident-related information requirements. The PIO develops accurate detailed information on the incident's cause, size, and current situation to include resources committed. This information may be used internally or externally. The PIO is responsible for monitoring public information. The Incident Commander must approve all information releases as previously stated.

The Safety Officer monitors the event operations and provides advice to the Incident Commander regarding operational safety, including the health and safety of staff. The Safety Officer is responsible for the system procedures that promote safety.

Medical/technical/specialist roles may assist the Safety Officer in their role of ensuring safety for the staff, visitors, and patients. Specialist may include experts in toxicology, who assist with defining medical decontamination needs, a radiation safety officer who assists in response standards for a radiation exposure, and infectious disease physicians, who assist in defining response standards to an infectious or contagious outbreak. All of these roles simply serve in an advisory capacity to the

Safety Officer. Their purpose is to provide an immediate assessment of potential risk, and to assist the command staff in developing and finalizing the response plan.

The Liaison Officer is the point of contact for representatives of other nongovernmental organizations, government agencies, and private entities. Representatives from assisting or cooperating agencies coordinate through the Liaison Officer. Organizational representatives assigned to an incident must have the authority to speak for their organization on all matters, following appropriate consultation with the organization's leadership.

The planning committee will define the targeted leaders for the command staff. These individuals must have a strong knowledge of the political and geographic environment, the surrounding EMS, local trauma system, and hospital capabilities. Shift coverage for the command staff and general staff is typically 12-hour shifts. A rotation schedule must be defined. Individuals targeted for this role should have a comprehensive knowledge of their system's disaster plan, the hospital, and defined NIMS and ICS courses (NIMS 700, ICS 100, and ICS 200).

The general staff comprised the incident management personnel who are the representative leaders for the major functional elements of the ICS. General staff includes the Operations Section Chief, Planning Section Chief, Logistic Section Chief, and the Finance/Administration Section Chief. Command staff and general staff must continually communicate and share information regarding the current and predicted future situation to develop recommended strategies and actions to the Incident Commander. Divisions are established to divide an incident into physical or geographic areas of operations. Groups are established to divide the incident into functional areas of operation. Branches are used to combine functional groups and geographic divisions. Branches may be used when the number of resources exceeds the recommended span-of-control.

Operation Section

The *Operations Section* directs and carries out all incident tactical operations. This section is responsible for tactical operations, participating in the planning process, and modifying the actions plan to meet contingencies. Operations will provide the information and data, or "intelligence," to the Planning Section and Command. It should be noted that the other sections are in place to support the Operations Section in carrying out its tactical objectives. In HICS IV, operations includes the hospital system's operations of medical care branch, infrastructure branch, business continuity branch, hazmat branch, security branch, and staging. Hospital current patients, routine emergency patients care and casualty care are the function of the medical branch.

The medical care branch oversees all emergency response casualty care from triage, treatment areas, inpatient areas, clinic sites, and clinical support services. The infrastructure branch is responsible for continuity of all facility utilities and management. This includes damage assessments and corrective tactical measures to restore utilities and facility infrastructure. The business continuity branch is responsible for the tactical operations of information technology management, medical records, and patient registration. The hazmat branch is responsible for the tactical operations of all potential decontamination response.

The security branch oversees all security operations to secure the facility, traffic control, and facility lockdown. The staging manager oversees the site where resources such as personnel, equipment, and resources are staged, waiting on a tactical assignment. Resources can be in one of three status conditions: assigned, available, or out-of-service. Resources in a staging area are available and ready for assignment. Resources out-of-service (resting, eating) are not located in the staging area.

Planning Section

The *Planning Section's* responsibilities focus on maintaining resource status, maintaining and displaying situational status, preparing the Incident Action Plan, developing alternate strategies for response, providing documentation services, and preparing for demobilization. One of the most important functions of the planning section is to look beyond the current and next operational period and anticipate event needs. The Planning Section Chief schedules routine update meetings with the other Section Chiefs to evaluate and define the response status and needs. This information is summarized and given to the Section Chiefs and Incident Commander. The Incident Commander redefines priorities from the situational assessment and defines incident objectives. The Planning Section defines the incident action plan to meet the incident objectives and shares this information with all Section Chiefs. This process continues throughout the duration of the response.

The resource unit leader is responsible for all check-in activity and for maintaining the status of all personnel and equipment resources assigned to the incident. The situation unit leader collects and processes information on the current situation, prepares situational displays and situation summaries. The documentation unit leader prepares the Incident Action Plan, maintains all incident-related documentation, and provides duplication services.

Logistics Section

The *Logistics Section* is responsible for all support requirements, including communication, medical support for the hospital responding staff, food for responding incident personnel, and supplies (medical supplies, equipment, and facilities). Logistics acquires the resources and turns all resources over to the Planning and Operations Sections. The functions in the Logistic Section are the service branch and support branch. The service branch consists of the following units: communications, medical, and food. The communication unit is responsible for developing plans for the effective use of incident communications equipment and facilities, installing and testing communication equipment, distribution of communication equipment, and maintenance of equipment.

The medical branch is responsible for the healthcare of employees. The food unit is responsible for supplying the food needs for the entire incident including remote off-campus locations.

The support branch includes the supply unit, facility unit, and ground support unit. The support branch is responsible for the labor pool, ordering equipment and supplies, receiving and storing all supplies, maintaining an inventory of supplies, services, and maintenance of nonexpendable supplies and equipment. The facilities unit is responsible for the layout and activation of incident facilities such as staging areas, staff sleeping areas, and sanitation facilities for increased staff resources. The ground service is responsible for supporting the out-of-service resources. This includes transporting personnel, supplies, food, and equipment as well as service maintenance and repair of vehicles and equipment.

Finance/Administration Section

The *Finance/Administration Section* is established when incident management activities require finance and other administrative support services. The Finance/Administration Section includes the time unit, procurement unit, compensations/claim unit, and cost unit. The time unit is responsible for recording and documenting equipment and personnel time. The procurement unit is responsible for administering all financial matters pertaining to vendor contracts, leases, and fiscal agreements. The compensations/claims unit is responsible for facility damage, response injuries, and responder fatalities from the event. The cost unit tracks and analyzes cost data, defining cost estimates and recommending cost-saving measures.

The hospital planning committee is responsible for defining and prioritizing educational programs and access to training for all hospital responders. Hospital staff needs access to the necessary NIMS and ICS courses. Systems to track NIMS element of performance must be implemented.

Triage

Disaster triage is a core function of the hospital's emergency response procedures. In a disaster response, the goal is to direct the limited resources to provide the *greatest good for the greatest number*, and *not* to focus on one patient's "standard of care." The goal is to identify the most *salvageable* critical injured casualties.[13] This requires that triage of the casualties be accurate, efficient, and that the most common triage errors be minimized. Disaster triage has become controversial regarding the triage classifications, triage tags, and who should be the triage officer. Best practice models have a regional system of triage process that is adopted by all responders and hospitals. This standardizes the process for the community. Typical hospital triage systems categorize the salvageable patients with immediate life-threatening injuries or illness as "immediate," patients that require interventions but are not in immediate danger as "delayed." These patients can typically wait an hour for medical care and interventions. Patients who have minor injuries or may even be well are triaged as "minimal." These patients are usually moved to alternate care sites to reserve resuscitation resources. Casualties whose prognosis is very poor and non-survivable are triaged as "expectant." These casualties receive comfort care.

Geographic effect refers to situations in which the nearest hospital to a disaster scene becomes inundated with the majority of casualties, preventing the delivery of effective medical care.[13] Studies have shown that 75% of all casualties in major disasters arrive at, and overwhelm, the nearest hospital to the disaster scene. Designating this facility as a *triage hospital,* which only functions as a central triage center rather than a treatment center, has been shown to improve the effectiveness of casualty flow. Casualties are only stabilized at the facility, then immediately transported for treatment to area hospitals in a systematic and sequential fashion according to their capabilities. This process is termed *leap-frogging.* This has the potential to maximize resources and maximize treatment area utilization in any given community. To be successful, this requires joint planning, common terminology, and that these facilities accept the concept of keeping the "family-unit" together. The planning committee defines the equipment and resources to be deployed for triage personnel.

The planning committee defines the rotation schedule and rest intervals for the triage team. If medical decontamination is required, the triage team will follow the established medical decontamination protocols. It should be noted that this is a high-risk area for stress and psycho-emotional trauma among medical providers. Every effort should be taken to decrease the psychological impact, and to provide crisis intervention for all staff members assigned to triage. (See Chaps. 13 and 14 covering medical decontamination in response to chemical and radiological exposure.)

Sustainability Planning

NIMS and the Joint Commission require hospitals to have a 96-hour sustainability plan. The hospital's HVA defines the system capabilities at greatest risk. The planning committee is challenged with creating backup systems of redundancy for medical supplies, medical equipment, pharmaceuticals, and utilities. The *just-in-time* inventory programs provide 12–24 hours of supplies. Mass casualty response consumes these resources in a short time. Mechanisms to replenish and stock the critical acquisition of supplies and resources must be implemented. A hospital inventory management system (NIMS and Joint Commission) will assist in defining the resources available, contact information for various backup vendors, and contract services. A house wide listing of all contract vendors and backup vendors used to provide routine service is critical. Database programs can assist as long as the technology system remains functional. It is recommended that hard copies of all vendor contracts be organized and kept on file for easy access. Hospitals must be cautious of vendors that have contracts with multiple hospitals in the region. These vendors may not be able to meet all demands of all hospitals in a disaster response in a timely manner due to these multiple commitments.

The planning process will define the agencies that have services available that require a signed "Memorandum of Sharing," or "Mutual Aid Agreement" to request resources.

These agencies may be other healthcare facilities, EMS agencies, or transportation agencies. These agreements require legal review. Agreements need to be logged into the inventory management system's contact list. Contact names and emergency numbers must be readily available to prevent resources delays.

Alternate Care Site Planning

Sustainability responses may require procedures to expand or to evacuate hospital patients to an alternate care site. The planning committee defines the potential alternate care sites and the resources required to convert these areas into clinical care areas. The acquisition of the equipment may require funding or reallocation of supplies and beds. Staffing patterns and staffing needs for the alternate care site are addressed in advance by the planning committee. Patient transportation mechanisms to off campus alternate care sites are addressed in the sustainability planning. This typically requires vendor contracts. Critical care monitoring and ventilatory capabilities in an alternate care site must be carefully planned.

Most situations attempt to keep all critical care patients at the hospital and move the noncritical to alternate care sites. Hospital areas such as GI labs, cardiac cath labs, radiology special procedures, postanesthesia care units, and day surgery units may be considered for ICU bed expansion or relocation areas. General patient care units may be relocated to areas such as cafeterias, lobbies, vacant units, and temporary spaces on existing units. Alternate care sites in the community, away from the hospital, may be appropriate for certain casualty care and needs, such as warehouses or sports stadiums. These areas may address nonurgent, chronic health, and behavioral healthcare needs.

Staff education, training, equipment, and resources for the alternate site are defined in advance by the planning committee. The organizational structure and communication systems for an off-site alternate care site are integrated with the ICS's established procedures. Security for the site and staff parking is included in the emergency response plan. Patient tracking, family notification, infection control procedures, and equipment tracking mechanisms are addressed through the incident objectives and incident action plan.

Evacuation Planning

Evacuation planning is very similar to the alternate care site planning. Hospital evacuation can be very calm or very chaotic, and may occur in an imminent danger situation. The HVA will define the hazards that pose threats that may lead to evacuation. Mitigation actions and will decrease the potential need for evacuation. Planning must cover simple, single unit horizontal evacuations to the most complicated and dangerous evacuations. The planning committee may choose categorization systems to designate the types of patient being evacuated, resources required to evacuate these patients, and equipment needs for evacuations. The equipment to support the evacuation process is defined by the planning committee. Funding required to purchase special equipment is addressed through the budget process. The planning committee will make recommendations for vendor and contract services with agencies to support the hospital's evacuation plan. These vendors may include EMS, patient transport vehicles, trucks to facilitate movement of patients with equipment, and critical care equipment and documents. Mutual Assistance Agreements are critical in the event of an evacuation. Trained personnel and long term acute facilities, may help the management of ventilated patients.

Patient tracking systems are an essential response tool. Mechanisms to notify the patient's family must be in the plan. The *safe harbor area*, or location that is designated as the place for staff and patients to go to in an imminent danger evacuation, is defined by the ICS. Communication to inform all staff is critical to patient, visitor, and staff safety.

Staffing Alterations

The Incident Commander will define the business priorities for the hospital and the hospital closures. Staff in the closed area assists with the other hospital functions. Most hospitals have established procedures that mandate that all staff automatically move to 12-hour shifts during a disaster response. The ICS address staffing resources and staff needs. Response plans must address department call-back procedures, team assignments, and communicate changes in staffing plans.

The Logistic Section will address the staff support needs. Family, childcare, or dependent care needs and pet care needs are addressed through this process. Guidelines that define how staff access these care support centers and what is needed to register their child/dependent individual and pet into these care centers are defined through the planning phases. The planning committee must develop the specific protocols to address these issues. Staff may also need special diets, sleeping arrangements, medications, or transportation assistance to maintain their schedules. The ICS's Logistic Section addresses this function.

Casualty Flow Planning

How the mass casualty response impacts the emergency department, operating suite, day surgery, special procedures, the ICUs, and general units is related to the event. How and when the system cancels elective surgeries to maximize resources is defined through the ICS. Procedures to address current patients must be addressed through the ICS's medical branch. The operational measures to address routine emergency patients that will continue to occur during a disaster, such as imminent labor, chest pain, abdominal pain, and routine motor vehicle trauma are specific to the event and addressed through the ICS.

Provisions to address surge capacity to expand capabilities of services to meet the needs of mass casualty response are addressed in the preparation and planning phases of the response. During the event, surge is addressed through the ICS, with specific response from each of the support sections. Surge capacity in the emergency department refers to the number of casualties arriving each hour. The planning activity established procedures for immediate availability of supplies and staff to address casualty influx, to maximize the surge capacity, and to promote acceptable standards of care in mass casualty events.

Inpatient units and ICUs define patients that may be discharge or moved to a less acute unit to address critical care capacity needs. ICU bed expansions may consider alternate areas with monitored beds. The general care units must have procedures that facilitate the movement of discharged patients to a discharge holding area to create capacity.

Hospitals that have outpatient clinics and other patient care services must have procedures in place to cancel patient care activities to utilize those resources for mass casualty response. These initial response procedures implemented by the Incident Commander enable an increase in surge capacity. The location for a discharge holding area, an admission holding area, and a transfer coordination center is defined in the emergency response procedures but should also be addressed through the ICS. Bed turn-around, bed assignment management, and patient tracking are also components of the emergency response procedure. Procedures to move essential equipment and supplies to these areas, and to areas that have changed their scope of responsibility, must be in place.

Casualty Patient Flow

The emergency department is the hub of the initial response. It is critical that this area rapidly prepare to receive casualties. The emergency response procedures identify the unidirectional flow from the EMS receiving area through the initial triage area to medical decontamination if activated, to the secondary triage area, to the resuscitation and treatment area. Unidirectional flow simply refers to the constant forward movement of the patients. Patients cannot be moved to the radiology department or elsewhere for special procedures and then returned to the resuscitation area. Experience with drills, medical controllers, and training facilitates the unidirectional flow. Minimal acceptable care standards replace the "standard of care" practice, to preserve resources and to ensure that all casualties are evaluated rapidly and moved to appropriate areas. These procedures ensure that the primary goal of mass casualty treatment – the greatest good for the greatest number – is achieved.

Hospital emergency response plans must define the role and have job action sheets for the patient flow coordinator and medical controller.[14] The medical controller is responsible for the oversight of the treatment area and patient triage into the treatment area. Resource utilization, capacity management, compliance to minimal care standards, and unidirectional patient flow are the medical controller's responsibilities. The patient flow coordinator oversees specific patients and limits the use of laboratory testing and radiographic imaging as much as possible during the period of acute casualty influx to conserve resources and maintain casualty output flow.

Casualties are rapidly moved to the admission holding areas for the operating suite, intensive care areas, and general units. The medical controllers in the receiving units of the OR, ICU, and general units will re-evaluate patients to define priorities and patient movement into their areas. Patients who are discharged are rapidly moved to the discharge holding areas where assigned staff complete the discharge instructions and family notification. The type of event will define if discharged patients are held to conserve traffic around the hospital or if it is appropriate to release patients at areas that are away from traffic flow. A system to coordinate patient transfer is initiated to create additional capacity. Priorities for transfer are ICU ventilated patients that clinically can be managed by skilled facilities or long-term acute care facilities. Established procedures combined with education and training must prepare the staff and system for these critical casualty flow functions of mass casualty management.

The OR's medical controller must ensure that minimal standards and patient outflow is addressed for the OR. This individual may initiate a casualty staging area in the OR to hold and prioritize patients (vs. immediate movement into the operating theater) until casualty priorities are evident. This ensures appropriate OR triage for the casualties, and optimizes OR utilization. A senior trauma surgeon or general surgeon is best assigned to this controller role due to knowledge of the systems capabilities and capacity. The OR medical controller establishes the priorities of damage control interventions. Patients that require life-saving procedures during the first wave of surgical intervention must have beds assigned to ensure ongoing patient movement. Neurosurgery, orthopedic, plastic, and thoracic surgery procedures will typically be completed in the second and third wave of surgical intervention on casualties in the delayed categories.

The medical controllers assigned to the ICU and general units ensure forward casualty patient movement and appropriate care. These controllers approve admission of a casualty to their area and establish priorities for medical management.

Modular team assignments to specific rooms, beds or stretchers in the ED, OR, ICU, and general unit organize the staff, ensure that each patient's needs are addressed, provide necessary documentation, and reduce the chaos of unnecessary communication and lingering in hallways. Patient acuity and staff resources will define the nurse and physician ratio of the modular team.

Morgue

A temporary morgue with defined procedures for tracking the deceased is a critical element of the emergency response procedures. If the deceased individual is not identified, then procedures to carefully photograph and describe the individual must be initiated. Any identifying marks such as tattoos, and comments from other casualties regarding the identification or location of the deceased, should be recorded. This information may assist the appropriate agencies with identification. Fingerprinting may be performed by the law enforcement agencies as available.

Protocols for body bags and movement to the medical examiner's office are essential elements of the response plan.

Agreements with vendors to expand refrigeration capacity for morgue care may be necessary. These agreements should be addressed in the planning phase of the emergency response procedure. In exposure events that require decontamination, an additional temporary morgue may be established outside of the hospital. The location, resources, supplies, infection control procedures, and coordination with the local medical examiner's office should be addressed in these established procedures.

The planning committee should consider the psycho-emotional impact that the temporary morgue will have on the casualties, staff, arriving families, and the opportunity for media exposure when defining the location for the temporary morgue. It is best to place the temporary morgue in an area not easily visible. Hospitals should collaborate with the local medical examiner to coordinate the movement of the deceased to the medical examiner's office. Attempts to identify the individual and to contact the family prior to movement to the medical examiner's office should be recorded. Logs defining the casualties placed in temporary morgues should be included in the formal business summary of the disaster response.

Documentation

The patient care documentation during a disaster response is as important as routine documentation. This documentation must be accurate and concise, to facilitate a coordinated continuity of care as the casualty moves through the system. The documentation provides the history and record of activity for the next provider. Documentation provides essential information that allows a critical review of the medical response. Essential documentation must include triage category, initial assessment, vital signs, interventions, Glasgow Coma Score, Revised Trauma Score, findings, and priorities of care. Providers in the echelon of care will continue to provide brief but pertinent documentation defining findings and the priorities of care to provide effective continuum of care. This enhances patient care, reimbursement, and provides an opportunity to report findings and improve response performance. The planning committee must establish procedures and tools to capture essential documentation.

Psycho-Emotional Care

The planning committee must establish procedures that offer provisions, immediate debriefings, and planned critical incident stress management (CISM) for all staff members (including medical staff) after the disaster event. This may require that designated staff be trained in critical incident stress debriefing. Each department should have procedures in place to screen staff for signs of stress and to make referrals for CISM. A posted schedule for the debriefing sessions should be in every area.

Casualty Family Center

Response plans must address the casualty's family needs. They should include a defined location with specific providers to assist in crisis intervention. In most disaster plans, behavioral medicine, chaplain services, and social services are targeted for this task. These individuals provide the organizational structure and management for the casualty's family center. Behavioral Health Services typically provide the crisis intervention and address psycho-emotional needs. The assigned providers serve as a liaison to assist with reconnecting the casualty's family with the casualty. Documentation tools for this area may include sign-in sheets with contact information. Defined tools to collect data that will assist in identifying the casualty should be available. These tools request information and specific descriptions of the individual, identifying marks, tattoos, and other specific information. Pictures may be attached to these documentation tools to assist in the identification process. Communication systems to assist with requests for information, and to assist the families by providing updates to other family members are critical.

Education

Every hospital employee should be introduced to the hospital's disaster plan. Their departmental orientation should include a review of their department's role and the employee's individual role in a disaster response. This information includes the expectations from departmental employees, whom they report to, and what schedule changes they may anticipate. The overview will include the role of employees that are off-duty, when they report back to the hospital, the return traffic route to the hospital, where they park, what entrance to use, where they report in, how employee validation occurs, and their required identification (hospital identification, drivers license, and/or professional license). The medical staff orientation should include the same information.

Community Volunteers

The planning committee should review the issues of volunteer registration with the hospital's legal services before developing their plan. The planning committee will define the type of screening information and identification that are required for both nonmedical and medical volunteers. The volunteers should be registered, provide their drivers license, professional license, and current employer identification badge. Their professional license, if any, must be validated. Legal counsel may request that security complete a background check using the individual's driver's license to screen out those with criminal records or outstanding warrants. The credentialing process for the medical volunteers should take every precaution to validate the professional licensure. Websites and pre-registration systems can assist with this process. The hospital's medical staff credentialing office can assist with the medical volunteer license validation process. Nursing administration can assist with the nurse's license validation and credentialing process. Communities may implement the Emergency System for Advanced Registration of Volunteer Health Professionals Program (ESAR-P), created by HRSA. This allows for advanced registration and credentialing of healthcare professionals needed to augment a hospital or other medical facility to meet increased surge capacity needs.

Performance Improvement

The planning process defines the outcome measures specific to emergency response. These performance measures are integrated with implementation of the incident command system, communication, provider response, resource availability, system integration, and patient outcomes. Facilities have specific exercise mandates by regulatory agencies. Exercises that test the facility's sustainability and community integration are mandated. Exercises are more effective when defined monitors evaluate the response procedures. These monitors are assigned to specific functions of the response to evaluate the response compliance to the written plan. Video records and photographs of the response are recommended to provide timelines and evidence of actual performance. These steps assist in identifying specific areas for improvement. Each exercise or drill must have a completed written critique and after action report.

The critique begins at the department level as each responder completes a shift. Questions regarding what worked and what needs improvement identify opportunities. Formal department critiques are completed immediately following the demobilization to capture pertinent information and data. A hospital wide critique must be completed to review the overall response. This critique or after action review is structured and must have minutes. This is a required standard. Hospitals then participate in community system-wide after action review. The after action reports of the hospital's response and system integration define actions needed to improve response. These actions should then be tracked for corrective actions. The revised plans must be tested in the next scheduled drill and monitored for improvement measures. This is an ongoing process designed to improve the overall response plans.

Conclusion

Hospital emergency operations plans are a key element of terror medicine. These require time, diligence, and committed providers to participate in the planning processes. Each phase of response is carefully reviewed comparing past experiences to published best practice reports to define opportunities to improve the plan. Hospital leadership commitment defines the expectations, budget, and operational support to develop an effective, efficient response plan. Regulatory requirements produced by accreditation agencies, State and Federal mandates, and requirements for reimbursement must be integrated into the response plans. Documentation to provide evidence of compliance to these requirements must be in place. A response plan is essential to effective hospital performance in the face of a terror attack or other mass casualty event.

References

1. Robert T. Stafford Disaster Relief and Emergency Assistant Act, as amended by Pub. 1. No. 106–390, October 30, 2000. Available at htpp://www.fema.gov/library/stafact. shtm.
2. Federal Emergency Management Agency. FEMA history. Available at: http://www.fema. gove/about/shtm.
3. US Department of Homeland Security. The Department of Homeland Security. Available at: http://www.dhs.gov/interweb/assetlibrary/book.pdf.
4. The White House Homeland Security Presidential Directive/HSPD-5. Available at: http://www.dhs.gov/dhs/dhspublic/disp;ay?theme = 42&content = 496.
5. US Department of Homeland Security. Emergencies ad disasters: planning and prevention: National Response Plan. Available at: http://www.fema.gov//rr/frp/.
6. US Department Homeland Security. National Incident Management System. Available at: http://www/dhs/gov/dhspublic/display?theme = 51&contnt = 3423.
7. Joint Commission Accreditation Standards. Available at: www.jcinc.com/ perspectivesspecialissue-26K.
8. The National Lessons Learned and Best Practices Information Network. Emergency Management Programs for Healthcare Facilities: Hazard Vulnerability Analysis: Comparing and Prioritizing Risk. Available at: http://www.llis.dhs.gov./grontpage.cfm.
9. Klein JS, Weigelt JA. Disaster management: lessons learned. Surg Clin North Am 1991;71:257–266.
10. Federal Communications Commission. Communicating during emergencies. Available at: http://www.fcc.gov/cgb/consumerfacts/emergenices/ergencies.html.
11. Ennis-Holcomb K. Disaster Communication. Disaster Medicine. Ciottone et al., Mosby: 2006: pp. 229–230.
12. Hospital Incident Command System. Available at: http://www.emsa.ca.gov/hics.asp.
13. Frykberg ER. Principles of mass casualty management following terrorist disasters. Ann Surg 2004;239(3):319–321.
14. Disaster Management and Emergency Preparedness Course. Hospital Response. American College of Surgeons.

9
Technology Opportunities and Challenges

Annette L. Sobel

The Global War on Terrorism represents a crossroads of globalization, radicalization, and technology. Ultimately, successful counter-terrorism operations begin at home and with human capability.

Natural threats have plagued human populations throughout the course of time. Emerging and reemerging infectious diseases coupled with the emergence of technologic capabilities, global information access, and terrorist motivations have converted the natural course of infectious disease emergence and virulence. The earliest recorded epidemics of bubonic plague and smallpox more than 2,500 years ago, and the 1918–1919 Spanish Flu, though naturally occurring events, shaped the course of history as does the recurrent threat of global terrorism. We now recognize the potential of unnatural scalability when measured in human effects and counter-measures capabilities necessary to effectively mitigate these threats. Technology growth begets technology growth and the potential opportunities to enhance society. However, we must be prepared as a global medical community to contain or eradicate these broad health threats, which could affect national and international security, stability, and even the future of civilization.

The purpose of this chapter is to describe the operational, policy, and technology landscape in the war on terror, and to specifically cull out medically relevant issues. The national leadership of the United States coined the term "Global War on Terror" (GWOT) in response to attacks of 9/11. The following objectives of the GWOT were issued by President George W. Bush in the 2006 National Security Strategy of the United States[1]:

- Prevent attacks by terrorist networks before they occur.
- Deny WMD (weapons of mass destruction) to rogue states and to terrorist allies.
- Deny terrorist groups the support and sanctuary of rogue states.
- Deny terrorists control of any nation they would use as a base and launching pad for terror.

The National Military Strategic Plan for the War on Terrorism similarly defines the framework and principle military objectives[2]:

S.C. Shapira et al. (eds.), *Essentials of Terror Medicine*, DOI: 10.1007/978-0-387-09412-0_9, Springer Science+Business Media, LLC 2009

- Protect and defend the homeland.
- Attack terrorists and their capacity to operate effectively at home and abroad.
- Support mainstream Muslim efforts to reject violent extremism.

The National Security Strategy document also expands the scope of GWOT missions beyond war-fighting missions to humanitarian assistance/disaster relief (HR/DR) to countering proliferation of unconventional threats such as biological, chemical, nuclear, and radiological threats.

Our understanding of the asymmetric threats we are currently facing globally has matured and we now recognize some similarities between the GWOT and the Cold War. For one, these periods of history contain "wicked problems" (continuously evolving and complex situations characterized by solutions that generate new problems). Additionally, our adversaries are smart, motivated, and have access to global technology and information. As global radial presence expands and the GWOT with associated anti-American sentiment continues, the pool of potential terrorist recruits increases. Economic disparity, regional instability, and reduced quality of life are powerful incentives for recruitment.

Background

The Threat Environment

The anthrax attacks of 2001 transformed the threat of a biological attack on the United States into a reality. What was previously considered a hypothetical "away game" in countries like Iraq took on grim new meaning and relevance in the lives of Americans. Terrorism was redefined in the minds of many Americans as a powerful, precision "weapon" of enormous potential to create fear and a sense of helplessness, and undermine confidence in government. This weapon possessed the same lack of respect for socioeconomic status and gender as other weapons. However, the ability of the US Government to respond effectively and protect and inform its citizens was only partially successful. Despite extensive investigations including forensic analysis, the perpetrators remained unidentified. Nor is it clear how well current measures of preparedness could effectively prevent a future attack.

Building a National and Global Strategy

The US National Strategy for Homeland Security was developed to "… provide a framework for the contributions we can all make to secure our homeland."[1] Proactive measures to eliminate and mitigate vulnerabilities will contribute to thwarting terrorist activities globally. When coupled with technology, these measures are a human capability "multiplier." Throughout medical operations, technology expands the ability to orient, observe, decide, and act to enhance both the individual and aggregate human condition.

When considering a holistic strategy for counter-terrorism, the work of the US Office of the Director of National Intelligence (ODNI) should be included. This Office is tasked with the mission of integration of transnational information to better understand and predict transnational threats, intensify the comprehensiveness of the analytic process, and improve the objectivity of "threat estimation" and human analytic performance (i.e., likelihood and confidence of an attack(s) occurring). These activities translate into medical intelligence, impacting all aspects of the medical mission. These mission areas include force protection; early warning and detection; prevention and containment/decontamination/quarantine; triage; diagnosis; treatment; transport and rehabilitation. These mission areas rely heavily upon the synergy between human and technology capabilities.

Command and Control in Counter-terrorism Medical Operations

A strategic plan for integrated command and control (C2) is essential to reaching full operational capability in response to an asymmetric terrorist attack. Unconventional attacks may be characterized by lack of early warning and possibly extended and unpredictable effects.

Biological Warfare Scenario and Requirement for Surge Capacity

Much of the tactical relevance of technology stems from the crossroads of technology and terror. The scenario for consideration focuses on anthrax, a naturally occurring bacterium that can be "weaponized" as a threat agent. Although considered a high-consequence, low-probability event, the location of such an attack in the continental United States would likely be in a densely populated urban setting. The optimal timing for such an attack is dusk, with an inversion layer, minimal winds, and delivery of a total effective dose 1 kg of weaponized anthrax via airborne means. This scenario would conservatively result in 100,000 lethal doses. This number assumes 8,000–10,000 spores per lethal dose. There could be 10,000 fatalities and 3.7 million infected. An estimated additional ten times the infected numbers will be categorized as "worried well."[3,4]

In this scenario, the primary response functions include medical, security, logistics, and communications. Each of these functions has associated enabling technologies. Some examples include medical functions enabled through new diagnostics and therapeutics; enhanced security functions through robotics; new advanced materials for personal protective gear; remote sensing capabilities for threat and environmental assessments; logistics through intelligent modeling and simulation; communications through ad hoc networking capabilities, thus allowing adaptive operational command and control.[5]

There are a number of opportunities and challenges in the development of counter-measures to biological agents. The 2001 anthrax contaminated letters generated fear, economic impact, and several deaths.[6,7] Despite the fact that these attacks were considered small in scale, these occurrences underscore the need for well-coordinated prevention and response efforts intertwined with deployment of counter-measures and medical surge capacity.

In the above hypothetical biological agent scenario, a systems approach may be very helpful. For example, the attack may have been detected and early warning may have occurred through either persistent or "triggered" data collection (surveillance) from a combination of pre-positioned and rapidly responsively stand-off and point sensors. Once fused with baseline medical epidemiologic and environmental data, anomaly detection software may be employed to determine whether a natural or manmade event may have occurred with high certainty. There are many challenges and potential pitfalls to this approach beyond the obvious lack of data and faulty assumptions. A detailed understanding of the biophysics of such events and a high fidelity baseline of population epidemiologic data and environmental factors affecting disease transmission is highly desirable, if not essential. This baseline will improve the fidelity of predictive analysis and the probability of favorable measurable outcomes likely to ensue from the analysis. In this scenario, the strategy with highest probability of success is early threat detection, containment, and eradication. The bio-effects of such an attack could have been mitigated though the use of new identification and early prevention and intervention therapeutic platforms against anthrax toxin.

Early detection and combined diagnostic/therapeutic strategies are among the most important thrusts in technology counter-measure development. Two major categories of research exist: study of large and small inhibitors. Large inhibitors include antibiotics and other nonfunctional proteins (decoys), and small inhibitors include peptides and nonpeptides. This taxonomy applies to ongoing work to counter such important toxin threat agents as anthrax toxin, botulinum neurotoxin, ricin toxin, and staphylococcal enterotoxin.[8]

Another major category of biological counter-measures research is therapeutics for viral infectious agents. This work is categorized as targeting the virus and its replication. This area of work and its application poses a number of opportunities and challenges. For example, viruses possess specific binding characteristics and may be removed either harmlessly through antibiotic use or destructively through destabilization by drugs or antibodies. Challenges exist in countering the natural variations in genotype, phenotype, and viral coats present in viral populations undergoing amplification.[7]

The Technologic Dilemma and Security

A natural conclusion of the technologic revolution is that technology may be simultaneously viewed as "dual-use," and thus a simultaneous enabler of extremist or disenfranchised populations. One would hope that sustained technology investment results in greater benefit to society, as measured by economic growth, scientific discovery, improved quality of life indicators, and regional coalitions and international stability. Technology innovation also results in improved counter-measures intended to pre-empt and mitigate potentially destructive activities.

The threats of unconventional weapons such as chemical, biological, radiological, and nuclear (with/without coupling to explosives), and cyber-weapons continue to loom on the horizon as radical movements such as al-Qaeda continue to acquire, organize, train, and equip with such weapons and advanced technologies.[8] The medical community must track the exponential growth of biological research and associated technologies, and be effectively organized, trained, and equipped to understand the threats and benefits of these advances.

A number of subject matter experts have voiced concerns over the past 30 years regarding the explosion of life sciences research and the concerns of "dual-use" of technologic advances. Epstein referred to the umbrella term of "contentious research" as an armament in the tug-of-war between much needed scientific advances and potential for proliferation of unconventional weapons.[9] In response to this challenge, the open source or public domain accessibility of complete genome databases for plague, botulism, hemorrhagic fever viruses (Ebola), smallpox, and anthrax was reviewed by the National Interagency Genomics Sciences Coordinating Committee (NIGSCC). This Committee considered its recommendations in the context of escalating research in this field, associated genetic engineering capability to produce enhanced pathogens, global data accessibility, and high fidelity analytic tools for modeling and simulation of biophysics and molecular interactions. Tracking of such research and limiting its dissemination is of importance due to the potential to engineer microorganisms that may directly affect transmissibility and virulence of naturally occurring pathogens.[10,11]

The National Academy of Sciences (NAS) subsequently chartered a study on "Countering Bio-terrorism: the Role of Science and Technology" to perform an in-depth study of afore-mentioned "dual-use" concerns. The study concluded that heightened awareness in the science and technology (S&T) community "… could reduce the inadvertent spread of knowledge that may aid terrorists …" and supported the concept of a global effort to confront bioterrorism through academic exchange and collaboration. The study recognized the pivotal functional roles of intelligence, detection, surveillance, and diagnosis and associated technologies in countering threats due to terrorism while emphasizing the concurrent role in public health emergencies and emerging infectious disease outbreaks.[12] The Academy also acknowledged the significant role of information technology in global monitoring and prevention of threat agent research and development and trafficking. The ensuing section will continue to address this paramount issue of information technology as a nonattributable weapon of proliferation of terrorism ideals, techniques, tactics, and procedures essential to form a global infrastructure of destruction.

Threats Posed by New Technologies

Proliferation of cyber-terrorism sites by radical organizations deserves special attention. As radicalization strengthens as a global (political) movement, use of the internet has become an effective "virtual weapons platform" for the sharing of information. The growing list of concerns that medical personnel need to remain abreast of includes the wealth of medical threat information freely available on the internet. This material includes sharing of techniques, tactics, and procedures for inflicting mass casualties including psychological casualties and "worried-well," recruiting terrorists, propagandizing anti-US sentiments, radical ideology legitimization, and movement of resources, to include financing. Each of these areas deserves international attention.

This chapter will further elucidate some of the roles that the scientific and academic communities have played in counter-terrorism and homeland security policy development, influencing strategic and tactical decision-making and assuring that healthcare providers possess, the minimum, intellectual situational awareness of this area of concern and the current and emerging threats.

The NAS took a bold step to enhance the ability of the academic and scientific communities to police themselves and become a full partner in the Global War on Terrorism. The NAS considers the balance of information dissemination and advance of science versus potential compromise of homeland or national security a very serious matter. Of course, science can also be a very powerful arrow in the quiver of national security and must not be deterred. The report entitled *Biotechnology Research in an Age of Terrorism* is a pivotal document, written by a committee of security experts and scientists.[13] The scientists recommended a system of self-governance, with special attention to the following topics: vaccine efficacy; antibiotic/antibiotic resistance: pathogen/nonpathogen virulence; denial and/or deception of sensor technologies; weaponization techniques, tactics, and procedures for biological agents or toxins. In addition, the National Science Advisory Board for Biosecurity (NSABB) was established in 2004 to provide advice and oversight of dual-use research of concern.[14]

A study submitted for publication that launched academic debate on this dilemma was a bioterror scenario postulated by Wein and Liu.[15] The article reviewed vulnerabilities of the supply chain of a single milk processing facility and the associated critical variables and uncertainties to the introduction of botulinum toxin into the nation's milk supply. This review assisted in enhancing security and robustness of the milk supply to attack or to inadvertent contamination.

Sequencing of the genetic code, and synthetic genomics capabilities, coupled with global accessibility via the internet is another example of the pivotal role of the scientific community in accelerating this debate. The dual-use aspect of technology is heightened by the ability to detect, track, monitor, and protect such data and associated technologies from terrorists or "would be" terrorists. The integration of such functions was initially recommended in a landmark study on countering bioterrorism.[12] These recommendations are summarized as follows:

- Inter-agency collaboration among all agencies charged with homeland security, to include public health, science and technology, and intelligence.
- Collaboration between federal agencies and the private sector in the rapidly advancing area of detection technology.

- Creation of a global biosurveillance network.
- Implementation of automation and pattern recognition software/classification algorithms to assist with diagnosis of ambulatory patients.
- Expansion of the roles of the US Department of Agriculture (USDA) in prevention and containment of threats to agriculture and plants.

The Counter-terrorism Technology Landscape

As we assess the counter-terrorism technology landscape, critical areas for investment emerge. General categories of enabling technologies include: more sensitive/specific sensors for detection/identification of biological agents, chemicals, toxins, radiological and nuclear materials; tools for rapid forecasting, analysis, and collaboration; interoperable communication platforms; and personal protective gear for response personnel. Additional high-payoff areas for medical and other operations are robotic systems for "far-forward" medicine; sustainable human performance methodologies for extreme environments; biotechnology to support new vaccines, adjuvant therapy. Desirable device characteristics, as applicable, include requirements for minimal training, power, equipment and software calibration, cost, disposability, information security, and noninvasiveness of use.

Unique Challenges of Stability, Security, Transition, and Reconstruction (SSTR) and HA/DR

The counter-terrorism environment poses unique challenges and opportunities for technology use. The medical end-user community is characteristically well educated and highly experienced, demanding technology that is robust, sustainable, and interoperable with pre-existing equipment. Systems must support collaboration. Training must be minimal, sustainable, and interdisciplinary in nature. For example, law enforcement, military personnel, medical and emergency response personnel support overlapping missions, and utilize functionally identical equipment, although they initially train in very different cultures and under very different stressors. Interoperability is further complicated by the dynamic, high operations tempo, and low tolerance for error in counter-terrorism operations.

These operations are high consequence and low probability when including unconventional threats, and thus, readiness requires these organizations to jointly organize, train, and equip to achieve seamless operations. During operations in response to large-scale disasters such as Hurricane Katrina or the 2004 Indonesian tsunami missions dynamically shifted. For example, units were tasked to form, reorganize, and disassemble to meet demand. A mission could shift from airlift to hauling supplies and potable water, to search and rescue operations, to emergency medical response, to imagery collection for bio-environmental and infrastructure assessments. All missions required reliable, sustained, secure communications and information management between agencies. Missions were tasked in an ad hoc manner and during a very compressed time frame. Complex emergency operations underscore the importance of seamless interagency communications and ad hoc networking and network adaptation as one of the pillars of homeland security, counter-terrorism, and HA/DR operations.[16]

Recognizing the vital role of the United States in SSTR globally, and the importance of these missions to the Global War on Terrorism, the US Department of Defense (DoD) published DoD Directive 3000.05 in an effort to provide guidance for military support to other nations. SSTR has significant overlap with Homeland Security and counter-terrorism operations, as noted above.[17]

Elements of Success

Measures of effectiveness and performance (MOEs and MOPs) are as myriad as there are types of missions. However, there is commonality and cross-domain issues exist among the response elements. Critical elements of mission success include clear lines of command and control; sustainable and interoperable communications; and delivery of timely, accurate information that is *actionable*.[18]

Information Sharing Environments

Effective command, control, communications, and information sharing are essential to mission success in counter-terrorism operations. As a corollary, the demand for timely, valid, actionable information is high across disparate communities responding to a Homeland Security or counter-terrorism event.

A national strategy for information sharing was released in October 2007 to address these crucial issues, especially access to timely, accurate information.[19] The guiding principles of this Strategy are

- Rapid identification of immediate and long-term threats;
- Identification of persons involved in terror-related activities;
- Implementation of information-driven and risk-based detection, prevention, deterrence, response, protection, and emergency management efforts.

Implicit in these strategic initiatives is the empowerment of newly established fusion centers across the United States. These centers are quite variable in staffing, expertise, and organizational structure, but have the singular goal of sharing information across federal, state, and local entities, the private sector, and foreign partners. For information fusion to matter, it must be cross-cutting and contextually germane to a wide community of interest, to include intelligence, diplomatic actors, homeland security, law enforcement, and defense personnel. This initiative provides teeth and specificity to the national implementation plan for the Information Reform and Terrorism Prevention Act of 2004.

The mission of information fusion centers may be enhanced through technology insertion. Nonetheless, technology and human factor challenges will continue to exist in efforts to seamlessly share across inter-agency silos and cultures, and across levels of classification. A major technology thrust area that has emerged to meet this need is the development of automated tools for information translation, detection, extraction, summarization, coupled with declassification algorithms. Early efforts such as the Defense Advanced Research Projects Agency's Translingual Information Detection, Extraction, Summarization program demonstrated the powerful utility of such multimedia tools to support humanitarian assistance/disaster response missions.[20] Such technology approaches are capable of redacting and filtering information according to predetermined rules or by self-learning software algorithms. By employing this strategy information transparency may be assured to end-users with a "need-to-know" and "need-to-share." In parallel, organizations can maintain appropriate operational security to enable mission success.

Among the greatest challenges is avoidance of information overload while optimizing and maintaining human performance. This end goal may be achieved through enabling access to all-source, mission relevant, timely, and actionable information. A number of technology tools exist to facilitate shared situation awareness within collaborative environments. The net result is a common relevant operational picture (CROP) that is shareable across the interagency community. One such tool is the Defense Advanced Research Projects Agency's Command Post of the Future.[21] Ideally, this CROP will include medical and medically relevant information that will assist in achieving positive effects-based operations. Medically relevant information is derived from such data categories as: geospatial, meteorological, demographic, epidemiological, population movement, social and cultural relationship networks, and historical data, to name a few.

Effective information sharing requires interoperable communications. In a Homeland Security event(s), first responders and federal, state, and local governments face the challenge of maintaining and sustaining interoperable and adaptive communications throughout the crisis.[3,17] This capability is vital not only to operational command and control but also to ensuring the public confidence is not lost. Similar challenges exist in the global counter-terrorism operational environment.

The Limitations of Technology Applied to Terror Medicine

The proposition of anticipatory medical training and planning for consequence or improved "effects-based" outcomes following low-probability/high-consequence events such as terrorist attacks has the primary priorities of saving life and property, mitigating irreversible damage, and promoting expeditious return to normalcy. Despite a focus on response and management of consequences through improved methodologies, systems analysis, and technology insertion, prevention is really the key to recovery and return to baseline of human function and government services. Hence, the real role of technology is the improvement of performance and measurable outcomes.[3]

In general, many tasks in counter-terrorism medicine can be performed without the use of technology. However, added value may be measured and is highly recommended when "effects-based" operations are desired. When determining when and where technology insertion is appropriate, objective measures of effectiveness and performance are highly desirable. For example, technologies for threat agent detection and identification add value through improving the timely and appropriate use of medical and protective counter-measures. Robotic and other unmanned vehicles may be used to assist (civilian and military) responders in early warning, and threat detection/mitigation, performance of high risk tasks such as urban search and rescue from confined spaces such as collapsed structures. Similarly, autonomous systems may be employed for remote sensing and verification, and imagery collection for time-critical tasks such as determination of infrastructure integrity (roads and bridges, water reservoirs, power grids, for example). Another medical management adjunct is use of self-learning tools for analysis and forecasting. These tools are among many methodologies that may assist with scarce resource deployment, and information management to include such tasks as rapid dissemination, assimilation, filtering, pattern recognition, change detection, and validation of actionable, timely information critical to mass casualty management.

Case Study: The Threat of Avian Influenza

Avian influenza viruses are known for their pandemic potential; most notably the Spanish Flu of 1918–1919 was possibly the most deadly infectious disease outbreak in history.[22] This naturally occurring disease is discussed here because of its potential as a weapon of terror and pandemic potential associated with a low barrier to transmission to humans.

Recent outbreaks of avian influenza in Asia re-energized fears of influenza pandemic in the near-term. If such a pandemic were to occur, epidemiologists predict that between 2 and 50 million people may be affected, depending upon virulence, availability of effective anti-viral therapy, transmissibility, geolocation of initial cases (urban vs. rural), etc.[23]

It is now understood that Avian influenza viruses are transmissible to humans via two pathways: through an intermediate host (pigs) or directly from infected birds or contaminated environments.[24] As a result of effective transmission, the threat of infection could result in mass chaos and terror, regardless of whether the event is natural or manmade and will stress surge capacity to its peak. As a result, scarce medical resources will be allocated through prioritized guidelines or randomly, resulting in dissatisfaction of some proportion of the population. Government and military capabilities could be undermined, as will all services necessary to mitigate further disease spread.

This scenario highlights the absolute necessity for civil–military cooperation and pre-emptive planning in close collaboration with the private sector. Public education and engagement in civil–military planning and reporting is an essential component of this preparation. One example previously stressed is the value of information sharing among local, state, and federal entities. Specifically, civil–military epidemic prevention and response systems must be modernized and routinely exercised among all sectors.[25] Technology may be of great value in accomplishing this end goal, through provision of robust communication infrastructure and interoperable communications systems.

Emerging infectious diseases and biological warfare agents alike respect no geographic boundaries and necessitate exquisite management of potential transnational disease spread. Within military theaters of operation, disease outbreaks must be carefully tracked and managed and patients monitored appropriately prior to return to the continental United States. Similarly, international transportation networks must fully cooperate with health authorities and establish checkpoints for early recognition and containment of potential infectious disease threats. Healthcare workers are a high-risk sector and should be monitored and subjected to stringent preventive medicine programs. Such an early warning and intervention process exists within the agriculture and animal disease sectors and should be equally enforced and standardized to prevent human-to-human disease transmission. Technology software that employs syndromic surveillance of disease outbreaks is one approach enabling earlier recognition, pathogen identification, and often, pre-emption of disease outbreaks. Such a methodology is adaptive to local, state, national, and international applications, and portrays the real-time, common operational picture, and actionable information needed in a terrorism event.[26]

Conclusion

Homeland Security and counter-terrorism operations require a unique blend of human capability, interagency cooperation, applied technology, and visionary leadership. Technology plays a key role in sensing and early warning, "sense making" of the environment to achieve situation understanding, and communicating actionable information that can save lives and prevent casualties. This chapter has attempted to provide the reader with a high-level overview of effective use of technology in medical aspects of counter-terrorism operations. These operations depend heavily on tracking indications and warnings of unconventional terrorist threats and accurately forecasting the epidemiology of agent spread, taking proactive measures to prevent, eliminate, or mitigate human bio-effects, and maintaining active, continuous situation awareness of a dynamic environment.

When prioritizing technology needs, real-time diagnostic capability is one of the most highly sought after classes of technology necessary for early intervention in a bioterrorism event. A number of diagnostic approaches are currently available for detection of pathogens in wounds and on environmental surfaces. In addition to point detection, the merit of stand-off (remote) sensing in a bioterrorism event is obvious. Beyond the task of initial detection, pathogen identification capability, and counter-measure susceptibility is essential. One must consider the technology –human system as a critical node in the intervention pathway of crisis and consequence management.

As previously stated, the most essential element of these operations remains the human capability–technology partnership. Whether building a national strategy or performing tactical pre-hospital planning for a bioterrorism event, the essential role of the human operator must be considered the critical element in countering terrorism.

References

1. George W. Bush. The White House. Washington, D.C., March 2006; 12.
2. General Peter Pace, USMC, Office of the Chairman, Joint Chiefs of Staff, Washington, D.C., February 1, 2006; 3.
3. Personal Communication with Dr. Richard Danzig; and Defense Advanced Research Projects Agency. Reload and the Post-Attack Environment. Arlington, VA, 2005.
4. NATO Guidelines for the Surveillance and Control of Anthrax in Humans and Animals, World Health Organization, 1998.
5. Homeland Security: Challenges in Achieving Interoperable Communications for First Responders, U.S. General Accountability Office, Washington, D.C., November 6, 2003.
6. Cole LA. *The Anthrax Letters: A Medical Detective Story.* Washington, DC: Joseph Henry Press/National Academies Press, 2003.
7. Burnett JC., Henchal EA., Schmaljohn AL., Bavari S. The evolving field of biodefence: therapeutic developments and diagnostics. *Nature Reviews Drug Discovery*, Vol. 4, April 2005; 281.
8. The Terrorist Threat to the U.S Homeland, National Intelligence Estimate, National Intelligence Council, July 2007.
9. Epstein GL. Controlling biological warfare threats: resolving potential tensions among the research community, industry, and the national security community, *Critical Reviews in Microbiology.* 27 (4): 321–354.
10. Lederberg J., Shope RE, Stokes SC., Jr., eds. *Emerging Infections: Microbial Threats to Health in the United States.* Committee on Emerging Microbial Threats to Health, Institute of Medicine, National Research Council. National Academies Press, Washington, D.C. 1992.
11. *Seeking Security: Pathogens, Open Access, and Genome Databases.* The National Academy of Sciences. Washington, D.C.: National Academies Press, 2004; 1–3.
12. *Countering Bioterrorism: The Role of Science and Technology.* National Academy of Sciences. Washington, D.C.: National Academies Press, 2002.
13. Fink GR., et al., *Biotechnology Research in an Age of Terrorism.* National Research Council. Washington, D.C.: National Academies Press, 2004.
14. National Science Advisory Board for Biosecurity. http://www.biosecurityboard.gov.
15. Wein LM., Liu Y. Analyzing a bio-terror attack on the food supply: the case of botulinum toxin in milk. *PNAS* 2005:102, 10.1073/pnas.0408526102
16. The National Strategy for Homeland Security, Office of Homeland Security, The White House, Washington, D.C., July 2002; 43.
17. U.S. Department of Defense. Directive 3000.05, Military Support for Security, Stability, Transition, and Reconstruction Operations, USD (P), Washington, D.C., November 28, 2005.
18. U.S. Department of Homeland Security. Challenges in Achieving Interoperable Communications for First Responders, U.S. Government Accountability Office, Washington, D.C., November 6, 2003.
19. George W. Bush. The White House. National Strategy for Information Sharing, Washington, D.C., October 31, 2007. http://www.whitehouse.gov/nsc/infosharing/index.html.
20. Defense Advanced Research Projects Agency. Translingual Information Detection, Extraction, Summarization (TIDES). October 5, 2007. http://www.darpa.mil/dar-patech99/presentations/scripts/ito/itotidesscript.txt.

21. Defense Advanced Research Projects Agency. Command Post of the Future. August 30, 2007. http://www.darpa.mil/sto/strategic/cpof.html.
22. Barry JM. *The Great Influenza: The Epic Story of the Deadliest Plague in History*. New York: Penguin Books, 2004; 96.
23. Enserink M. WHO adds more "1918" to pandemic predictions. *Science*, December 17, 2004, Vol. 206; 2025.
24. Centers for Disease Control and Prevention. Transmission of Influenza A Viruses Between Animals and People. http://www.cdc.gov/flu/avian/gen-info/transmission.htm. Modified Oct. 17, 2005.
25. Thompson DF., Swerdlow JL., Loeb CA. The bug stops here: force protection and emerging infectious diseases. Monograph. Center for Technology and National Defense Policy, National Defense University. Washington, D.C., November 2005.
26. Alan Zelicoff, personal communication on Syndrome Reporting Information System (SYRIS) experience in Texas, 2006.

Part III
WEAPON ETIOLOGIES

10
Epidemiology of Terrorism Injuries

Limor Aharonson-Daniel and Shmuel C. Shapira

Terrorism attacks occur at unexpected times and locations, resulting in large variations in victim profiles. Population characteristics will differ among casualties injured on commuter buses or trains, in family restaurants, schools, shops, market-places and dancehalls. Nevertheless, these populations also have much in common and there is a great deal to be learned from the cumulative experience of treating casualties of terrorist attacks on civilian populations.

Terrorist attacks are generally divided into conventional terror, chemical terror, biological terror and radiological terror. There may be a combination of weapons (i.e. conventional + non-conventional) and the volume may vary from an attack on an individual, to mass conventional attacks, to a mega terror assault such as that which took place on 11 September 2001 in New York City and Washington, DC.

Conventional Terror

Conventional terror involves different mechanisms such as causing penetrating injuries with various instruments, including bullets, which are symmetrical projectiles, or shrapnel and metal debris, defined as asymmetrical projectiles. Knives cause penetrating injuries that are associated with a different pathophysiology.

Stoning and intentional road accidents may be other forms of conventional terror, associated with blunt injuries. Explosions involve other mechanisms of injury such as blast and blunt. These may be associated with hurling. While the flexibility to choose the time and place of the attack is likely to contribute to the effectiveness of the explosion, it is not the sole factor affecting higher efficiency compared to known tactics of conventional terror. The addition of metal fragments to the explosives, together with the ability to choose confined crowded locations, makes these attacks particularly devastating.[1-3] Other known effects of explosions include burns from the flash and hot gasses, blasts (described as brief and extreme change in environmental pressure) that cause damage by abrupt changes in pressure, mainly in hollow viscous organs (tympanic membrane, lungs and bowel), displacement by mass movement of air and impact of rigid objects, and injuries from flying objects.[4,5]

S.C. Shapira et al. (eds.), *Essentials of Terror Medicine*,
DOI: 10.1007/978-0-387-09412-0_10, Springer Science+Business Media, LLC 2009

Recent terror attacks have almost always been implemented with conventional weapons. The two notable exceptions were the anthrax letters mailed in 2001 in the United States and the release of the nerve agent sarin in 1995 in the Tokyo subway by the Aum Shinrikyu cult.

It is also important to note that the practice of suicide bombing as a mechanism of conventional terrorism is not a new phenomenon. In 1983, the building accommodating the US Marines peacekeeping force in Beirut was destroyed by a suicide bomber and ever since, this method has been used widely by many terrorist organizations. Recently, because of its effectiveness, suicide terrorism seems to be on the rise. During the 1980s, most suicide attacks took place in Lebanon and Sri Lanka, but since the year 2000, suicide bombers have attacked in Israel, Iraq, India, Pakistan, Chechnya, Indonesia, Yemen, Algeria, Turkey, Afghanistan, England and Spain.

Chemical Terror

Chemical terror attacks, such as the Matsumoto and Tokyo subway attacks of 1994–1995 with the organophosphate nerve agent sarin, are also a major terrorist threat. The Tokyo subway sarin attack was the first large-scale disaster caused by nerve gas. A religious cult, Aum Shinrikyu, released sarin gas into subway commuter trains during the morning rush hour. Twelve passengers died and more than 1,000 people were harmed. Sarin is a highly toxic nerve agent that can be fatal within minutes to hours.[6] It is worth mentioning that 20% of the casualties were non-protected first responders.

Failure to identify the nature of the attack caused a delay in the adoption of personal protective measures and decontamination of the victims. Delayed effects were reported in addition to the acute consequences of organophosphates. A recent study published in *Annals of Neurology* examines 38 victims of the sarin attack, 5 years after the assault, concluding that sarin intoxication might be associated with structural changes in specific regions of the human brain, including those surrounding the insular cortex.[7]

Biological Terror

Biological warfare agents have been used sporadically, most notably with the anthrax letters in the United States in 2001. The use of contagious or non-contagious biological agents (microorganisms or toxins) is a real threat that the medical community has to prepare for by training and establishing surveillance systems and drills.[8]

Radiological Terror

An improvised radiological dispersing device is a leading form of threat. The assassination of Litvinenko by polonium 210 ingestion demonstrates the devastating effects of lethal doses of radiation. As in other forms of weapons of mass destruction (WMD) anxiety and stress reaction may be disproportional to actual damage.[9]

In this chapter, we characterize the common patterns of injury caused by conventional terror attacks. We identify the unique profile of terror-related injury and discuss how it differs from other modes of trauma. Finally, we try to summarize the knowledge gained into practical conclusions for enhanced preventive measures, for preparedness and for management of potential future attacks. The accumulation of various information from a multitude of sources, from pre-hospital to debriefing, facilitates a broad overview of events which serves as the basis for standard operating procedures (SOP).

Epidemiology

Unique Characteristics of Terrorism Injuries: Arrival and Injury Patterns

In the past, it was assumed that terrorism casualties would show patterns similar to victims of war injuries. However, quite early on, it was clear that this was not the case. While wars are rarely conducted in urban centers, within minutes from major hospitals, terrorism often strikes right at the hub of the city. Wars are continuous, thus sometimes an injured soldier will not be evacuated until rescue forces are safe. Terror attacks, however, are usually incidental strikes that allow rescue attempts and evacuation to begin almost immediately. Because the location of terror attacks is usually crowded urban environments, for the victims of terror, the duration of evacuation from the place of injury to hospital is significantly shorter, increasing chances of immediate survival and also altering the presenting condition profile. Unless shattered by the blast or injured directly in vital organs, critically injured terrorism victims usually arrive at the hospital in time for resuscitative attempts. In contrast, casualties of war commonly result from exsanguination.

Unlike war situations, terror attacks will find a civilian population in its everyday living environment; therefore, people will not be wearing protective gear. As a result, there will be relatively more trunk and head injuries in comparison to soldiers.[10,11] The age range and gender of victims will vary as well, as civilians include people from infants to the elderly, males and females, and the ill and healthy, while soldiers are usually males, mostly young and healthy.

Lastly, injury in most wars is caused by fragments and high velocity bullets. Recent terror attacks have been characterized by bombs fortified with metal debris exploding in confined spaces, causing injuries by shrapnel, combined with severe blast effects. Suicide bombers who usually detonate these bombs choose the exact timing and location for the explosion to cause the most extensive harm.

To understand that terrorism-related injuries are very different from war injuries necessitates their independent characterization.

Arrival Patterns

Terrorism injuries have been shown to have a unique epidemiology – unique distributions of age, gender, mechanism, pathophysiology, injury patterns and more.[12,13] But first, we must recognize that terrorism injuries also have a different pattern of arrival. According to a study conducted by Magen David Adom (MDA, Israel's Emergency Medical Services, EMS), there was an average of 45 casualties per event.[14] Good triage is aimed at distributing the load to decrease the number of casualties per hospital, and to avoid overburdening hospitals nearest to the mass casualty incident.[15] Overcrowding of patients in hospitals near the event and a recognition of the need to send patients to other medical facilities was nevertheless identified, which is consistent with studies following the Oklahoma City bombing[16] and others.[17,18]

Injury Mechanisms

As described in the Introduction, there are various injury mechanisms associated with conventional terrorism attacks including stabbing, stoning, deliberate running-over by a vehicle, overtaking and crashing public busses, sniper shooting, high-velocity gunshots, conventional bombs and the relatively novel "suicide bomber" detonating bombs with metal debris including nails, screws, bolts, ball bearings, etc.

The different periods of terrorism and the various geo-political scenes are characterized by assorted events. Depending on culture, resources, targets and organizational characteristics, terrorism patterns vary in different parts of the world. It appears that the most recent terrorism uprising in Israel, since September 29, 2000, has involved mainly suicide bomber explosions (54% of the hospitalized victims) and gunshots (36% of the hospitalized victims).[12] However, this impression reflects the severity of the damage sustained by these events, and not their frequency, as reported in Israeli Defense Forces data.[19] In 2000–2004, suicide bombers comprised less than 1% of attacks but caused 47% of the fatalities. In Jerusalem though, the majority of patients (60%) hospitalized at Hadassah University Hospital were injured by gunshot rather than explosion.[20] Nevertheless, explosion victims present with more complex, challenging, resource-consuming conditions. The severe outcome of these injuries justifies the focus on the most injurious and fatal mechanisms rather than on the most frequent attacks.

Some explosives such as trinitrotoluene TNT-trinitrotoluene, nitroglycerin and dynamite produce a "blast wave" (supersonic over-pressurization shock wave), while others, known as low explosives, create a subsonic explosion and lack the over-pressurization wave. Injury intensity depends on the degree of over-pressure.

Primary blast injuries are typically pulmonary, auditory and gastrointestinal (mainly with underwater explosions). Amputations may occur, mainly due to the blast wind, as well as multiple penetrating injuries, most severe when involving the abdominal cavity or blood vessels. Injuries to solid organs such as the liver or spleen, and serious intracranial injuries are also often recorded. In bombings that occur in confined spaces such as buses and closed halls, there is a higher incidence of pneumothorax, blast lung injury, and tympanic membrane rupture, as well as burns, and hepatic or splenic injury. In open air explosion events, the predominant injury is penetrating soft tissue injury caused by shrapnel.[21] Inhalational injury might also be associated with closed space explosion. In bombing incidents that include structural collapse, patients may further experience crush injuries and fractures.[22,23] (For more information on blast injury classification, see Chap. 11 and Table 19.1)

Recent terrorist attacks in Israel have resulted in victims sustaining injuries that are more complex and more severe than in earlier periods of terrorist activity.[24,25] The literature describes some syndromes of combined primary and high-magnitude secondary blast injury,[26] and discusses the mechanisms of multilevel injuries.[13]

Shrapnel Wounds

In addition to the main blast effect, new injury mechanisms introduced by terrorism included penetrating injuries by shrapnel – small metal pieces, such as nails, screws, pellets and bolts, that are inserted into the bomb and fly with extreme force upon explosion. Many such metal pieces, penetrating an individual simultaneously, result in challenging injuries. The ability to identify penetrations that often leave only minor entry wounds, concealed by hair or clothes, is limited. These obscured wounds might seem minor, but are often associated with severe internal damage. Diagnostic imaging is necessary to map the routes and the extent of injury. Furthermore, debridement of each and every entry wound is time-consuming and may not always be justified, especially when taking into account the limited resources at the time of a large influx of patients. The decision either to delay treatment of the minor injuries or transfer these patients to other facilities has to be made.

Despite the recommendation that triage should be precise to identify minor (if any) visible entry wounds caused by nails and bolts included in explosives, some authors suggest the use of some external markers to predict the occurrence of blast lung injuries and intra-abdominal injury.[27] The significance of these signs needs to be validated before they are incorporated into triage protocols and used to direct victims to the appropriate level of care, both at the scene and in the hospital.

Gunshot Wounds

Gunshot wounds during this period in Israel came mostly from snipers shooting at pedestrians or drivers in isolated areas or at similar targets. As such, these shootings are well aimed at vital organs such as the head and the chest and are often fatal. The patients who arrive alive at the hospital after a shooting incident have usually survived a longer transportation process in comparison to victims of explosion attacks. The chances for patients with gunshot wounds to die in the pre-hospital setting are therefore greater. A study of gunshot casualties treated in a level I trauma center in

Jerusalem reports that the vast majority of those inflicted with injuries from gunshots were young (60% aged 19–30 years) and were men (90%). This is explained by the fact that members of the main group injured by this mechanism were soldiers (34.4%), drivers or hikers in isolated regions.[20]

Patient Profile

Because of the different scenarios and the unexpected occurrence in terms of time and place of terrorist attacks, the population affected will be variable and will include (depending on the location) infants, children, youth, young mothers, pregnant women, elderly people, disabled people and others. Each population group will have different needs in terms of care and support. This will result in specialized personnel and equipment being needed (e.g. pediatric surgeons and equipment). During a mass-casualty event (MCE), infants and young children are often separated from injured parents and may therefore experience anxiety and have difficulty in describing their injuries.

Pregnant women involved in blast injuries will warrant special attention by an obstetrician. Injuries to the placenta, such as shearing injuries and placental abruption, are possible and must be detected; fetal monitoring, as well as a pelvic ultrasonic screen and an obstetric-gynecologic consultation, is necessary. Elderly casualties often have co-morbidity and therefore are at a higher risk of extended hospitalization and mortality. Orthopaedic injuries in these patients may be more numerous due to a decrease in bone density and reduced body mass.

The majority of patients injured by terrorist attacks are males. The exact percentage varies according to the time and type of attack, but generally males comprise 60–70% of the injured population, as reported in all studies. This percentage is higher among gunshot victims than among casualties of explosion.[20,25] Patients injured in explosions included a higher proportion of children and elderly than gunshot patients. Most patients treated were between 15 and 29 years of age (Fig. 10.1). Both age and gender distributions were similar to data cited in the terrorist attacks in Spain in 2004.[17]

Injury Profile

When an explosive device detonates, a small volume of explosive is rapidly transformed into a large volume of gas. A high-pressure blast wave quickly expands outward, and its interaction with the body causes primary injuries (mainly at air-filled and hollow organs such as the lung, ear and bowel). Often, the consequent blast wind propels solid particles from the immediate environment, embedding them in the patient (secondary injury) or hurling the patient into solid matter (causing tertiary injury) and covering the explosive. Quaternary injury is caused by crush, heat, flames, or the inhalation of smoke and hot gasses. Confined spaces worsen such effects: surface reflections amplify and prolong the blast wave, the blast wind is channeled, and heat and gases are contained. The severity of injuries and the resultant mortalities are thus greater.[28,29]

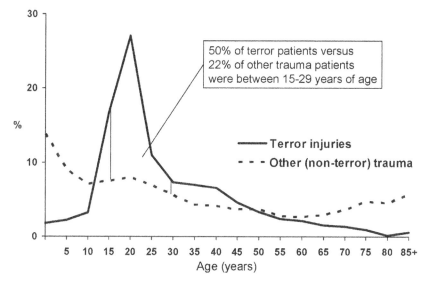

FIG. 10.1. Age distribution of terror versus other (non-trauma) trauma casualties. Israel National Trauma Registry Data, 10/2000–12/2003, 69,877 patients 1,789 (3%) terror injuries. The lines illustrate the age distribution of terror versus other (non-trauma) trauma casualties, the gap is largest between ages 15 and 29: half of terror patients compared with only 22% of other patients were in this age group.

Injury Severity

Several factors influence the impact of explosion, the number of casualties, and corresponding outcomes. The magnitude of the blast and the composition of the bomb have significant consequences. The presence of shrapnel is known to increase the complexity and severity of injury. The contamination of a bomb with chemical, biological or radiological materials could further complicate matters. The environment of the blast is also important – explosions in open spaces have less severe blast effects. Explosions in buses have been associated with the most severe outcomes[27,28] and high scene mortality rates. Barriers such as seats sometimes protect passengers from shrapnel and roofs that detach and allow for blast wind to exit the bus, reduce the blast impact. Distance between the victim and the blast is of utmost importance. Buildings that collapse or furniture and fixtures that fly may cause further damage through crush injuries or injuries from flying objects. Rapid evacuation in most events helps to prevent deterioration of patient status. Preparedness and capacities of the admitting hospital are the final external factors that affect injury outcome. Efficient and accurate triage, good skills, available medical resources and good flow through the system may help to increase patient survival, in spite of severe injuries.

Table 10.1 describes the distribution of injury indicators in hospitalized victims of suicide bomber explosions. Severe to critical (Injury Severity Score, ISS* ≥ 16) injuries were suffered by 29.3% of the casualties. These proportions are nearly three times higher than in trauma not related to terrorist explosions[29] and are similar to those recorded in hospitalized patients following the Madrid bombings.[17] Systolic blood pressure below 90 mmHg was present in 6.1% of suicide bomber explosion victims, Glasgow Coma Scale of 3 (in emergency department, ED) was noted in 7.8% of suicide bomber explosion patients and finally a third of the patients had injuries to multiple body regions, complicating care and increasing severity.

Body Regions Injured

The number of persons in danger is increased by detonation in a rush hour commuter environment. As described following the London attack in 2005,[18] among the survivors, traumatic tympanic perforation was common. Secondary injuries, including penetration by biologic material, were frequent, as were traumatic amputation and smoke inhalation. These phenomena have been described earlier in Israel, for example, in a case in which a woman was injured by a chip of bone from a hepatitis B carrier terrorist.[31] More details are provided in the "Perpetrator Bone Fragments" section.

A report on the patients cared for at a central hospital in Madrid following the 2004 explosion of ten bombs simultaneously, killing 191 and injuring 2000, gave an account that among the 243 victims with moderate-to-severe trauma, tympanic perforation occurred in 41%, chest injuries in 40%, shrapnel wounds in 36%, frac-

TABLE 10.1. Injury characteristics of 1,155 hospitalized terror explosion victims

Injury Severity Score (ISS)	N	%
Minor injury (ISS 1–8)	593	52.7
Moderate injury (ISS 9–14)	202	18.0
Severe injury (ISS 16–24)	123	10.9
Critical injury (ISS 25+)	207	18.4
Three or more body regions injured	332	29.5
Intensive Care Unit (ICU) (% stay)	306	26.6
Surgery	598	51.8
Total length of stay >14 days	221	1+9.4
Median (interquartile range)	5 days	(2–11) days
In-patient mortality		
In all patients	74	6.4
In severe/critical (ISS* 16+) patients	69	20.9
Death within 24 h	74	6.4

From Aharonson-Daniel et al.[29] Reprinted with permission from Lippincott Williams & Wilkins.

---

* ISS – Injury Severity Score is calculated by summing the squares of the Abbreviated Injury Scale (AIS) severity score for the three most severely injured body regions in one patient. It is a common method for representing the overall severity of injury.

tures in 18%, first-degree or second-degree burns in 18%, eye lesions in 18%, head trauma in 12% and abdominal injuries in 5%.[17]

A recent paper on bombing casualties in Israel[29] reports that 32% of the hospitalized casualties suffered internal injuries, 59% had open wounds and 17% had burns, while 8% had injuries to blood vessels and nerves. While this proportion is low, it is noteworthy that these injuries are very rare – in other trauma cases, less than 1% have these conditions. The practical implication of this finding is the need to staff ED with vascular and plastic surgeons ready to treat blood vessel and nerve injuries upon the occurrence of a mass terrorist event.

Nearly 18% of the patients suffered traumatic brain injuries, more than 80% of them with an injury in another body region. In certain cases, there were multiple injuries that required competing forms of treatment, such as burns and blast lung. Burns were present in 16.6% of suicide bomber explosion casualties; in 70.5% of them, another penetrating or blunt injury was also found.

Brief reviews and comments from the literature on the frequency of various typical injuries are given here.

Lung and Chest Injuries
Blast lung injury is a major cause of immediate death and morbidity. Blast lung injury can occur without external chest wall injury, caused by the very high-pressure primary blast wave pushing the chest wall towards the spine, causing transient high intrathoracic pressure.[32] Among the casualties recorded in Israel as suffering an injury from bomb blasts, 21% had a lung injury – 17.5% severe (AIS 3 or above) and 3.7% of minor severity. In the Jerusalem terrorist attacks, one medical center reports that more than half (52%) of the patients in the intensive care unit (ICU) had lung injuries[33] while in another medical center, 70% of the ICU patients had blast lung,[34] 21% had combined chest and head injuries and 11% had combined chest and abdominal injuries. Blast lung is a very complex injury to handle and demands advanced critical care ability and especially advanced ventilation capabilities to balance between low-pressure ventilation and acceptable oxygenation.

Brain Injuries
Brain injuries were present in 44 of the 101 patients in the ICU in Jerusalem following a bombing MCE.[33] Overall, 16.1% of the patients had a head injury with an associated AIS score of 3 or above and another 6.5% had a head injury of lesser severity (AIS 1–2).[29] Most (78%) traumatic brain injuries were related to penetrating, secondary, metal junk shrapnel or to bullets, but some (22%) were related to blunt trauma induced by hurling or by heavier flying debris. Of the hospitalized patients with brain injuries, 26% suffered both blunt and penetrating brain injuries (Table 10.2).

Abdominal Injuries
Of all the patients recorded in the Israel National Trauma registry as suffering from abdominal injuries (15.2%), more than half (8.6%) had severe (AIS ≥ 3) injuries. Nearly a third of the patients in the ICU had suffered an abdominal injury.[33] Abdominal injuries were most often (96%) caused by penetration of shrapnel or bullets. Only a small portion of them were solely secondary to blast or blunt

injuries (4%), while 21% were a combination of blunt and penetrating injuries (Table 10.2). Most patients with significant abdominal trauma underwent explorative and/or curative laparotomy. Only a minority were placed under observation.

Orthopedic Injuries

Skeletal injuries inflicted by terrorism are described by Weil,[35]who has specified several modes of severe penetrating injuries causing high-grade open fractures. Gunshot wounds and multiple shrapnel injuries caused by terrorism produce severe penetrating long bone injuries, often associated with multiple trauma. In a study of 85 orthopedic patients from 33 recent terrorist attacks in Jerusalem, 113 long bone fractures caused by penetrating gunshot and shrapnel injuries were recorded. There were 36 femoral fractures, 50 tibial fractures, 5 humeral fractures and 24 forearm fractures. Thirty-six per cent of the patients had multiple fractures, while 43% suffered from significant associated injuries, mainly vascular damage and/or nerve injury to the fractured extremity.[33]

Other (Minor) Injuries

In many terrorist bombings, there is an overwhelming predominance of relatively minor injuries that are not life threatening.[35-38] These are usually caused by secondary and tertiary blast effects and are typically soft tissue and skeletal injuries that nevertheless tend to be extensive and contaminated and require multiple procedures. After the terrorist attacks in Madrid in 2004, soft tissue, musculoskeletal and ear blast injuries predominated in up to 80% of the cases but were mostly noncritical in severity and contributed little to mortality.[17] The main problem with these minor injuries is that the multiple-contaminated wounds contain various debris and fragments. The wound debridement in these patients is necessary to prevent infection. In Spain,[17] such injuries accounted for more than a third of all operations performed in the first 24 hours. Standard procedure in Israel is to avoid the chase for each piece of shrapnel. Shrapnel fragments are removed if they are found during some necessary exploration, or if their close proximity to a vital organ may carry potential danger or may cause some irreversible damage.

TABLE 10.2. Distribution of type of injury by body region

| Body region | Head | | Chest | | Abdomen | |
Type	N	%	n	%	N	%
Blunt	58	21.64	9	5.00	7	4.24
Penetrating	139	51.87	122	67.78	131	79.39
Blunt & penetrating	71	26.49	49	27.22	27	16.36
	268	100	180	100	165	100

Patients hospitalized at Hadassah University Hospital, 10/1/2000–12/ 31/2005, Hadassah Trauma Registry. The figures in table cells are the count and percent of patients with injuries of the type specified in the row title, for each body region as noted in the column title. Patients may have other injuries as well.

Perpetrator Bone Fragment Injuries

Braverman et al.[31] report on yet another injurious element – the penetration of bone fragments from the human suicide bomber. In this report, the perpetrator had hepatitis B and the bone fragments were positive for hepatitis B surface antigen HbsAG– Hepatitis B Surface Antigen, resulting in the need to administer active immunization against hepatitis B for all the patients injured in the attack. Such consequences necessitate a review of the protocols for hospital preparedness. Current protocol is that in each case of suicide bombing, all victims are vaccinated for hepatitis B.

Psychological Effects

Emotional shock is a common consequence of terrorist bombings. Although it is not as lethal as physical injury, there is significant potential for long-term psychological disability. It should be considered in the same category as other major injuries that need treatment. Recent attacks have exposed large parts of the civilian population to horrors. People who witness the devastation of a terrorist attack develop a panic response that needs medical attention.[39] The number of people presenting with acute- and post-traumatic stress disorder may be larger than the physically wounded. In some instances, the number of people presenting with the psychological effects of terrorist attacks was ten times larger than those physically wounded. Once the system recognized the situation, special areas, sometimes detached from the hospital, were set aside for treating people with mental instability.

Solomon[40] examined gender differences in post-traumatic vulnerability in the face of terrorist attacks and found that women were more susceptible to post-traumatic and depressive symptoms than men and that, generally, the odds of their developing post-traumatic stress symptoms were six times higher than those of men.

Pre-Hospital Issues

A retrospective analysis of medical evacuations performed by the Israeli National Emergency Medical Services rescue teams from MCE focused on 33 MCEs and 1,156 casualties.[15]

Twelve of these events occurred within the metropolitan area of one of the three largest cities in Israel. In these cities, evacuation options included a trauma center as well as other medical centers. Twelve other incidents occurred in smaller cities with a relatively large population but with only medical centers in close proximity. Only nine events occurred in rural regions: either in sparsely populated areas or in towns with a small population and an evacuation time to a medical center greater than 20 minutes. For these events, 1,123 ambulances were available and mobilized, yet 506 ambulances sufficed to provide 612 patient evacuations.

In a bus explosion occurring on January 29, 2004 in an urban setting (bus #19 in Jerusalem), 38 casualties and 11 fatalities were reported. Within 4 minutes after the explosion, 4 ambulances arrived. Within 22 minutes, 48 ambulances had arrived, bringing to the scene 15 paramedics, 3 physicians and 85 emergency medical technicians (EMT-1).

In a rural event on November 28, 2002 in Beit Shean, the first ambulance arrived 3 minutes after the event, 2 more ambulances arrived 11 minutes after the event and within 26 minutes, 22 ambulances were present, with 4 physicians, 17 paramedics and 54 EMT-1. National data show that on an average, rescue teams arrived on the scene within 5 minutes and evacuated the last urgent casualty within 15–20 minutes. The majority of the patients were transported to medical centers close to the event. Less than half the urgent casualties were evacuated to more distant trauma centers.[15] Since Israel is a small country, air evacuation has a limited role in preliminary triage, but it is often used for secondary triage.

Among 869 patients hospitalized at Hadassah University Hospital, 91 pre-hospital intubations were preformed (10.5%). The protocol for pre-hospital care in MCE is rapid assessment and *scoop and run*, which includes provision of airway, manual ventilation when needed, a needle application for tension pneuomothorax and control of external bleedings. This protocol and the fact that most victims (81%) were injured in urban settings explain the relatively low-field intubation rate. The provision of airway was often managed manually until arrival at the hospital.

Hospital Issues

A study of 33 MCEs during the first 2 years of the recent terrorism wave found that hospitals nearest to the event played a major role in trauma patient care.[15] Despite recommendations for sending patients to several trauma centers, the nearest hospital has to be prepared at full capacity once a terrorist event has occurred.

After a terrorist attack, there is a brief latent period, lasting ~20 minutes, in which events take place outside the hospital.[41] The optimal SOP is the initial report by the EMS dispatch center. This can be enforced by listening to the EMS radio channels trying to estimate the rough number of victims and the possible severity of their injuries. Data regarding the location and extent of injuries can sometimes be supported by initial media reports. In accordance with the ED checklists, during this latent phase, lower-intensity care areas of the ED should be cleared of patients. Patients in the ED should be quickly triaged, admitted to a ward or discharged. The attending professional in the ICU can use this period to quickly review the patients in the ICU, to identify potential available beds.[33]

Preparedness for Mass Arrival

Explosions occurring in closed areas, detonated at a choice of timing – when perceived as most effective – result in MCE. As a result, the nearest hospital will suffer a sudden surge of patients within the first 30 minutes of the attack. A study of attacks taking place in Jerusalem over 3 years found that the first casualties arrived at the hospital as soon as 11 minutes following the assault and 80% of the victims arrived within the first hour. The median time to arrival was 36 minutes overall, while among explosion events, 60% of the patients arrived within 30 minutes.[42]

A national study of bombing during the same period[43] confirms these findings, further reporting that 34% of the patients arrived within 10 minutes of the first patient's arrival and 65% within 30 minutes.

One of the first lessons learned was that hospitals in the vicinity of the attack should immediately get ready to manage an MCE. This preparation should follow the predetermined SOP and the checklist and should involve all the medical and administrative teams.

The intensity of events in Israel was high during 7 months in 2001; in one block in Jerusalem, eight suicide bombers had exploded. In March 2002, there were 17 terrorist attacks (11 suicide bombers) in Israel, resulting in 91 dead and 574 injured. Such frequent events challenge even the most well-organized system. In order to maintain fresh, emotionally capable and alert forces for the yet-unknown, guidelines for on-call staff were rehearsed. During the first attacks, all the staff would rush to hospital (causing havoc beside the MCE and sometimes turning it into a "mass health care providers event"). Only people who are on the MCE networks are supposed to arrive during an event, and if the incident is limited, some of them would be relieved by the event manager. This arrangement freed access by reducing the number of employee vehicles that were trying to access the hospital concurrently. It also helped maintain the necessary staffing level and put personnel on reserve, rather than work double and triple shifts for days in a row. It is worth mentioning that during extreme and prolonged events, protocols allow the change of shifts from 8 to 12 hours. This can increase the available manpower by 33%, excluding physicians, who do not work in shifts.

Patient Care and Service Utilization

Of the 1,155 cases of victims of suicide bomber explosions recorded in the Israel National Trauma registry, 27% were treated in the ICU. A detailed documentation of ICU care can be found in a recent paper by Aschkenasy.[33] Of about 12,000 hospitalization days, 1,965 days were in the ICU (until the end of 2004), the range was 1–8, median 3 and the mean 8.3 days per person.

High rates of immediate surgery and ICU utilization were reported in suicide bombing events recorded in the Israeli national trauma registry.[29] These have important effects on the hospital. Operating rooms and ICU are expensive and limited resources that function at high utilization rates. There is a clear need to create space for emergency cases, and to mandate protocols and contingency plans. This SOP should also be rationalized to minimize harm to patients who are already in the hospital and to optimize care for emergency patients when such an event occurs.

The number of surgical procedures conducted in the operating theater, such as thoracotomies, laparotomies, craniotomies and fracture management, is detailed in Table 10.3, showing the statistics for the entire patient population and separately for the severely or critically injured victims. Compared with non-terror-related trauma, all types of surgical procedures were significantly more frequent among patients affected by suicide bomber explosions.[29] Most significant is the difference in vascular surgery and laparotomies.

Intubation in the ED

The proportion of patients intubated in the ED among explosion victims was six times higher than in other trauma. According to Hadassah data, 10.5% (91 of 869 patients) of terror-related hospitalizations were intubated in the pre-hospital setup and 14.2% (123/869) in the ED. The proportion of ED intubations is augmented by the fact that explosions are frequently MCEs, so evacuation teams are less likely to intubate at the scene and often manage the airway manually, leaving more patients to be intubated in the ED. Perhaps pre-hospital intubation should be administered more generously, though certainly in some cases, especially for short evacuations, the airway can be maintained efficiently by manual maneuvers.

Thoracotomies in the ED

Nearly 4% of severely injured patients had ED thoracotomies (Table 10.3). This rate is significantly higher than in other patients with trauma. Data from Hadassah University Hospital report a relatively high rate of 2.3% (20 of 869 patients).

Ultrasound Scanning and Diagnostic Imaging

Ultrasound was used to detect free peritoneal or pericardial fluid to identify the source of haemodynamic compromise, or as a screening test for peritoneal or pericardial penetration. Despite the limitations of ultrasound in penetrating injuries, its mobility, reproducibility and immediate results made this modality a valuable and effective tool in MCEs.

TABLE 10.3. The proportion of hospitalized patients undergoing procedures, by injury severity

	%	
	Among all (N = 1,155)	Among severe (ISS 16+) (N = 329)
In the emergency department		
Intubation	12.2	32.4
Chest decompression	5.9	17.9
Thoracotomy	1.2	3.6
Arteriograms	2.9	5.8
Computed tomography (CT)	36.6	59.7
Ultrasound scan	26.8	47.0
X-ray	53.2	60.0
In the operating room		
Thoracotomy	6.2	20.3
Laparotomy	12.9	33.9
Vascular	4.5	12.1
Craniotomy	6.7	20.6
Fracture management	21.8	33.6

From Aharonson-Daniel et al.[29] Reprinted with permission from Lippincott Williams & Wilkins.

One major change that took place following the introduction of metal pieces within explosives and their detonation by suicide bombers is the frequent use of imaging in the triage process.[1–3,44] Sixty per cent of all severe casualties underwent computerized tomography (CT) scans in the ED (37% in all patients). In one case, a penetrating wound was located inside the mouth and completely invisible. The CT scan disclosed a nail nested in a 14-year-old girls' brain. Therefore, seemingly stable bombing casualties should be reassessed for concealed injuries. This could be done by a CT scan or whole body scout radiographs. This shift in triage process implies heavy loads on hospital imaging resources, requiring a well-planned sequence of procedures for patients.

Additional Contributors to Shifting Patterns of Hospital Utilization

Two major factors affect the triage demands in a terrorist-related MCE – one, mentioned above, is the mass arrival of patients with a unique injury pattern of concealed fragments and the other is the individually motivated arrival of masses who sustained minor injuries.

A corollary of the need for triage to be more sensitive is an increase in routine use of CT to find foreign metal bodies. As terrorist explosions have the potential to inflict multisystem, life-threatening complex injuries on many people simultaneously, there will be an urgent need to do mass screening, possibly causing the formation of bottlenecks at radiology and presenting other manpower demands.[32,45]

In a study that documented terrorist explosion events in Israel, the proportion of patients who had a CT scan performed in the ED was 36.6% in suicide bomber explosions; 26.8% had ultrasound scanning and 53.2% had X-rays in the ED.[29]

Utilization of Operating Rooms

A study of 325 casualties admitted following 32 mass casualty suicide bomber events and recorded in the national trauma registry, suggested guidelines for hospital organization during terror-related MCEs, based on the experience of six level-I trauma centers.[43] This study presents the proportion of patients entering surgery during each time interval by ISS (Fig. 10.2). In the first hours, it is clear that there is predominance of the more severe (ISS 16+) injuries; this proportion, as denoted by the arrow, decreases with time. The majority of patients entering surgery within the first 2 hours were severely injured (Fig. 10.2).

During the first hours, initiation of abdominal, thoracic and vascular surgical procedures predominated, and most patients entering surgery required two or more surgical teams working in parallel. After several hours, the proportion of procedures being started for patients with lesser injuries gradually increased (Fig. 10.3). Orthopedic and plastic surgery predominated at this time and an increased demand for these surgeons and anesthesiology services continued for more than 24 hours.[43]

A recent paper [47] reports a study of the role of the surgeon during terrorist-related multiple-casualty events. Based on interviews with 60 hospital physicians with experience in MCEs, the paper concludes that the physician's role expands beyond providing traditional trauma care. During MCEs, surgeons fill pivotal roles in hospital command and control and hands-on clinical care.

Beyond the need for ED preparedness and organization, ICU and operating theaters, hospitalization rates in terrorism mass casualty incidents are expected to be higher than among routine trauma incidents, requiring preparation of hospital capacity accordingly. A study of 17 suicide bomber attacks in Jerusalem reports that of 430 patients evaluated in the ED of the Hadassah University Hospital, Ein Kerem Campus, 157 patients (36.5%) were hospitalized.[27]

Outcomes

Mortality from Terrorist Attacks

A study of all terrorist attacks in the Jerusalem district between September 2000 and September 2003 found that 83% of deaths occurred immediately at the scene. Of the remaining 17% who died in hospital, half died within the first 4 hours of arrival, a quarter died between 5 and 24 hours and one quarter suffered a late death (after 24 hours).[43] The overall approximate in-hospital mortality rate of suicide

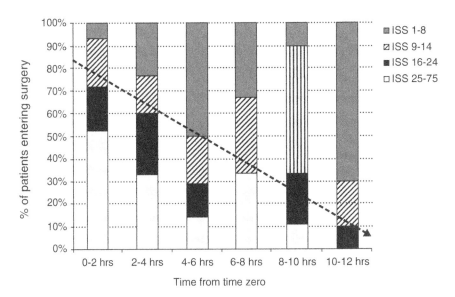

Fig. 10.2. Per cent of patients entering surgery during each time interval by Injury Severity Score (ISS). Percent of patients entering surgery during each time interval by ISS. Time is calculated from the time of arrival of the first admitted patient ("time zero"). Note the predominance of severe injuries (ISS > 16) in the first hours. The arrow denotes the decreasing portion of high ISSs. From Eniav S, et al.,[46] with permission from Lippincott Williams & Wilkins©.

bomber casualties is more than three times higher than that of non-terrorist-related trauma. Since these are more severe injuries, a comparison was made with in-patient mortality of patients injured severely by non-terrorist mechanisms, yet mortality from suicide bomber explosions remains higher in patients with ISS 16 or above (21.7% vs 13.0%).[25] A study on the care of patients injured in the March 2004 terrorist attack in Madrid reported 17.2% in-patient mortality for patients with critical injuries.[34] The overall mortality recorded in Madrid (8%) was similar to the percentage in the attack on London in 2005, where four suicide bombers had left ~700 persons injured and 56 (8%) dead.[30] In both attacks, most of the deaths occurred at the scene. Among patients who died in hospital, nearly half (47%) suffered injuries to multiple body regions including the head (51%), thorax (49%) and abdomen (54%).[43]

These figures highlight the natural triage occurring for victims who make it alive to the hospitals and also indicate that resuscitation attempts are usually not futile.

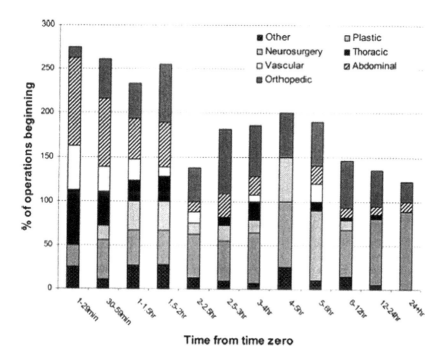

FIG. 10.3. The percent of surgical procedures commencing over time. The percent of surgical procedures commencing, by time elapsed from "time zero" (defined as the time of arrival of the first admitted patient). Subdivisions denote the surgical specialties performing the procedures. A large number of patients underwent multidisciplinary surgery, yielding a proportion of procedures per patients greater than 100% (e.g. 2.75 procedures/ patient in the initial 0–30-min time frame). $N = 196$. Note the duration of surgery is not shown. From Eniav S, et al.,[46] with permission from Lippincott Williams & Wilkins©.

Discussion

Terrorism injuries have a unique form of epidemiology. The uniqueness can be noted at almost all levels of injury characteristics – from the circumstances and environment, to the population profile, the medical distinctiveness, care needs and consequences. In terms of circumstances and environment, terrorism attacks usually affect people in crowded and public places. It may be a bus, a restaurant, a shopping mall, a market or a wedding hall – all places where the potential damage is large can attract terrorist activity. The population affected is therefore usually young and healthy, capable of moving around and being in public places. The patient profile of casualties injured in terrorist attacks indeed shows that more than half of them were aged between 15 and 29. This distribution is different from that of other injury types as demonstrated in Fig. 10.1. Places that match potential criteria for terrorist attacks, by definition, will most likely be in urban areas. The frequent occurrence of terrorist attacks in urban centers has implications for both evacuation and preparedness of hospitals. Understanding patterns of injury is essential for optimal preparedness in hospitals. The studies described above can help to anticipate the workload, the number of specialists and space necessary to provide care after the event. A sufficient amount of organizational resources should be made available to provide an adequate response in case an attack takes place. Data of the sort presented above are crucial for such planning and organization.

The range of insights gained by this data creates an informative picture of the characteristics of injury and care in an MCE. While this is interesting and challenging in terms of care, the ultimate goal of this data collection is to define and build SOPs that will enable the optimal functioning in the unfortunate event of a new terrorist attack. Building SOPs has great importance anywhere, but for these scenarios it has added value. Terrorist attacks occur at the most unexpected times and locations. The victims are often innocent citizens, children and mothers. The initial period after the attack is characterized by panic and frenzy, sometimes impairing the ability to function optimally. The availability of SOPs to act upon can help improve efficiency. In Israel, unfortunately, we have had so much experience in recent years that systems have been developed for routine practices. In other countries, however, for those who have suffered sporadic attacks and those who have been fortunate enough not to have been attacked, practice has to be based on theoretical knowledge and drills. Figure 10.4 demonstrates how data from the various sources can be used to build SOPs.

Data from various care providers, such as EMS, hospitals and forensic institutes, have been added to data from other bodies such as municipal services and fire squads. Debriefing sessions are conducted for all rescue forces and hospitals and summaries are distributed to all providers involved in the chain of care. Literature reviews and data analysis support evidence-based conclusions, all coming together in the formation of SOPs. Efficient and accurate triage, good skills, available medical resources and a good flow through the system may help to increase patient survival. Up-to-date, comprehensive SOPs are a useful tool for reaching these goals.

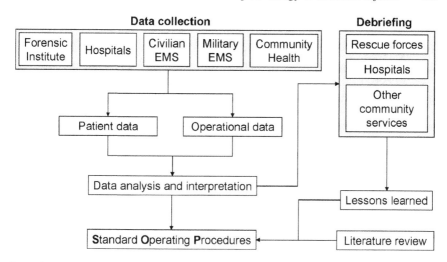

FIG. 10.4. The development of standard operating procedures (SOP) for medical care in terror situations. Data are collected from various sources that provide medical care in terror situations. Debriefing sessions provide an understanding of processes and identify flaws. A combination of data analysis and interpretation and evidence from the literature are the basis for the development and construction of SOP.

Conclusion

From the information presented, we can summarize the following lessons learned from the epidemiology of terrorism medicine. SOPs for MCEs related to terrorism should be prepared and rehearsed in all hospitals. It is recommended that hospitals near the attack site should be ready to manage an MCE, based on practiced SOP, within 10–20 minutes after attack. Every SOP should include protocols for clearing ED waiting areas, diagnostic imaging facilities, operating rooms and wards from routine workload without causing harm to other patients in the chain.

In addition to the usual and reserve staff, at the time of a terrorist MCE, readily available staff should include vascular surgeons. All medical and administrative teams assigned to tasks in an MCE should arrive promptly, but additional staff should be urged not to come. Finally, for medical staff who act as the first response, it is critical in these scenarios that triage should take into account concealed injuries caused by shrapnel.

References

1. Stein M, Hirshberg A. Limited Mass Casualties Due to Conventional Weapons A Daily Reality of a Level 1 Trauma Center. In: Shemer J, Shoenfeld Y eds. Terror and Medicine. Pabst Science Publishers, Berlin, 2003:385.
2. Kluger Y. Bomb explosions in acts of terrorism—detonation, wound ballistics, triage and medical concerns. IMAJ 2003;5:235–240.

3. Almogy G, Belzberg H, Mintz Y, Pikarsky AK, Zamir G, Rivkind AI. Suicide bombing attacks: update and modifications to the protocol. Ann Surg 2004;239(3):295–303.
4. Philips YY. Primary blast injuries. Ann Emerg Med 1986;15:1446–1450.
5. Frykberg ER, Tepas JJ. Terrorist bombings lessons learned from Belfast to Beirut. Ann Surg 1988;208(5):569–576.
6. Tokuda Y, Kikuchi M, Takahashi O, Stein GH. Prehospital management of sarin nerve gas terrorism in urban settings: 10 years of progress after the Tokyo subway sarin attack. Resuscitation 2006;68(2):193–202.
7. Yamasue H, Abe O, Kasai K, Suga M, Iwanami A, Yamada H, Tochigi M, Ohtani T, Rogers MA, Sasaki T, Aoki S, Kato T, Kato N. Human brain structural change related to acute single exposure to sarin. Ann Neurol 2007;61(1):37–46.
8. Bigalke H, Rummel A, Medical aspects of toxin weapons, Toxicology 2005;214: 210–220.
9. Waselenko JK, MacVittie TJ, Blakely WF, Pesik N, Wiley AL, Dickerson WE, Tsu H, Confer DL, Coleman CN, Seed T, Lowry P, Armitage JO, Dainiak N. Strategic national stockpile radiation working group. Medical management of the acute radiation syndrome: recommendations of the Strategic National Stockpile Radiation Working Group Ann Intern Med 2004;140(12):1037–51.
10. Peleg K, Rivkind A, Aharonson-Daniel L. Does body armor protect from firearm injuries? J Am Coll Surg 2006;202:643–8.
11. Kosashvili Y, Hiss J, Davidovic N, et al. Influence of personal armor on distribution of entry wounds: lessons learned from urban-setting warfare fatalities. J Trauma 2005;58:1236–1240.
12. Peleg K, Aharonson-Daniel L, Stein M, Shapira SC. Patterns of injury in hospitalized terrorist victims. Am J Emerg Med 2003;21:258–62.
13. Kluger Y, Peleg K, Aharonson-Daniel L, Mayo A. ITG, The special injury pattern in terrorist bombings. J Am Coll Surg 2004;199(6):875–879.
14. Feigenberg Z. Multi-casualty incidents caused by terrorist bombing explosions treated by Magen David Adom in Israel. (Abstract), 11th World Congress on Emergency and Disaster Medicine www.pdm.medicine.wisc.edu/wademtoc.htm#medical.
15. Einav S, Feigenberg Z, Waisman C, Zaichic D, Caspi G, Kotler D, Freund HR. Evacuation priorities in mass casualty terror related events: implications for contingency planning. Ann Surg 2004;239(3):304–310.
16. Hogan DE, Waeckerie JF, Dire DJ, Lillibridge SR. Emergency department impact of the Oklahoma city terrorist bombing. Ann Emerg Med 1999;34(2):160–167.
17. de Ceballos JP, Turegano-Fuentes F, Perez-Diaz D, Sanz-Sanchez M, Martin-Llorente C, Guerrero-Sanz JE. 11 March 2004: The terrorist bomb explosions in Madrid, Spain—an analysis of the logistics, injuries sustained and clinical management of casualties treated at the closest hospital. Crit Care 2005;9(1):104–11.
18. Ryan J, Montgomery H. The London attacks—preparedness: Terrorism and the medical response. N Engl J Med 2005;353(6):543–5.
19. Israel Defense Forces Web site. Available at: http://www.idf.il/. Accessed September 30, 2008.
20. Sheffy N, Mintz Y, Rivkind A, Shapira SC. Terror-related injuries: a comparison of gunshot wounds versus secondary-fragments—induced injuries from explosives. J Am Coll Surg 2006;203:297–303.
21. Arnold JL, Tsai MC, Halpern P, Smithline H, Stock E, Ersoy G. Mass casualty, terrorist bombings: epidemiological outcomes, resource utilization and the time course of emergency needs (part I). Prehospital and Disaster Medicine 2003;18(3):220–234.

22. Better OS, Stein JH. Early management of shock and prophylaxis of acute renal failure in traumatic rhabdomyolysis. N Engl J Med 1990;322(12):825–9.
23. Michaelson M. Crush injury and crush syndrome. World J Surg 1992;16(5):899–903.
24. Mintz Y, Shapira SC, Pikarsky AJ, Goitein D, Gertcenchtein I, Mor-Yosef S, Rivkind A. The experience of one institution dealing with terror: the El Aqsa Intifada riots. Isr Med Assoc J 2002;4:554–6.
25. Peleg K, Aharonson-Daniel L, Stein M, Michaelson M, Kluger Y, Simon D, ITG, Noji E. Gunshot and explosion injuries: characteristic, outcome and implications for care of terror-related injuries in Israel. Ann Surg 2004;239(3):1–8.
26. Ad-El DD, Eldad A, Mintz Y, Berlatzky Y, Elami A, Rivkind AI, Almogy G, Tzur T. Suicide bombing injuries: the Jerusalem experience of exceptional tissue damage posing a new challenge for the reconstructive surgeon. Plast Reconstr Surg 2006;118:383.
27. Almogy G, Mintz Y, Zamir G, Bdolah-Abram T,Elazary R, Dotan L, Faruga M, Rivkind AI. Suicide bombing attacks can external signs predict internal injuries? Ann Surg 2006;243:541–546.
28. Katz E, Ofek B, Adler J, et al. Primary blast injury after a bomb explosion in a civilian bus. Ann Surg 1989;209:484–488.
29. Aharonson-Daniel L, Klein Y, Peleg K. Suicide bombers form a new injury profile. Ann Surg 2006;244:1018–1023.
30. Chaloner E. Blast injury in enclosed spaces. BMJ 2005;331:119–20.
31. Braverman I, Wexler D, Oren M. A novel mode of infection with Hepatitis b: penetrating bone fragments due to the explosion of a suicide bomber. IMAJ 2002;4:525–529.
32. Hare SS, Goddard I, Ward P, Naraghi A, Dick EA. The radiological management of bomb blast injury. Clin Radiol 2007;62(1):1–9.
33. Aschkenasy-Steuer G, Shamir M, Rivkind A, Mosheiff R, Shushan Y, Rosenthal G, Mintz Y, Weissman C, Sprung CL, Weiss YG. Clinical review: the Israeli experience: conventional terrorism and critical care. Crit Care 2005;9(5):490–9.
34. Avidan V, Hersch M, Spira RM, Einav S, Goldberg S, Schecter W. Civilian hospital response to a mass casualty event: the role of the intensive care unit. J Trauma 2007;62(5):1234–9.
35. Weil YA, Petrov K, Liebergal, M, Mintz Y, Mosheiff R. Long bone fractures caused by penetrating injuries in terrorists attacks. J Trauma 2007;62:909–912.
36. Feliciano DV, Anderson GV, Rozycki GS, et al. Management of casualties from the bombing at the Centennial Olympics. Am J Surg 1998;176:538–543.
37. Brismar B, Bergenwald L. The terrorist bomb in Bologna, Italy, 1980: an analysis of the effects and injuries sustained. J Trauma 1982;22:216–2204.
38. Frykberg ER. Medical management of disasters and mass casualties from terrorist bombings: how can we cope? J Trauma 2002;53:201–212.
39. Shalev AY, Freedman S. PTSD following terrorist attacks: a prospective evaluation. Am J Psychiatry 2005;162:1188–1191.
40. Solomon Z, Gelkopf M, Bleich A. Is terror gender-blind? Gender differences in reaction to terror events. Soc Psychiatry Psychiatr Epidemiol 2005;40(12):947–54.
41. Shamir MY, Weiss YG, Willner D, Mintz Y, Bloom AL, Weiss Y, Sprung CL, Weissman C. Multiple casualty terror events: the anesthesiologist's perspective. Anesth Analg 2004;98:1746–1752.
42. Shapira SC, Adatto-Levi R, Avitzour M, Ivkind AI, Gertsenshtein I, Mintz Y. Mortality in terrorist attacks: a unique modal of temporal death distribution. World J Surg 2006;30:1–8.
43. Einav S, Aharonson-Daniel L, Freund H, Peleg K. Hospital organization and management during multiple casualty events. Ann Surg 2006;243:533–40.

44. Shaham D, Sella T, Makori A, Appelbaum L, Rivkind AI, Bar Ziv J. The role of radiology in terror injuries. IMAJ 2002;4:564–567.
45. Hirshberg A, Stein M, Walden R. Surgical resource utilization in urban terrorist bombing: a computer simulation. J Trauma 1999;47:545–550.
46. Eniav S, et al. Hospital organization and management during multiple casualty events. Ann Surg 2006;243:533–540.
47. Einav S, Spira RM, Hersch M, Reissman P, Schecter W. Surgeon and hospital leadership during terrorist-related multiple-casualty events: a coup d'état. Arch Surg 2006;141(8):815–22.

11
Explosions and Blast Injury

Eric R. Frykberg

The strategy of terrorism is to intimidate populations through the ruthless and random infliction of violence upon innocent civilians, for the purpose of advancing political or ideological agendas.[1] The two primary goals to achieve this strategy are the maximizing of casualty generation, and maximizing the lethality among those casualties.[2] There is a general perception that the classic *weapons of mass destruction* (WMD) of biological, chemical, and radiological agents pose the greatest risk for achieving widespread injury, infrastructural damage, and death by terrorists. However, these agents are in fact quite difficult to weaponize for this level of destruction, and require substantial money and training to properly implement. This is most clearly confirmed by the rarity of WMD terrorist attacks over the past several decades. Although preparation for WMD disasters is important, the actual level of threat they pose is far below the level of funding and concern for this possibility that has been garnered in the media, government, and general population.[3]

Explosive agents are by far the most common cause of terror-inflicted mass-casualty events globally, which is evident in even the most cursory review of daily news reports over the past 40 years.[2,4–7] Between 1968 and 1980, there was a tenfold increase in terrorist bombings worldwide, with 3,689 deaths and 7,991 injuries documented in over 5,000 incidents.[8] Of the 93 terrorist attacks throughout the world from 1991 to 2000 that resulted in at least 30 casualties, 88% involved explosions.[9,10] Over 17,000 terror-related explosive and incendiary incidents occurred on US soil alone from 1988 to 1997, causing 427 deaths, 4,063 injuries, and $680 million in property damages, and the number of actual and attempted bombings increased by 127% during this same period.[11] These numbers continue to rise exponentially, largely because of how successfully explosions have achieved terrorist aims at relatively little cost and training. There is no need for the expense and complexity of classic WMD agents. Explosions should clearly be recognized as the *fourth* WMD, and as the most likely mass-casualty threat that health care providers will face, and for which they must train, in the foreseeable future. A review of the history, epidemiology, physics, and pathophysiology of explosive blasts should facilitate an understanding of how to most appropriately evaluate and treat the mass casualties that typically result from this mechanism, and how to best develop a rational and effective medical response to these disasters.

S.C. Shapira et al. (eds.), *Essentials of Terror Medicine*,
DOI: 10.1007/978-0-387-09412-0_11, Springer Science+Business Media, LLC 2009

History of Explosive Disasters

Since the Chinese developed gunpowder in the eleventh century AD, explosives have played a major role in violent acts both in warfare and in terrorism. The first recorded application of a major explosion to terrorist aims occurred in Antwerp, Belgium in 1585,[2] when 7 tons of gunpowder were floated on two barges under a bridge on the River Schelt and detonated. The bridge was destroyed, and there was a report of 1,000 soldiers being killed, among whom "...some dropped dead without any wounds, sheerly from concussion." This appears to be the first description of *primary blast injury* (PBI). The full destructive capabilities of major blasts came to fruition during the twentieth century, in the settings of armed conflict, terrorism, and industrial accidents.

Two of the most powerful man-made explosions in world history occurred in major urban areas within the past 100 years. Both were accidental, and both demonstrated several lessons that can be applied to understanding the patterns of injury and destruction resulting from blasts, which can further advance an understanding of the principles of casualty management in these events.

On December 6, 1917, the Belgian ship Imo collided with the French munitions ship Mont Blanc in the harbor of Halifax, Nova Scotia, which ignited 35 tons of benzene into a major fire on the top deck of the Mont Blanc. This brought the city's firefighters and hundreds of onlookers to the harbor shore to help and watch, and hundreds more residents in their homes overlooking the harbor came to their windows to watch. About 15 minutes later, the fire spread below decks to ignite its cargo of 2,300 tons of picric acid, 10 tons of gun cotton, 300,000 rounds of ammunition, and 200 tons of trinitrotoluene TNT-trinitrotoluene, to cause the largest man-made explosion ever recorded to that time. The ship was vaporized, and burning pieces of its metal hull rained down on the city for the next hour. The smoke plume rose 4 miles into the air, and the ship's 2-ton anchor was found 2 miles away. The blast shattered windows 100 km away, and was heard in Boston. The surrounding city was leveled by the blast and a subsequent 150-foot high tidal wave, and the hundreds of first responders and onlookers to the initial fire were wiped out. There were 2,000 deaths and 9,000 injuries, and 20,000 left homeless in a city of only 50,000 population. Most serious injuries involved lacerations from shattered glass among the many who watched in front of windows.[12]

On April 16, 1947, a fire broke out on the top deck of the cargo ship Grand Camp in the port of Texas City, Texas. Approximately 20 minutes later, after the city's entire fire and police departments, and hundreds of onlookers, flocked to the scene, the fire spread below decks to ignite a cargo of several hundred tons of ammonium nitrate fertilizer. This resulted in a massive explosion that shot a column of smoke 2,000 feet into the air, and hurled the ship's 1.5-ton anchor 2 miles away. Several days were required to bring the fires under control and the city was largely destroyed. A 150-foot high tidal wave engulfed much of the city shortly after the blast. Many thought they had been attacked by an atomic bomb. There were 600 deaths in a city of 16,000 population, including, once again, all the first responders and onlookers who had rushed to the initial fire.[13]

Both of these accidental disasters of the twentieth century demonstrate the extensive destructive potential of major explosions on civilian populations and societal infrastructure, and how effectively they can achieve the terrorist aims of casualty generation and lethality if deliberately inflicted. The loss of life in both cities was equivalent to about 300,000 deaths in a city the size of New York. Medical resources were wiped out in both cities, and would have been overwhelmed in any event by the casualty load, resulting in ongoing loss of life beyond the direct effects of the blast. Outside help was required for medical care but could not arrive for several days. Furthermore, the Texas City explosion demonstrated how great a magnitude of energy can be unleashed from inexpensive and readily available materials such as simple fertilizer (ammonium nitrate). In both disasters, the explosions occurred within the confined spaces of the lower decks of the ships, to greatly magnify their destructive force beyond that of open-air blasts. The survivors of these events were afflicted with severe injuries from scattered debris set into motion by the blast, most commonly from glass fragments that were hurled from shattered windows.

One important pattern demonstrated in both of these disasters was the *second hit phenomenon*. This refers to a second, usually more deadly, event that follows an initial event (i.e., the fires aboard the ships) by enough of a time interval to allow large numbers of medical first responders, firefighters, law enforcement, and curious onlookers and volunteers to rush to the scene to help. This results in these first responders and volunteers also being killed, thus further depleting the already scarce rescue and medical resources, compounding the level of injury and death over and above the initial event. Delayed structural collapse of damaged buildings, delayed explosions from leaking gas mains, multiple tsunamis following the first, and after-tremors following major earthquakes are examples of Second hit events that emphasize the dangers and inherent instability of disaster scenes, and how the desire to help, and who should have access to the scene, must be carefully assessed following any disaster.

Lessons Applied in Terrorist Bombings

All of these observations and patterns have been consistently reproduced in major terrorist bombings of the past 40 years, indicating that terrorists have studied the effects of major explosions such as these, and have exploited them very effectively to maximize terror, destruction, and death. Thousands have been killed or injured in these incidents (Table 11.1).

Ammonium nitrate preparations (i.e., fertilizer) have caused major accidental blasts, as occurred in the Texas City disaster, and in the explosion of a train carrying a cargo of fertilizer in Ryongchon, North Korea in 2004 that killed 54, injured 1,249, and destroyed over 8,000 homes. This material has also been used in several major terrorist bombings, causing thousands of deaths and injuries, in view of how readily available and easy to use it is (Table 11.2). Immense destructive energy can be created by soaking fertilizer with fuel oil, and incorporating this into a fuel-air explosive device to create a chain reaction of detonations that can achieve blast magnitudes of several tons of TNT equivalence.[2,7,14–16] The Khobar Towers terrorist

TABLE 11.1. Major global terrorist bombings

Event	Year	Total casualties (deaths)
Train terminal, Bologna[a]	1980	291 (85)
US Marine barracks, Beirut[b,a]	1983	346 (241)
World Trade Center, New York City[a]	1993	1,042 (6)
AMIA, Buenos Aires[b,a]	1994	286 (85)
Murrah Building, Oklahoma City[b]	1995	759 (168)
Centennial Olympics, Atlanta	1996	111 (2)
Khobar Towers, Saudi Arabia	1996	574 (20)
US Embassies, Tanzania and Kenya[b]	1998	4,100 (223)
USS Cole, Yemen	2000	52 (17)
World Trade Center, New York City[b]	2001	2,839 (2,819)
Shopping mall, Helsinki[a]	2002	166 (7)
UN Headquarters, Baghdad[b,a]	2003	100 (17)
Train terminals, Madrid[a]	2004	2,092 (191)
Subways and bus, London[a]	2005	>700 (55)

[a]Confined space explosions
[b]Involved some element of building collapse

TABLE 11.2. Major explosive disasters caused by ammonium itrate (fertilizer) explosive

Event	Year
Texas City harbor explosions	1947
Beirut suicide bombing	1983
AMIA, Buenos Aires	1994
Oklahoma City truck bombing	1995
Khobar Towers, Saudi Arabia[a]	1996
Helsinki shopping mall suicide bombing	2002
UN Baghdad Headquarters suicide bombing	2003
Ryongchon, North Korea train explosion	2004

[a]Tanker truck with raw sewage

bombing of US military personnel in Saudi Arabia in 1996 was caused by a tanker truck filled with a similar material, simple raw sewage, which when appropriately detonated achieved an estimated blast energy of 10 tons of TNT equivalent.[6]

Several terrorist bombings have been deliberately detonated indoors and in confined spaces, usually when large crowds are present, to greatly magnify the destructive force and casualty load.[17–19] The casualty numbers and immediate death rates of confined-space explosions are substantial (see Table 11.1). These rates of injury and death can be further enhanced by an explosive that is powerful enough to collapse a major building into which it is introduced, explaining why terrorists always try to put their bombs indoors (see Table 11.1).[4,15,16] Glass fragmentation remains a common cause of severe injury among casualties of terrorist bombings, especially indoor bombings when windows are shattered, as occurred in the Halifax disaster.[20] Knowledge of these patterns provides an opportunity to mitigate deaths and injuries from bombings, with such simple measures as barriers to prevent vehicles or unauthorized people from entering buildings, and shatterproof glass. Although the intent behind the 1995 Oklahoma City terrorist bombing was to drive the truck bomb loaded with a fertilizer-fueled device into the Murrah Federal Building to maximize casualties, concrete barriers prevented this, and clearly saved hundred of lives as the bomb (2-ton TNT equivalent) had to be detonated outdoors as an open-air blast.[15]

The second hit phenomenon that was so well demonstrated in the Halifax and Texas City disasters has been deliberately used in terrorist bombings quite effectively. Suicide bombing events in Israel have commonly been followed by a second delayed blast 15–20 minutes later to injure and kill the first responders who flock to the scene to help.[21,22] A delayed building collapse can accomplish the same purpose, as was demonstrated in the World Trade Center Towers collapse about 60–90 minutes after the initial airliner crashes in New York City on September 11, 2001, which killed over 400 first responder firemen and policemen in addition to the thousands of building occupants. Falling rubble from the building damaged in the Oklahoma City bombing in 1995 killed a nurse who had run from her hospital to this scene to "help" in rescue efforts. Nine days after a mine collapse in Utah in 2007, three rescuers were killed in a secondary collapse of a rescue tunnel they were digging. This emphasizes the importance of protecting resources, especially medical assets, in these events by restricting access to the scene of a bombing, or any disaster, to all but those specifically trained and authorized for this.

Blast Physics

An effective medical response to terrorist bombings requires a thorough understanding of these lessons and patterns. This is best accomplished through education in the physics and pathophysiology of explosions and blast injury. An explosion is the sudden release of energy from the conversion of solids and liquids into gas. Low-energy explosives, such as gunpowder, release energy relatively slowly through a process called *deflagration*. This imparts a pushing effect, and these agents are commonly used as propellants. High-energy explosives (TNT, Semtex, C-4, dynamite) are very destructive and are the type commonly used in terrorism. These are characterized by a virtually instantaneous transformation of solids or liquids into gas in the process of *detonation*, filling the same condensed volume, and therefore under very high pressures. This creates an intense pressure wave as the surrounding medium is compressed by a rapid outward expansion, termed the *blast wave*, which spreads radially at supersonic speeds of 3,000–8,000 m/s. This instantaneous (lasting 2–10 ms) rise in surrounding pressure at the site of the blast is called the *peak overpressure*, the magnitude of which is dependent on the strength of the explosion. The leading edge of the blast wave is the *blast front*, which has a shattering ability called *brissance* that low-energy explosions do not have. Blast waves are propagated in water three times more powerfully and more distant than in air, due to the greater density and lesser compressibility of water. High-energy explosions are also characterized by an initial thermal burst, or *fireball*, as a result of the high magnitudes of energy released.[23–28]

176   E.R. Frykberg

The blast wave rapidly dissipates in air according to the cube of the distance from the blast, so that moving three times further away reduces the magnitude of energy by 27-fold. The peak overpressure is followed by a more gradual ebbing of pressure that lasts up to ten times longer to the point of falling below ambient atmospheric pressure, resulting in a negative pressure phase known as *underpressure*, which creates a relative vacuum. Ultimately, as surrounding air returns to ambient pressure, the blast wave deteriorates into acoustic waves, providing the sound of the explosion (Fig. 11.1). The underpressure phase explains why *implosive* effects are often seen following major explosions, and why blasts in coastal areas near large bodies of water, such as Halifax and Texas City, may be followed by tidal waves. Blast wind refers to these rapid and powerful back and forth movements of air, which can reach hurricane strength following high-energy blasts, and has great ongoing destructive potential.

Blast waves within buildings and other confined spaces are more powerful and destructive than in open air, as they are magnified, rather than dissipated, by reflection off of walls, floors, and ceilings. This creates a more complex blast wave than in open air that has three components: the incident wave, a disorganized collection of reflected waves, and the static pressurization of the confined space. This results in a much greater degree of structural damage, and physical injury among people in the structure, than that occurs in open-air blasts. The intensity and duration of this pressure wave depends on the blast magnitude, the volume of the confined space, and the degree of venting and decompression allowed by open doors and windows.[27] This explains why terrorists often detonate their bombs within buildings and confined spaces, especially when crowded with people, such as nightclubs, trains, and buses, as the casualty load and mortality substantially exceed those of open-air blasts. A further rationale for placing bombs in buildings is that, with a

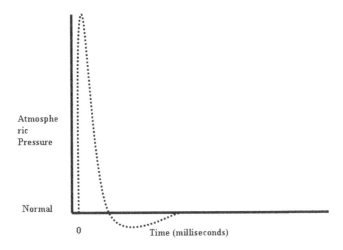

Fig. 11.1. Graphic representation of pressure changes over time resulting from high-energy explosions.

powerful enough blast, the building may collapse and still further magnify injury and death (see Table 11.1).[15,29] Suicide bombings in Israel have frequently occurred in crowded buses, in which setting the mortality rate approaches 50%, compared with 8% in open-air blasts.[17]

The terrorist bombing in Helsinki, Finland, in 2002 occurred in a relatively open shopping mall, with only a 3% immediate death rate (7/166).[7] The Khobar Towers bombing in Saudi Arabia in 1996 involved an open-air bombing of an estimated power of 10 tons of TNT in front of a dormitory building that did not collapse, with only a 3% immediate death rate.[6] In the Centennial Olympics bombing in Atlanta in 1996, the open-air explosion killed only one person immediately.[30] All 163 immediate deaths among the 759 total casualties of the Oklahoma City terrorist bombing in 1995 occurred in occupants of the partially collapsed Murrah building, with no deaths among the casualties outside the building. Even among the 361 casualties within the building, only 3% of those in the uncollapsed portion died, compared with a 42% mortality in the collapsed portion. Ninety-four percent of all immediate deaths were in the collapsed portion of the building.[15]

There are three recognized components of blast waves. *Stress* waves have a velocity similar to sound waves but with a higher amplitude; *shock* waves have higher pressure and amplitude than do sound waves; and *shear* waves have lower velocity and longer duration and distance than do sound waves, but travel in a transverse axis that severely disrupts tissues and materials in their path. The orientation of objects and bodies to the blast wave is a major factor in their level of destruction and injury.[27] All of these characteristics of blast waves cause significant disruptive forces in the surrounding medium that result in destruction of exposed organic tissues. Forcible rapid expansion and contraction of the blast wave leads to shearing of tissues through the generation of high-pressure differentials and inertial mismatches. *Spalling* refers to the disruptive movements of fluid, especially at air:liquid interfaces, due to the differences in compressibility of these two mediums. This explains the profound effects of blast on the human body.

Blast Pathophysiology

The characteristics described above make it clear why major blasts result in greater numbers, severity, and complexity of injuries than do the standard forms of blunt and penetrating trauma seen in routine daily practice. Reports of terrorist bombings and blast-related burns in Israel have documented significantly younger victims (and higher percentages of females and children among those victims), higher levels of injury severity (30% with Injury Severity Scores [ISS] > 15 vs 10%), more complex injuries involving more than three body regions (28% vs 6%), greater percentages of injuries requiring major operations (23% vs 4.5%), longer average intensive care unit (ICU) stays (5 days vs 3 days), and higher mortality (6% vs 2%) among victims of terror-related blasts and burns than among nonterror-related trauma victims.[31–36] A collective review of over 3,300 terrorist bombing victims from 220 incidents worldwide[37] documents that most immediate deaths are due to lethal injuries of the head, chest, and abdomen. Most (80–95%) survivors are afflicted with noncritical soft tissue and skeletal injuries, but the minority of survivors with major abdominal, thoracic, and head injuries and traumatic amputations account for virtually all late deaths (Table 11.3).

There are four categories of blast injury, each with distinct etiologies and implications for medical care: primary, secondary, tertiary, and quaternary.

Primary Blast Injury

This form of injury is caused by the destruction of tissues that results solely from the passage of the blast wave through the body. The greater the magnitude of a high-energy explosion, the more powerful is this blast wave. It causes the greatest damage to air-containing organs such as the lungs, the hollow viscera of the abdomen, and the ears through the effects of spalling at air:liquid interfaces. In fact, tympanic membrane (TM) rupture is a sensitive marker of exposure to the blast wave, though it does not reliably correlate with lung injury or severity of injury.[7,38] TM rupture requires about 20–50 lb per square inch of pressure, and is not always present in victims who were close to the blast. In the 2004 Madrid train bombings, less than 50% of hospitalized survivors (240/512) had TM rupture, and the majority of these were not severely injured.[39]

The pressure wave causes implosive effects in these organs, which compresses tissues and causes the inertial mismatches between the differing densities of air and water that lead to spalling, disrupting the tissues. Solid organs tend to be relatively spared of PBI due to their homogeneous densities. The lung is most commonly afflicted by PBI in open-air blasts, while the bowels are most commonly injured in underwater blasts.[23,24,27,28]

Blast lung injury (BLI) is characterized by loss of the integrity of alveolar and pulmonary microvascular basement membranes, resulting in a high incidence of cerebral and coronary air embolism, which is a common cause of immediate death

TABLE 11.3. Patterns of injury and mortality in 3,357 victims of terrorist bombings

Specific injury	Incidence in immediate deaths (%)	Incidence in survivors (%)	Specific mortality(%)[a]	Survivor deaths with specific injury (%)[b]
Head	71	31	1.5	52
Chest	25	2	15	21
Blast lung	47	0.6	11	4
Abdomen	30	1.4	19	21
Traumatic amputation	–	1.2	11	10
Skeletal	–	11	0	0
Soft tissue	–	55	0	0

Adapted from Frykberg et al.,[37] with permission from Lippincott, Williams & Wilkins.
[a]Percentage of all survivors with specific injury who died of that injury
[b]Percentage of all late deaths among survivors who had specific injury

among victims very close to the blast. In the past, less than 1% of survivors of terrorist bombings have had BLI due to the rapid dissipation of the blast wave in air (see Table 11.3). A recent analysis of the patterns of injury following the Madrid train bombings in 2004 showed a higher incidence of BLI among hospitalized survivors than in past bombings (2.4% vs 0.6%), although their ultimate mortality was also higher (18% vs 11%). This was attributed to the rapid pre-hospital response that allowed mortally injured casualties to reach the hospital alive who in the past died before reaching medical care.[39] Those close enough to major blasts to be affected by PBI generally have multiple severe body system injuries that are immediately lethal. However, those few survivors with BLI are at significant risk of mortality (see Table 11.3), emphasizing the need to recognize these quickly and provide urgent treatment.

The clinical and radiological presentations of BLI are similar to those of pulmonary contusions. A scoring system for recognition and prognosis that is based on the chest X-ray findings has been reported.[40] However, the management of BLI is very challenging because of its pathophysiological complexity, consisting of combinations of barotrauma, bronchopleural and alveolar-venous fistulae, pneumothorax, penetrating fragment injuries, inhalation injuries, and shock, many of which may require contradictory therapies. While the respiratory insufficiency generally requires higher ventilatory pressures to expand functional residual capacity, this may aggravate air leaks and promote air embolism, requiring judicious ventilatory support.[20,21,27,41,42] Adding to these therapeutic challenges is the tendency for BLI to develop symptoms gradually over several hours or days after exposure to the blast, predisposing these casualties to be overlooked initially and assigned to less urgent care where they may suddenly deteriorate in an unmonitored environment.[43,44]

Bowel injuries from PBI have two major etiologies. There may be direct damage to the bowel wall that leads to intramural microcirculatory disruption and eventual infarction and perforation. The blast wave may also cause lacerations of the bowel mesentery, impairing the blood supply and eventually leading to infarction. In both cases, like BLI, the casualty may initially present without symptoms or physical findings, and deteriorate hours to days later with increased risk of mortality if not monitored carefully.[40]

Another recognized consequence of PBI is traumatic amputation of long bones of the extremities. Anatomic and computer modeling studies have shown that this clearly results from the direct coupling of the blast wave into extremity tissues, which weakens the bone through the exertion of powerful axial stresses. The subsequent blast wind then causes flailing of the limb with bone fracture and tearing of the soft tissues to complete the amputation, which occurs through the shaft of long bones and not through joint disarticulation. This injury is another reliable marker of exposure to the blast wave and the potential for critical life-threatening status among that small minority (about 1.2%) of survivors who have suffered this. Again, most casualties with this devastating injury are killed immediately due to the close proximity to the blast that is necessary to suffer this level of energy (see Table 11.3).[21,45]

Research has shown that the brain and spinal cord may also suffer severe tissue disruption from PBI, which is characterized by abnormal mental status and electroencephalographic EEG-electroencephalogram activity. Air emboli to the central nervous system from BLI can contribute to this condition with ischemic neurologic deficits. It is likely that the classic manifestations of "shell shock" in combat veterans, as well as chronic conditions, such as posttraumatic stress disorder, have an organic basis from exposure to explosive blast waves, in addition to their psychological components. A rapid resolution of spinal cord deficits, especially in the absence of skeletal vertebral injuries, is a marker of PBI, contrasted with the permanent deficits that would be expected from air emboli or direct trauma to the spinal cord. Such "spinal shock" from PBI was documented in 1.6% (8/512) of hospitalized survivors of the Madrid train bombings in 2004.[39]

Spinal vertebral fractures are another recognized consequence of PBI, which tend to occur in unusual locations and at multiple levels in this setting when compared to routine forms of blunt trauma. These were noted in close to 5% (25/512) of hospitalized survivors of the Madrid train bombings, and 65% of these were in the upper thoracic spine. These injuries were also associated with severe torso trauma.[39]

Effective body armor against blast injury has been developed as a result of understanding the relationship between blast physics and its pathophysiology, to augment the normal protection against blast provided by the chest wall. The use of materials that specifically resist and degrade the effects of the stress, shock, and shear components of the blast wave significantly reduce torso injuries from PBI.[28,46]

Secondary and Tertiary Blast Injury

Secondary blast injury refers to the physical damage caused by debris and objects set in motion by the blast wind that impact the body. It includes the effects of *primary fragmentation* of the material that makes up the bomb, as well as *secondary fragmentation* created by pieces of other objects propelled by the blast or primary fragments (i.e., chips of wood from trees or wooden structures).[47] Glass shards from shattered windows are a common mechanism of severe wounding from secondary fragmentation, as was seen in survivors of the Halifax and Khobar Towers explosions.[6,20] These forms of blast injury are found in the great majority of survivors of major explosions.

Terrorist bombings have increasingly involved the addition of destructive metal fragments in the explosive device to cause severe high-energy penetrating wounds as another form of secondary blast injury.[30] One bizarre twist on such secondary fragmentation is that body parts of suicide bombers or other casualties are increasingly recognized as secondary missiles (*human remains shrapnel*) that further magnify casualty injuries and terror beyond the effects of the blast alone, especially with the finding that these body parts have been infected with such chronic diseases as hepatitis or HIV.[48–50]

Tertiary blast injury refers to physical damage from the body itself being thrown against other objects and structures by the forces of the blast. Children tend to be more prone than adults to tertiary blast injury due to their lighter weight.[51]

Both secondary and tertiary blast injuries result in standard forms of blunt and penetrating trauma and impalement, though the injuries tend to be more severe and complex than seen in routine surgical practice. Most of these injuries involve soft tissue and skeletal wounds that are not critical or life-threatening (see Table 11.3). This emphasizes the importance of surgical capability in the medical response to explosive disasters, and of surgeons being in leadership positions in the response, as that minority with critical injuries require immediate surgical attention to optimize their outcome.[3,4,14,18,21,30,31,34,37,52]

Quaternary Blast Injury

These are also termed *miscellaneous* blast injuries, resulting from indirect consequences of a blast. This category includes thermal burns, crush injuries from structural collapse secondary to a blast, and inhalation injuries from dust and toxic chemicals in the wake of a blast. The terrorist bombing event with the highest rate of acute and chronic inhalation injuries among casualties (93%) was the 1993 World Trade Center bombing in New York City.[10] Inhalation injuries continue to afflict rescue workers involved in the site clearing of Ground Zero following the collapse of the World Trade Center towers in New York City in 2001, due to inadequate use of personal protection. Building collapse is a result of a major confined-space explosion, and may occur immediately with the blast (Beirut 1983,[14] Asociación Mutual Israelita Argentina [AMIA] in Buenos Aires 1994,[16] Oklahoma City 1995[29,30]), or after a period of time after the explosion as a result of structural instability (World Trade Center 2001). These mechanisms clearly increase the level of injury, long-term disability, and death over and above the effects of the blast alone.

Burns are a severe form of quaternary blast injury following high-energy explosions, which result from exposure to the intense thermal energy in the immediate vicinity of the blast. Severe burns therefore serve as a marker of proximity to an explosion, and of the likelihood of multiple other critical injuries. Terror-related burns from bombings afflict older age groups, and tend to be more extensive and with significantly greater mortality than nonterror burns.[35] They are more common in confined-space explosions than in open-air incidents.[37] Following the 1983 suicide bombing of the US Marine barracks in Beirut, 57% of late deaths were due to burns.[14] Among 512 hospitalized survivors of the 2004 Madrid train bombings, 89 (17.4%) suffered thermal burns, of which 64% were extensive second and third degree.[39]

The dissemination of toxic biological, chemical, or radiological agents through explosive devices, or *dirty bombs*, is another form of quaternary blast injury. These have also been termed *combined* blast injuries.[52] Often these agents are destroyed by the blast, and cause little if any harm to casualties beyond the effects of the blast itself. The bomb causing the 1993 World Trade Center explosion contained enough cyanide to have contaminated a large area of lower Manhattan, but the blast destroyed it. Even if not destroyed, there is unlikely to be any substantial contamination from these agents. Their presence in explosions causes terror more through hysteria and panic than through actual injuries and deaths, and for this reason such dirty bombs have been called *weapons of mass disruption.*

Psychological sequelae of terrorist bombings are also a form of quaternary blast injury, and affect both surviving casualties and responders who participate in the search and rescue and site clearing efforts following these disasters. These problems may begin with acute stress reactions to witnessed horrors, which are aggravated by such factors as personal fatigue and death of friends and family members. Underlying psychoemotional disturbances will also aggravate this condition. If the acute symptoms of anxiety, insomnia, withdrawal, and altered personality are not recognized and addressed early, this may progress to chronic problems such as posttraumatic stress disorder.[53]

Implications for Mass-Casualty Management

The great magnitude of explosive force that can currently be achieved widely and commonly with relatively simple materials explains why major bombings virtually always result in mass-casualty events, especially when they occur in crowded settings. Knowledge of the physics and pathophysiology of explosions allows an understanding of the consistent patterns of injury they create, which can lead to effective planning and preparedness, and an effective medical response, for these disasters.

Injury Patterns

Terrorist bombings result in well-established patterns of injury and mortality. The number of casualties who are immediately killed at the scene is related to the magnitude of the blast, the extent of secondary blast injury by primary and secondary fragmentation, and the occurrence of building collapse.[4,15,17,29,37] Most survivors of these events are not critically injured, because most of those with critical injuries typically die immediately. The rate of critical injuries among survivors ranges from 5% to 25%, and late mortality occurs within this group. The incidence of late mortality is primarily influenced by the rapidity of the medical response and how quickly survivors, especially those critically injured, reach medical care from the scene of the blast. The most accurate measure of the success of a medical response following explosive disasters, and most other disasters, is the mortality among the critically injured casualties who are most at risk of death, known as the *critical mortality rate.*[4,19,37] The overall mortality rate based on all surviving casualties is artificially diluted by that great majority of survivors who are not seriously injured and not at risk of death (see Table 11.3). The longer it takes critical casualties, who have life-threatening injuries requiring immediate care, to reach medical facilities and receive care, the greater is the critical mortality. Following the 1983 suicide bombing in Beirut, in which it took at least 12 hours for most casualties to reach definitive medical care at American hospitals in Germany, the critical mortality rate was 37%. Following the terrorist bombing of the Murrah Federal Building in Oklahoma City in 1995, where medical care was only minutes away within a major city, the critical mortality rate was under 10%.[4]

The magnitude of the injuries in casualties of terrorist bombings and other explosive disasters is generally far greater than among routine victims of trauma in the civilian sector, and even greater than among combat injuries in soldiers of past wars. The ISS, the number of body systems injured, hospital and ICU length of stay, and mortality all tend to be significantly higher among bombing victims.[33,34] These have been termed *multidimensional injuries* in view of the complexity of the injuries, and of the decision-making and organization of medical care required.[5]

Triage Implications

Triage is the sorting and prioritizing of patient care based on the severity of injury and urgency of treatment needs. In a mass-casualty setting following major explosions, the added factor that must be considered in triaging casualties is *salvageability*. The extent of the limited resources that would have to be applied to any given casualty, and how much of these resources would be diverted from other more salvageable and less resource-intensive casualties, becomes an essential consideration that normally never comes into play in the care of emergency patients. The *greatest good for the greatest number* must prevail over our usual treatment principle of the greatest good for each individual, in view of the scarcity of resources that characterizes a true mass-casualty event. This *rationing* of resources to those most likely to survive, and the necessary denial of care to those with the most extensive injuries (i.e., *expectant* casualties who are expected to die) so as not to jeopardize the availability of these resources to most casualties is morally antithetical to the standard ethics and principles of medical care. However, it is essential that such *altered standards of care* be rapidly and strictly adopted in a mass-casualty disaster if overall casualty salvage is to be maximized.[4,5,21,36,37,54–57]

Triage is the essential process that governs the movement of casualties through the many echelons of medical care in any disaster medical response, and where medical providers may have the most direct impact on casualty outcomes. The basic challenge of triage in mass-casualty events is to rapidly identify that small minority of surviving casualties, who are critically injured and require immediate care, from among the majority who do not. The greater the number of noncritically injured casualties who are allowed to overwhelm medical facilities, the longer it will take to sort out the truly critically injured, leading to the triage error of *overtriage*. The assignment of expectant casualties to immediate care also should be considered an overtriage error.[36] Overtriage has been shown to directly correlate with the critical mortality of terrorist bombing victims for this reason (Fig. 11.2).[4,7,37] *Undertriage* is the assignment of critically injured casualties to delayed care, which also leads to delay in immediate treatment and mortality. *Triage accuracy*, or the minimizing of both overtriage and undertriage, is essential for optimal casualty outcomes in mass-casualty events. This requires that the triage officer who performs this task fully understand the nature of the anticipated injuries, and be trained in the unique decision-making skills and rapid assessments required in a mass-casualty setting.[7,58]

Judgments as to casualty disposition must be rapid to see all incoming casualties, and this requires that decision-making be based on a quick clinical assessment only.[21,59,60] There can be no time for extensive diagnostic imaging or laboratory testing. Knowledge of the clinical presentation and external markers of blast injury, and those injury patterns that correlate with a high risk of death, facilitate such judgments. Among immediate survivors of major blasts, blunt or penetrating torso injuries, skull fractures, traumatic amputations, extensive and deep burns, and respiratory insufficiency suggestive of BLI are all markers of life-threatening injuries regardless of hemodynamic stability.[21,55] TM rupture and even mild thermal burns correlate with exposure to the primary blast wave and proximity to the explosion, which should prompt a high index of suspicion for critical injuries, and assignment to a monitored care area for at least close observation. A high index of suspicion must also be applied to victims of confined-space explosions.[35] These markers will also assist in the triage of unsalvageable casualties to expectant care so as to only apply the limited resources to the most salvageable casualties. Which casualties should be expectant can only be defined at the time of the event, as it depends on the magnitude of the casualty burden and the resources available.[21,36,56,58]

Cumbersome triage schemes that require tallying up several clinical parameters in each casualty simply do not work in a true mass-casualty setting.[21,61,62] This emphasizes again how important the triage officer is to the success of a medical response. However, errors in triage decision-making must be anticipated in major blast disasters with large casualty loads, even with the most highly trained triage officers. The consequences of these errors should be mitigated by an *error-tolerant*

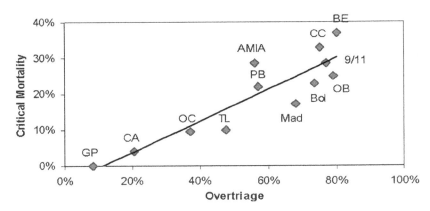

FIG. 11.2. Relation of overtriage to critical mortality in 12 major terrorist bombing incidents from 1969 to 2004. Linear coefficient (*r*) = 0.92. *GP* Guildford pubs, UK, *CA* Craigavon, Northern Ireland, *OC* Oklahoma City, *TL* Tower of London, UK, *BP* Birmingham pubs, UK, *Mad*, Madrid, *Bol* Bologna, Italy, *AMIA Asociación Mutual Israelita Argentina*, Buenos Aires, *9/11* Bellevue Hospital, New York City, *OB* Old Bailey, UK, *CC* Cu Chi, Vietnam, *Be*, Beirut. Adapted from Frykberg,[4] with permission from Lippincott, Williams & Wilkins.

system of casualty care. This involves such elements as multiple levels of triage to sequentially screen out noncritical and expectant casualties from overloading the limited resources of hospitals, thus minimizing the effects of overtriage, as well as clinical monitoring of delayed care areas to rapidly detect those who deteriorate and require upgrading to immediate care, thus minimizing the adverse effects of undertriage errors.[58,63]

Pre-hospital Casualty Handling

The top priority for the first responders who arrive at the scene of a major blast is to assure protection for themselves. This requires tight restriction of access to the scene to all except those specifically trained for its dangers and assigned to this duty. Unstable structures, leaking gas lines, downed power lines, toxic fumes, radiological contamination, and the possibility of a deliberately delayed blast that is an established terrorist tactic, all may lead to a second hit event that threatens first responders.[21] The presence of any toxic contamination of the scene must be determined at this time, and personal protection gear be donned and decontamination facilities then set up in appropriate locations. Hospital-based medical personnel do not belong at the scene, as there is little they can offer in this environment and they are not trained for these hazards.

Once responder safety has been assured, and the scene has been stabilized, attention should be directed to the evaluation and evacuation of casualties. The only attention that should be provided to casualties at the scene is to rapidly determine who is alive and who is dead, and expeditiously transport those alive to a nearby casualty collection area (CCA). This removes them from ongoing dangers. Ideally, casualties should not be transported directly to hospitals so as to allow the necessary screening and filtering to prevent hospital overload. CCA's should be located far enough from the scene to be safe, upwind and uphill from the scene, but near enough for easy accessibility. Decontamination should take place at CCA's. At the CCA a more thorough but still rapid evaluation of casualties must be done to simply determine who needs hospitalization and who does not. The dead and nonurgent casualties should be kept back and assembled in separate areas, preferably outside the hospital, to be monitored for any physiological deterioration and thus correct undertriage errors. "Triage at the scene" is largely a misperception, as *evacuation* must be the priority in the pre-hospital setting. It is unrealistic to think that the use of time-consuming protocols, formulas, and color tags have any benefit in the massive chaos of a mass-casualty event in a dangerous zone where only a few seconds can be spent on any given casualty.[5,21,54,61,62]

An imminent threat to area hospitals in the immediate aftermath of an explosive disaster is being overwhelmed by an uncontrolled influx of casualties, most of whom self-transport to the nearest hospital with a perception of this being a safe haven. Pre-hospital providers often aggravate this problem by transporting all casualties to the nearest hospital. This *geographic effect* of initial casualty flow consists largely of noncritical injuries that are able to mobilize on their own, and must be kept out of the hospital. This can be accomplished at the hospital by an immediate hospital *lockdown* to keep out this first wave of casualties who do not require hospitalization, saving the limited resources for the later waves of critical injuries who most require hospital care. Another mechanism to avoid the geographic effect is to control casualty flow from the scene by pre-hospital providers, who should systematically distribute casualties among all available hospitals from the scene. This prevents any one facility from being overloaded, and allows the distribution of casualties to the most appropriate facility for their specific needs, a process known as *leap-frogging*.

If the nearest hospital to the scene does become overloaded and cannot carry out its treatment mission, this hospital should then become a *triage hospital*, otherwise known as an *evacuation*, or *ground zero* hospital, converting its mission to one of distributing the casualties among the remaining area hospitals. This essentially extends the disaster scene to this nearest hospital, requiring it to do what should have been done at the scene, and thus delaying the ultimate care provided to casualties.[54]

Those casualties who ultimately arrive at the hospital should only be those requiring hospital care. Triage at the hospital entrance should again be carried out to once again ascertain that all require hospitalization, and to avoid admitting a potentially contaminated individual into the hospital. Once in the hospital, triage continues in an iterative fashion, determining who needs the operating room (OR), who needs the ICU, and who can wait for their care for optimal conservation of resources.

No casualty should get into the hospital before first being triaged, and if necessary, decontaminated. With the exception of quick and simple life-saving interventions, such as pressure on external hemorrhage, or covering open wounds, no treatment should be rendered to casualties through the pre-hospital phase. Even in the hospital, *minimal acceptable care* should be provided to all but the most severely injured who require immediate care and who most merit utilization of the limited resources.[21]

Hospital Resource Utilization

The extensive literature on terrorist bombings reviewed above documents the major prognostic factors that affect casualty outcome (Table 11.4). This permits a reasonable anticipation of the hospital resources required to manage blast mass casualties, which can be incorporated into effective planning. A discrete-event computer simulation of the impact on a hospital of an urban terrorist bombing attack[64] has shown that the number of surgeons, OR's, emergency department (ED) staff, and the level of triage expertise needed for mass-casualty care is typically overestimated in hospital plans. This is due to the small number of critical casualties in these events, and the smaller percentage of them that require urgent operations (only three ORs need to be available for every 100 casualties). Also the surgical operations done should be abbreviated according to *damage control* principles, leading to rapid turnover and ready availability of rooms during the acute casualty influx.[33]

TABLE 11.4. Terrorist bombings: Factors with adverse impact on casualty outcome

Blast-related factors
    Large magnitude of explosive energy
    Close proximity to blast
    Extensive primary and secondary fragmentation
    Biological, chemical, or radiological dissemination
    Occurrence of building collapse
Environmental factors
    Surrounding medium – underwater vs air
    Confined space explosion
    Rural or isolated locale – poor resource availability
    Toxic fumes, dust, and debris
Anatomic and physiological injuries
    Multiple body systems injured
    Injury severity score > 15
    Age < 60, multiple comorbidities
    Primary blast injury
        Tympanic membrane rupture
        Blast lung injury with respiratory failure
        Bowel injury
        Brain injury
        Spine and spinal cord injury
        Traumatic amputation
Secondary and tertiary blast injury
    Blunt and penetrating torso injuries
    Impalement
    Skull fractures
    Glasgow Coma Score < 10
    Foreign body implantation (metallic, glass, human remains)
Quarternary blast injury
    Extensive and deep burns
    Crush injuries
    Toxic inhalation injuries
    Biological, chemical, radiological exposure/contamination/ingestion
Casualty management factors
    Hospital overload
    Treatment delay
    Triage accuracy
    Disorganized casualty flow
    Absence of surgical capability

Typically underestimated in hospital disaster plans are the number of ED beds needed to accommodate the incoming casualties, the number of medical provider volunteers who tend to rush uninvited into the ED to help, and the extent to which imaging, especially CT scanning, is overutilized to create a potentially dangerous bottleneck in casualty flow. These data demonstrate the importance of rapidly clearing the ED of existing patients to develop a surge capacity of space for casualties,[57] of restricting access to the ED and OR to all but essential personnel to avoid a "mass provider" incident that worsens the actual disaster, of *not* requiring only the most senior and experienced surgeons to do triage who may be more effective in other roles, and of strictly limiting the degree to which diagnostic imaging and laboratory testing are permitted during the acute casualty influx to maximize smooth and always forward casualty flow.[41,57]

The hospital resources in highest immediate demand in explosive mass-casualty events are the ED, OR, and ICU. In one study of casualty flow following terrorist bombings in Israel,[65] 65% of 325 casualties from 32 incidents arrived in the ED within 30 min, and 36% were transported directly from the ED to the OR for urgent surgery. Multidisciplinary surgical teams are typically required for the multidimensional injuries of these victims, with abdominal, neurosurgical, thoracic, and vascular surgeons being required in the initial hours, and orthopedic and plastic surgeons predominating later for less urgent injuries.[7] Anesthesiologists are required continually during the event. A policy of *surgical conservatism* was adopted, in which operations on the incoming casualties are withheld as long as possible to conserve the available ORs for those with the most urgent needs. This was found to most effectively match resources to casualty needs, preventing a premature overloading of the OR with cases that could be delayed, to allow the most urgent cases immediate use. The tendency to rush casualties to the OR as they arrive should be restrained.

Another study of suicide bombing events in Israel[60] showed that the ICU is the hospital resource most in demand following explosive disasters, and is very resource-intensive with 73% of admissions requiring mechanical ventilation. One-third of hospitalized casualties were admitted to the ICU, 31% of these directly from the ED. One idea for expanding the surge capacity of the ICU is to use the OR recovery room (postanesthesia care unit, PACU-Postanesthesia Care Unit) as the ICU for postoperative patients requiring critical care, thus alleviating the bed strain in the actual ICU.

Senior ED physicians, surgeons, and intensivists are utilized as *controllers* in their respective clinical areas. These positions do not participate in medical treatment, but oversee the entire operation of casualty care to assure efficient and rapid casualty flow, brief surgery, avoidance of traffic gridlocks, and the appropriate disposition of casualties from the ED to the OR and ICU with a minimum of unnecessary evaluation, imaging, and laboratory testing. This function further contributes to error tolerance by serving as a safety net, to assure that triage, treatment, and disposition errors are corrected at each successive echelon of care, and do not impact casualty outcomes.[21,60]

There will always be a point at which casualty flow into a hospital will overwhelm its resources and its capability to provide optimal care for each individual patient, as medical providers normally practice. It is at this point that the paradigm change in medical care must occur to provide the greatest good for the greatest number to optimize overall casualty salvage.[10] Altered standards of care involving rationing of resources must occur.[56] A computer modeling study using data from 22 suicide bombing events in Israel shows that this "tipping point" in casualty care is reached at only 4.6 critical casualties arriving per hour with the resources normally available in an American trauma center.[66] Effective planning and preparedness, and efficient and accurate triage, can increase this capability for optimal care of mass casualties.

Conclusion

Like most disasters of all kinds, major explosions result in bodily injury to its victims. Surgeons and their teams must therefore be leaders in disaster planning and preparedness.[4,21,67] In particular, trauma surgeons should be integrally involved in these efforts, as they have experience and training to manage large numbers of seriously injured patients, to make rapid decisions with limited information, and to understand the organizational management of a hospital disaster response.[68] This requires active involvement in the multidisciplinary hospital disaster planning process that is the essential component of disaster preparedness.[69] Furthermore, coordination of health care providers over large regions that are subject to similar disaster threats promises to enhance the success of a regional medical response in geographically extensive disasters.[70]

Trauma centers should likewise be the foundation of any local, regional, or national disaster system. There are already state and national trauma systems in place in the United States. Trauma centers and systems already have resources in place to manage large numbers of severely injured patients, and they have the liaisons with the emergency medical services (EMS), emergency management, and public health infrastructure, transportation and communication assets, other hospitals, and relief agencies, which are so necessary in a disaster response.[4,18,71-74]

Education and training are necessary to successfully participate in the response to an explosive or any other form of disaster. However, blast injury and disaster management principles are not routinely taught in medical or nursing schools or residency training, resulting in poor preparation to respond to mass-casualty events.[75] There also exists a major disconnect in training and engagement between the medical sector and the nonmedical government-controlled disaster response infrastructure, even though both must function seamlessly in an actual disaster response. These hurdles must be overcome through a concerted educational campaign among acute care providers to understand the physics and pathophysiology of blast, and the approach to its diagnosis and treatment in the context of the unique challenges of the medical response to a mass-casualty event.

References

1. U.S. Department of State. International Terrorism. Selected documents, No. 24. Washington, D.C.: U.S. Government Printing Office; 1986.
2. Slater MS, Trunkey DD. Terrorism in America: An evolving threat. Arch Surg. 1997;132:1059–1066.
3. Frykberg ER. Principles of mass casualty management following terrorist disasters. Ann Surg. 2004;239:319–321.
4. Frykberg, ER. Medical management of disasters and mass casualties from terrorist bombings: How can we cope? J Trauma. 2002;53:201–212.
5. Kluger Y. Bomb explosions in acts of terrorism–Detonation, wound ballistics, triage and medical concerns. Isr Med J. 2003;5:235–240.

6. Thompson D, Brown S, Mallonee S, Sunshine D. Fatal and non-fatal injuries among U.S. Air Force personnel resulting from the terrorist bombing of the Khobar Towers. J Trauma. 2004;57:208–215.

7. Torkki M, Koljonen V, Sillanpaa K, et al. Triage in a bomb disaster with 166 casualties. Eur J Trauma. 2006;32:374–380.

8. Rignault DP, Deligny MC. The 1986 terorist bombing experience in Paris. Ann Surg. 1989;209:368–373.

9. Terror Attack Database. International Policy Institute for Counter-Terrorism. http://www.ict.org.il. Accessed February 16, 2008.

10. Arnold JL, Tsai M-C, Halpern P, Smithline H, Stok E, Ersoy G. Mass-casualty, terrorist bombings: Epidemiological outcomes, resource utilization, and time course of emergency needs (Part I). Prehospital Disaster Med. 2003;18:220–234.

11. Federal Bureau of Investigation. 1997 Bomb Summary. Bomb Data Center. Washington, D.C.: U.S. Department of Justice; 1998.

12. Macdonald LM. The Curse of the Narrows: The Halifax Disaster of 1917. New York, NY: Walker Publishing Company, Inc.; 2005.

13. Stephens HW. The Texas City Disaster, 1947. Austin, TX: University of Texas Press; 1947.

14. Frykberg ER, Tepas JJ, Alexander RH. The 1983 Beirut airport terrorist bombing: Injury patterns and implications for disaster management. Am Surg. 1989;55:134–141.

15. Mallonee S, Shariat S, Stennies G, et al. Physical injuries and fatalities resulting from the Oklahoma City bombing. JAMA. 1996;276:382–387.

16. Biancolini CA, Del Bosco CG, Jorge MA. Argentine Jewish Community Institution bomb explosion. J Trauma. 1999;47:728–732.

17. Leibovici D, Gofrit ON, Stein M, et al. Blast injuries: Bus versus open-air bombings–A comparative study of injuries in survivors of open-air versus confined-space explosions. J Trauma. 1996;41:1030–1035.

18. Guiterrez de Ceballos JP, Turegano-Fuentes F, Perez-Diaz D, et al. 11 March 2004: The terrorist bomb explosions in Madrid, Spain–An analysis of the logistics, injuries sustained and clinical management of casualties treated at the closest hospital. Crit Care. 2005;9:104–111.

19. Aylwin CJ, Konig TC, Brennan NW, et al. Reduction in critical mortality in urban mass casualty incidents: Analysis of triage, surge, and resource use after the London bombings on July 7, 2005. Lancet. 2006;368:2219–2225.

20. Wightman JM, Gladish SL. Explosions and blast injuries. Ann Emerg Med. 2001;37:664–678.

21. Stein M, Hirshberg A. Medical consequences of terrorism: The conventional weapons threat. Surg Clin North Am. 1999;79:1537–1552.

22. Jacobs LM, Ramp JM, Breay JM. An emergency medical system approach to disaster planning. J Trauma. 1979;19:157–162.

23. Clemedsson CJ. Blast injury. Physiol Rev. 1956;36:336–354.

24. Candole CA. Blast injury. Canad Med Assoc J. 1967;96:207–214.

25. Rawlins JSP. Physical and pathophysiological effects of blast injury. Injury. 1977;9:313–320.

26. Hill JF. Blast injury with particular reference to recent terrorist bombing incidents. Ann R Coll Surg Engl. 1979;61:4–11.

27. Cooper GJ, Maynard RL, Cross NL, Hill JF. Casualties from terrorist bombings. J Trauma. 1983;23:955–967.

28. Phillips YY. Primary blast injuries. Ann Emerg Med 1986;15:1446–1450.
29. Glenshaw MT, Vernick JS, Guohua L, Sorock GS, Brown S, Mallonee S. Preventing fatalities in building bombings: What can we learn from the Oklahoma City bombing? Disast Med Pub Health Preparedness. 2007;1:27–33.
30. Feliciano DV, Anderson GV, Rozycki GS, et al. Management of casualties from the bombing at the Centennial Olympics. Am J Surg. 1998;176:538–543.
31. Kluger Y, Peleg K, Daniel-Aharonson L, et al. The special injury pattern in terrorist bombings. J Am Coll Surg. 2004;199:875–879.
32. Peleg K, Aharonson-Daniel L, Stein M, et al. Gunshot and explosion injuries: Characteristics, outcomes, and implications for care of terror-related injuries in Israel. Ann Surg. 2004;239:311–318.
33. Shamir M, Weiss YG, Willner D, et al. Multiple casualty terror events: The anesthesiologist's perspective. Anesth Analg. 2004;98:1746–1752.
34. Almogy G, Rivkind AI. Surgical lessons learned from suicide bombing attacks. J Am Coll Surg. 2006;202:313–319.
35. Haik J, Tessone A, Givon A, et al. Terror-inflicted thermal injury: A retrospective analysis of burns in the Israeli-Palestinian conflict between the years 1997 and 2003. J Trauma. 2006:1501–1505.
36. Shapira SC, Adatto-Levi R, Avitzour M, et al. Mortality in terrorist attacks: A unique modal of temporal death distribution. World J Surg. 2006;30:2071–2079.
37. Frykberg ER, Tepas JJ. Terrorist bombings: Lessons learned from Belfast to Beirut. Ann Surg. 1988;208:569–576.
38. Leibovici D, Gofrit ON, Shapira SC. Eardrum perforation in explosion survivors: Is it a marker of pulmonary blast injury? Ann Emerg Med. 1999;34:168–172.
39. Turegano-Fuentes F, Caba-Doussoux P, Jover-Navalon JM, et al. Injury patterns from major urban terrorist bombings in trains: The Madrid experience. World J Surg. 2008;32(6):1168–1175.
40. Pizov R, Oppenheim-Eden A, Matot I, et al. Blast lung injury from an explosion on a civilian bus. Chest. 1999;115:165–172.
41. Halpern P, Tsai M-C, Arnold JL, Stok E, Ersoy G. Mass-casualty, terrorist bombings: Implications for emergency department and hospital emergency response. Prehospital Disaster Med. 2003;18:235–241.
42. Steuer G, Goodman S, Levin P, et al. Acute lung injuries among survivors of suicide bomb attacks. In: Shermer J, Shoenfeld Y, eds. Terror and Medicine: Medical Aspects of Biological, Chemical and Radiological Terrorism. Lengerich, Germany: Pabst Science Publishers; 2003:420–432.
43. DePalma RG, Burris DG, Champion HR, Hodgson MJ. Blast injuries. N Engl J Med. 2005;352:1335–1342.
44. Born CT. Blast trauma: The fourth weapon of mass destruction. Scand J Surg. 2005;94:279–285.
45. Hull JB, Cooper GJ. Pattern and mechanism of traumatic amputation by explosive blast. J Trauma. 1996;40(suppl):S198–S200.
46. Phillips YY, Mundie TG, Yelverton YT, Richmond DR. Cloth ballistic vest alters response to blast. J Trauma. 1988;28(suppl):S149–S152.
47. Sheffy N, Rivkind AI, Shapira SC. Terror-related injuries: A comparison of gunshot wounds versus secondary-fragments-induced injuries from explosives. J Am Coll Surg. 2006;203:297–303.
48. Braverman I, Wexler D, Oren M. A novel mode of infection with hepatitis B: Penetrating bone fragments due to the explosion of a suicide bomber. Isr Med Assoc J. 2002;4:528–529.

49. Leibner ED, Weil Y, Gross E, Liebergall M, Mosheiff R. A broken bone without a fracture: Traumatic foreign bone implantation resulting from a mass casualty bombing. J Trauma. 2005;58:388–390.

50. Wong JM, Marsh D, Abu-Sitta G, et al. Biological foreign body implantation in victims of the London July 7th suicide bombings. J Trauma. 2006;60:402–404.

51. Amir LD, Aharonson-Daniel L, Peleg K, Waisman Y, and the Israel Trauma Group. The severity of injury in children resulting from acts against civilian populations. Ann Surg. 2005;241:666–670.

52. Ciraulo DL, Frykberg ER. The surgeon and acts of civilian terrorism: Blast injuries. J Am Coll Surg. 2006;203:942–950.

53. Galea S, Ahern J, Resnick H, et al. Psychological sequelae of the September 11 terrorist attacks in New York City. N Engl J Med. 2002;346:982–987.

54. Waeckerle JF. Disaster planning and response. N Engl J Med. 1991;324:815–821.

55. Almogy G, Luria T, Richter E, et al. Can external signs of trauma guide management? Lessons learned from suicide bombing attacks in Israel. Arch Surg. 2005;140: 390–393.

56. Phillips SJ, Knebel A (eds). Mass Medical Care with Scarce Resources: A Community Planning Guide. Prepared by Health Systems Research, Inc., an Altarum company, under contract No. 290-04-0010. AHRQ Publication No. 07–0001. Rockville, MD: Agency for Healthcare Research and Quality; 2007.

57. National Center for Injury Prevention and Control. In A Moment's Notice: Surge Capacity for Terrorist Bombings. Atlanta, GA: Centers for Disease Control and Prevention; 2007.

58. Frykberg ER. Triage: Principles and practice. Scand J Surg. 2005;94:272–278.

59. Rignault DP. Recent progress in surgery for the victims of disaster, terrorism and war. World J Surg. 1992;16:885–887.

60. Avidan V, Hersch M, Spira RM, Einav S, Goldberg S, Schecter W. Civilian hospital response to a mass casualty event: The role of the intensive care unit. J Trauma. 2007;62:1234–1239.

61. Asaeda G. The day that the START triage system came to a STOP: Observations from the World Trade Center disaster. Acad Emerg Med. 2002;9:255–256.

62. Richards ME, Nufer KE. Simple triage and rapid treatment: Does it predict transportation and referral needs in patients evaluated by Disaster Medical Assistance Teams? Ann Emerg Med. 2004;44(suppl):S33–S34.

63. Ashkenazi I, Kessel B, Khashan T, et al. Precision of in-hospital triage in mass-casualty incidents after terror attacks. Prehospital Disaster Med. 2006;21:20–23.

64. Hirshberg A, Stein M, Walden R. Surgical resource utilization in urban terrorist bombing: A computer simulation. J Trauma. 1999;47:545–550.

65. Einav S, Aharonson-Daniel L, Weissman C, et al. In-hospital resource utilization during multiple casualty incidents. Ann Surg. 2006;243:533–540.

66. Hirshberg A, Scott BG, Granchi T, et al. How does casualty load affect trauma care in urban bombing incidents? A quantitative analysis. J Trauma. 2005;58:686–695.

67. Ciraulo DL, Barie PS, Briggs SM, et al. An update on the scope and depth of practice to All-Hazards emergency response. J Trauma. 2006;60:1267–1274.

68. Lennquist S. Management of major accidents and disasters: An important responsibility for the trauma surgeons. J Trauma. 2007;62:1321–1329.

69. Hammond JS. Mass casualty incidents: Planning implications for trauma care. Scand J Surg. 2005;94:267–271.

70. Mattox K, McSwain N, Frykberg ER, et al. Position statement from the steering committee of the Atlantic-Gulf States Disaster Medical Coalition: Integrated collaborative networks will facilitate mass casualty medical response. J Am Coll Surg. 2007;205:612–616.

71. Frykberg ER. Disaster and mass casualty management: A commentary on the American College of Surgeons position statement. J Am Coll Surg. 2003;197:857–859.

72. Ammons MA, Moore EE, Pons PT, et al. The role of a regional trauma system in the management of a mass disaster: An analysis of the Keystone, Colorado chairlift accident. J Trauma. 1988;28:1468–1471.

73. Champion HR, Mabee MS, Meredith JW. The state of US trauma systems: Public perceptions versus reality—Implications for US response to terrorism and mass casualty events. J Am Coll Surg. 2006;203:951–961.

74. Treat KN, Williams JM, Furbee PM, Manley WG, Russell FK, Stamper CD. Hospital preparedness for weapons of mass destruction incidents: An initial assessment. Ann Emerg Med. 2001;38:562–565.

75. Ciraulo DL, Frykberg ER, Feliciano DV, et al. A survey assessment of preparedness for domestic terrorism and mass casualty incidents among Eastern Association for the Surgery of Trauma members. J Trauma. 2004;56:1033–1041.

12
Biological Agents and Terror Medicine

Meir Oren

In the last decade, terror has become an increasingly global problem. More people have become radicalized, the know-how to use weapons of mass destruction (WMD) is easily accessible by Internet and electronic media, and precursors and basic ingredients are easily purchased. Terrorists are innovative and we now face a new era of nonconventional terrorism: chemical, biological, radiological, nuclear (CBRN), as well as cyber terrorism.

The deliberate use of (WMD–CBRN) by hostile states or terrorists and of naturally emerging infectious diseases that have a potential to cause illness on a massive scale could pose a national security threat.[1] Resulting panic and economic damage could paralyze a country.

Terrorists can act as independent groups or individuals, or can be sponsored, directed, and motivated by states. The use of bioagents intended to harm people, environments, or governments may also be deemed a biocrime. Assessing the threat of bioterrorism and its potential outcome was evaluated in tabletop exercises and mathematical modeling. TOPOFF 2 tested the scenario of a chemical attack in New Hampshire, a radiological event in Washington DC, and a biological event (plague) in Denver, Colorado.[2] Dark Winter exercise (2001–2002) tested a scenario of simultaneous spread of smallpox in Pennsylvania, Georgia, and Oklahoma.[3] TOPOFF 3 (April 2005) tested the scenario of a chemical attack in Connecticut, a bioterror event (pneumonic plague) in New Jersey and international involvement in United Kingdom and Canada.[4]

Bioterrorism has been described by the Center for Disease Control and Prevention (CDC) as "the deliberate release of viruses, bacteria, or other germs (agents) used to cause illness or death in people, animals, or plants. These agents are typically found in nature, but they could possibly be changed to increase their ability to cause disease, make them resistant to current medicines, or to increase their ability to be spread into the environment. Biological agents can be spread through the air, through water, or in food. Terrorists may use biological agents because they can be extremely difficult to detect and do not cause illness for several hours to several days. Some bioterrorism agents, like the smallpox virus, can be spread from person to person and some, like anthrax, cannot."[5]

The use of bioagents by military forces in battlefield conflicts has occurred throughout history.[6] It is generally assumed that only state-sponsored terrorists have

S.C. Shapira et al. (eds.), *Essentials of Terror Medicine*,
DOI: 10.1007/978-0-387-09412-0_12, Springer Science+Business Media, LLC 2009

the technical and scientific capability to weaponize biological agents. While it is questionable how effective terrorists can be in manufacturing or producing a bio-weapon, we should be aware that the advanced biological warfare (ABW) agents, including classical agents that could be genetically manipulated or engineered, pose a new and complicated challenge.[7] (Table 12.1)

The biological weapons system comprises four components:

1. *The biological material* consisting of the infectious agent or a toxin produced by bacteria, plants, or animals is the payload.
2. *Munitions* are the agents that carry, protect, and maintain the virulence of the payload during delivery.
3. *The delivery system* can range from a missile, a vehicle (aircraft, boat, auto-mobile, or truck), an artillery shell, an expendable soldier, or martyr, to mailed letters, as was the case with the 2001 anthrax incidents.
4. *The dispersion system* ensures dissemination of the payload at and around the target site among susceptible populations.[9–11]Potential methods of dispersion include aerosol sprays, explosives, and food and water contamination. Aerosol sprays are the most likely method to be used in a potential bioterrorism attack because they are the most effective means of widespread dissemination.[12]

The anthrax attack also demonstrated the effectiveness of the postal system as a facilitator of dispersion.[13]

TABLE 12.1. Case definitions of suspected or confirmed cases due to deliberate release

Deliberate release of anthrax
  • ≥1 confirmed case of inhalation anthrax.
  • ≥1 confirmed case of cutaneous anthrax arising in individuals who do not routinely have contact with animals or animal hides.
  • ≥2 suspected cases of anthrax that are linked in time and place, especially geographically related groups of illness following a wind direction pattern.
Deliberate release of smallpox
  • A single confirmed case.
Deliberate release of plague
  • A single confirmed case in the European Union must be regarded with a high degree of suspicion of deliberate release.
  • A confirmed case of plague in a person without history of being outdoors or having contact with animals.
  • ≥2 suspected cases of plague that are linked in time and place, especially to a particular pattern.
Deliberate release of tularemia
  • Single confirmed case of indigenously acquired tularemia NOT explained by occupational expo-sure.
Deliberate release of botulism
  • Clusters of >2 cases of acute flaccid paralysis with prominent bulbar palsies, especially where there are common geographic factors between cases, but no common dietary exposure or injected drug use.
  • Multiple simultaneous outbreaks with no obvious common source.
  • Cases of botulism with an unusual toxin type (type C, D, F or G or E not acquired from an aquatic food).

Source: From Bossi et al.,[8] reprinted with permission from Springer Science + Business Media.

The Centers for Disease Control and Prevention places the bioagents into three categories (A, B, and C), depending on how easily they can be spread and the severity of illness or death they cause (Table 12.2). Category A agents are considered the highest risk and Category C agents are those that are considered emerging

TABLE 12.2. Critical biological agent categories for public health preparedness

Biological agent(s)	Disease
Category A	
Variola major	Smallpox
Bacillus anthracis	Anthrax
Yersinia pestis	Plague
Clostridium botulinum (botulinum toxins)	Botulism
Francisella tularensis	Tularemia
Filoviruses and Arenaviruses (e.g., Ebola virus, Lassa virus)	Viral hemorrhagic fevers
Category B	
Coxiella burnetii	Q fever
Brucella spp.	Brucellosis
Burkholderia mallei	Glanders
Burkholderia pseudomallei	Melioidosis
Alphaviruses (VEE, EEE, WEE)	Encephalitis
Rickettsia prowazekii	Typhus fever
Toxins	
(e.g., Ricin, Staphylococcal enterotoxin B)	Toxic syndromes
Chlamydia psittaci	Psittacosis
Food safety threats (e.g., *Salmonella spp.*, *Escherichia coli* O157:H7)	
Water safety threats (e.g., *Vibrio cholerae, Cryptosporidium parvum*)	
Category C	
Emerging threat agents (e.g., *Nipah virus*, hantavirus)	

Venezuelan equine (VEE), Eastern equine (EEE), and Western equine encephalomyelitis (WEE) viruses.[14]

A recent publication by the US Department of Health and Human Services, [1] based on a list of Material Threat Determinations (MTDs) determined by the Department of Homeland security, describes the agents.

Material Threat Determinants (MTDs) and Population Threat Assessments
    (PTAs) issued to date by the Department of Homeland Security:
Bacillus anthracis (ANTHRAX)
Botulinum toxins (BOTULISM)
Burkholderia mallei (GLANDERS)
Burkholderia pseudomallei (MELIODOSIS)
Ebola virus (HEMORRHAGIC FEVER)
Francisella tularensis (TULAREMIA)
Junin virus (HEMORRHAGIC FEVER)
Marburg virus (HEMORRHAGIC FEVER)
Multidrug resistant B. anthracis (MDR ANTHRAX)
Radiological/nuclear agents
Ricketsia prowazekii (TYPHUS)
Variola virus (SMALLPOX)
Volatile nerve agents (PTA only)
Y. pestis (PLAGUE)

TABLE 12.3. Characteristics of category A agents

- They can be easily spread or transmitted from person to person.
- They result in high death rates and have the potential for major public health impact.
- They might cause public panic and social disruption.
- They require special action for public health preparedness.[5]

threats for disease. In this chapter, we will touch primarily on the medical aspects and main points concerning those agents that are categorized as Category A biological agents with relevance to bioterrorism. Specific attributes of these agents are listed in Table 12.3.

The pediatric age group in relation to bioterrorism deserves special attention.[15–17] Children may be more vulnerable than adults to biological agents because of their higher metabolic and respiratory rates, their proximity to the ground, and their frequent hand–mouth contact. In addition, they may act as vectors through nuclear and extended families, day care, and school systems.

Early attribution of a cluster of febrile, respiratory illnesses to an intentional release of a bioagent might be difficult in children because children are prone to respiratory symptoms with common colds more often than adults, and they cannot easily report the subtleties of their own symptoms.[18] Strict isolation is complicated in children. Young patients might need to be sedated, especially if isolated in negative pressure tents or rooms. Parents might need to remain with their children in isolation, which could expose them to the infectious agents.

Anthrax

Anthrax is a spore-forming gram-positive bacillus considered to be one of the most likely biological agents for use as a weapon. *Bacillus anthracis* spores can even be transmitted by aerosolization.

The name has its origin in the Greek word for coal, *anthracis*, after the characteristic black skin lesion it produces.[19] Anthrax is primarily a zoonotic disease of sheep and cattle. Spores can remain viable in the soil and infective to grazing livestock for many decades.[20] Humans get infected through skin contact and ingestion or inhalation of spores, typically from infected animals or animal products. Person-to-person transmission has not been documented.

Once introduced into the body, the spores are ingested by macrophages and travel to draining lymph nodes, where they germinate to their vegetative bacillary forms. The bacillus then produces an antiphagocytic capsule and three proteins: protective antigen, lethal factor, and edema factor. These act in binary combinations to form toxins. The protective antigen binds with the lethal factor to form lethal toxin and binds to the edema factor to form edema toxin, both of which play key roles in the pathogenesis of the disease.[21]

Cutaneous Anthrax

Approximately 95% of naturally occurring human anthrax is cutaneous and occurs when spores encounter openings in skin. Within 1–12 days after exposure to the spores, a susceptible patient develops a pruritic macule or papule. This progresses to a vesicle in 1–2 days and is followed by erosion, leaving a necrotic ulcer with a small painless, depressed black eschar. Diagnosis is often confused by its similarity to insect bites. The patient may also have symptoms of fever, malaise, headache, and lymphadenopathy. The case fatality rate is up to 20% without therapy and less than 1% with antibiotic treatment.[22]

Gastrointestinal Anthrax

This form of anthrax is rare and is the consequence of eating undercooked, contaminated meat. The incubation period varies from 1 to 7 days. Gastrointestinal anthrax is characterized by acute inflammation of the intestinal tract. Symptoms include fever, abdominal pain, anorexia, nausea, and vomiting. Bloody diarrhea and hematemesis frequently accompany the symptoms. The case fatality rate is unclear but is thought to range from 25% to 60%.

Inhalational Anthrax

Deliberately aerosolizing dry spores could induce widespread inhalation anthrax, the most lethal form of the disease. The spread of anthrax through the US mail in 2001 heightened concern about the feasibility of large-scale dispersal of bioagents by terrorist groups. *B. anthracis* was delivered by mail to various recipients and chiefly intended to cause inhalational anthrax disease. Twenty-two cases were identified, 11 of them inhalational associated with 5 fatalities, 7 confirmed as cutaneous, and 4 suspected cutaneous cases.[23]

Aerosolized anthrax spores of 2–3 μm can pass through the bronchi to the alveoli and be transported via the lymphatics to the hilar and mediastinal lymph nodes, where germination to the bacillary form may occur.[8] Spore may not immediately germinate and may continue to vegetate in the host for several weeks after inhalation. After alveolar macrophages incorporate the spores, the spores germinate and begin replication. That replication releases several toxins, leading to hemorrhagic thoracic lymphadenopathy and mediastinitis, edema, and necrosis. Hemorrhagic meningitis frequently develops and can be observed in up to half of patients. The median incubation period from exposure to the onset of symptoms is 4 days (range 1–7 days), but cases that occurred from 2 to 43 days after exposure have been reported in humans. This period seems to be inversely related to the dose of spores. It is assumed that a dose of 8,000–50,000 spores is sufficient to cause inhalational anthrax.[24]

Early diagnosis is essential for saving lives. The clinical presentation of the disease is classically biphasic. It starts with nonspecific symptoms of sore throat, mild fever, and muscle aches. The patient may also present nonproductive cough, dyspnea, headache, vomiting, chills, weakness, abdominal pain, malaise, and chest pain.[20,8,24] Physical examination is usually unremarkable, but chest examination can reveal bilateral decreased breath sounds, rhonchi, and/or inspiratory rales.

The illness progresses to the second phase within 2–3 days. In some patients, a brief period of clinical improvement follows, making it even harder to diagnose the disease. Usually, the second phase begins abruptly with sudden fever and chills, acute dyspnea, retrosternal chest pressure, diaphoresis, cyanosis, and shock.[25] At this stage, a chest X-ray most often shows a widened mediastium consistent with mediastinal lymphadenopathy and hemorrhagic mediastinitis, pleural effusion, and progressive bilateral perihilar infiltrates. CT scan of the chest can demonstrate parenchymal infiltrates or consolidation, large bilateral pleural effusions, pericardial effusions, and a widened mediastinum with a complete infiltration of the mediastinal fat planes, bronchial mucosal thickening, encasement, and compression of the hilar vessels, and hemorrhagic lymph nodes[25] (Table 12.4).

Treatment may be successful in the early stages, but by the time respiratory symptoms develop it is too late for it to have any effect, and death usually occurs within 24–72 hours in almost 90% of cases despite aggressive treatment.[23,28] Death usually occurs 7 days after the onset of symptoms. (Experience with the 2001 attacks suggests outcomes may be less dire since 6 of the 11 inhalation cases survived, and all had respiratory symptoms before treatment.[13]) Person-to-person transmission of inhalation anthrax has never been reported.

Diagnosis

Given the rarity of anthrax, especially the inhalation type, making a diagnosis can be difficult. Early diagnosis and effective antibiotic treatment are essential and are the only way to reduce mortality. Table 12.1 defines the recommended parameters for case definition.

It is very important to take samples before treatment since even one dose of antibiotics may cause sterilization of cultures. Sterilization would negate the chance to grow the organism in a standard blood culture, a traditional test to confirm the presence of the bacterium. Gram stain of vesicular fluids from cutaneous lesions, pleural effusions, CSF Cerebral Spinal Fluid, and ascites are essential for diagnosis. In case of cutaneous anthrax, punch biopsy may also be performed for immunohistochemistry.

Organisms must be tested for sensitivity to antibiotics for natural existence or resistant species and possible genetic manipulation before the deliberate release. Sputum culture and Gram stain are unlikely to be diagnostic of inhalational anthrax given the frequent lack of frank pneumonia.

Rapid identification of *B. anthracis* can be made by direct fluorescent antibody testing and gamma-phage lysis. Confirmatory diagnostic tests such as polymerase chain reaction (PCR) can also be used and may help in early diagnosis.[24] Antibody testing by enzyme-linked immunosorbent assay (ELISA) may yield positive results in convalescent serum specimens. Therefore, serologic testing is useful only retrospectively.

TABLE 12.4. Inhalation/intestinal anthrax

Postexposure prophylaxis (60 days)	Treatment of suspected or confirmed clinical cases of inhalation/intestinal anthrax (60 days)	Target population	
– Ciprofloxacin: 500 Mg per os bid	– Ciprofloxacin: 400 mg IV bid followed by 500 mg os bid	First line	Adults (including pregnant women) It is recommended, when possible, to cease breastfeeding
– Ofloxacin: 400 mg per os bid	– Ofloxacin: 400 mg IV bid followed by 400 mg per os bid	Alternative to ciprofloxacin	
– Levofloxacin: 500 mg per os once a day	– Levofloxacin: 500 mg IV once a day, followed by 500 mg per os once a day		
– Doxycycline: 100 mg per os bid	– Doxycycline: 100 mg IV bid followed by 100 mg bid per os	Alternative first-line treatment and follow-up when susceptibility is confirmed	
– Amoxicillin: 500 mg per os 3 times daily	– Penicillin G: 2.4–3 million units IV, 6 times daily		
	– Amoxicillin: 1 g IV 3 times daily, followed by 500 mg per os 3 times daily	Alternative first-line prophylaxis if susceptibility is confirmed	
– Ciprofloxacin: 10–15 mg/kg per os bid	– Ciprofloxacin: 10–15 mg/kg IV bid followed by 10–15 mg/kg per os bid	First line	Children
– Doxycycline >8 years and >45 kg or >8 years 2.2 mg/kg per os bid (max 200 mg/d)	– Doxycycline: >8 years and >45 kg: adult dose >8 years and <45 kg or <8 years 2.2 mg/kg IV bid followed by 2.2 mg/kg per os bid (max 200 mg/d)	Alternative first-line treatment and follow-up when susceptibility is confirmed	
	– Penicillin G: >12 years: 2.4–3 million units IV, 6 times daily <12 years: 30 mg/kg IV, 4 times daily	Alternative first-line prophylaxis if susceptibility is confirmed	
– Amoxicillin: 80 mg/kg per os daily in 3 divided doses	– Amoxicillin: 80 mg/kg daily in 3 divided doses, followed by 80 mg/kg per os daily in 3 divided doses		

Source: Data from: Bossi et al.,[8] Jernigan et al.,[24] the European Agency for the Evaluation of Medicinal Products,[26] and the Centers for Disease Control and Prevention[27]
IV intravenous, *bid* twice daily

The predictive value of nasal swab test for the diagnosis following exposure to *B. anthracis* spore is unknown. A negative result does not indicate that the patient has not been exposed to *B. anthracis*.

In inhalational anthrax, postmortem findings are thoracic hemorrhagic necrotizing lymphadenitis and mediastinitis, pleural effusions and, in 50% of cases, hemorrhagic meningitis. Usually, there are no signs of pneumonia.

Treatment

Many guidelines have been published on treatment and prophylaxis for anthrax.[20,23,24,26] There is no need to isolate patients with inhalational anthrax. In the case of cutaneous anthrax, health care workers should apply standard precautions with gloves. In the past, penicillin was the drug of choice for inhalational anthrax. It can still be considered as an option only if the strain is susceptible to this drug. Since there have been reports of resistant strains and it is not complicated to induce resistance to penicillin, doxycycline, chloramphenicol, macrolides, and rifampicine,[29] ciprofloxacin is currently the recommended first-line treatment as described in Table 12.4. Moreover, recommendations include administering one or two additional antibiotics in the case of inhalational anthrax, for example, rifampicin, chloramphenicol, clindamycin, or vancomycin.[23,26,30] For inhalation anthrax, the duration of treatment is at least 60 days. For cutaneous anthrax, duration of treatment is 7–10 days. The same antibiotics are recommended for postexposure prophylaxis as for treatment of the disease. Oral ciprofloxacin is also recommended as a first choice for prophylaxis for those who are at risk, and must be taken for at least 60 days. Starting antibiotic treatment within a day after exposure to a bacterial aerosol can provide protection against infection.

Vaccines for use against anthrax are licensed in the UK and the US.[31,32] These are considered to be first generation, and clinical trials on the safety and efficacy of a new recombinant protective antigen (rPA)-based anthrax vaccine have recently been initiated in the US.[33] The US vaccine is administered in a series of six subcutaneous injections: after the initial dose, injections are given at 2 weeks, 4 weeks, 6 months, 12 months, and 18 months, respectively. The UK vaccine is given in a series of four intramuscular injections at 0, 3, 6 weeks and a fourth booster at 6 months after the third dose, followed by annual boosters.

Smallpox

Smallpox is a viral infection caused by the variola virus, which belongs to the family of Poxviridae, which includes monkeypox virus, vaccinia virus, and cowpox virus.[34] It is a single, linear, double-stranded DNA virus. The disease was eradicated worldwide by the World Health Organization (WHO) in 1980 and last endemic case was reported in Somalia in 1977.[35,36] The last fatal reported case was in 1978 due to a laboratory-acquired infection in the UK. Variola virus is seen as one of the most likely viruses to be used as a biological weapon because of the properties of the virus: aerosol infectivity, high mortality, and stability.[34,37] Two different strains of variola virus are known and associated with smallpox: variola major and variola minor.

Clinical Features

Person-to-person transmission is the most common route of transmission but requires close contact.[35] Patients are not infectious during the asymptomatic incubation period (4–19 days; mean 10–12 days) before fever occurs. Smallpox is mostly contagious during the first week of rash, corresponding to the period when the lesions of the enanthem are ulcerated. At this stage, aerosol droplets from oropharyngeal lesions increase the likelihood of person-to-person transmission.

After aerosol exposure, the virus infects regional lymph nodes around the respiratory tract and in other lymphoid tissues such as the spleen, liver, bone marrow, lung, and other lymph nodes and causes the first wave of viremia. After a second viremia period, the virus localizes in small blood vessels of the dermis and in the oral and pharyngeal mucosa and proceeds to infect adjacent cells. Viruses remain present in the lesions until all scabs have been shed following recovery. At this stage, while viruses are enclosed within hard dry scabs, infectivity is lower than in the initial stage of the disease. Historically, it has been estimated that 30% of susceptible household members became infected when smallpox was endemic. Variola virus is stable and it has been estimated that it can be viable in certain conditions for up to a year in dust and cloth.[35]

Variola Major (Classical Smallpox)

The most virulent strain of variola virus causes variola major. Five clinical forms of variola major which differ in prognosis are described.[27,35]

Ordinary-Type Smallpox

This is the most common form and occurs in 90% of cases. The prodromal phase (2–3 days) has an abrupt onset and is characterized by severe and generalized headache, fever (>40°C), extreme prostration, intense, ill-defined pain in the back, chest or joints, intense anxiety, and occasionally abdominal pain. Children may have convulsions, and some adults are delirious. The fever subsides over a period of 2–3 days. Then, enanthem appears over the tongue, palate, mouth, and oropharynx. Usually, a day after, exanthema begins as a small reddish maculopapular rash on the face and forearms and spreads gradually with a centrifugal distribution within 24 hours to the trunk and legs and then to all parts of the body, including the palms of the hands and the soles of the feet. Within 1–2 days, the rash becomes vesicular (diameter of vesicle 2–5 mm), and then pustular.

The pustules, which are round, tense, and deeply embedded in the dermis, remain for 5–8 days, followed by umbilication and crusting. The lesions may vary in number and can be confluent or discrete. A second, less prominent spike of fever can be noted 5–8 days after the onset of the rash. Lesions are generally synchronous in their stage of development, not as in varicella. This characteristic also provides the main distinguishing feature from monkeypox. In the case of monkeypox, there is also remarkable enlargement of inguinal and cervical lymph nodes. Secondary pyogenic infection of the skin may occur, and other complications like panophtalmitis, keratitis, osteomyelitis, arthritis, orchitis, pneumonitis, pulmonary edema, and so on.

Death may occur in the first 48 hours, before any feature of smallpox has appeared. Most fulminant cases of death occur by the 4th or 5th day, and many others die between the 8th and 15th day. Mortality rate is 30% in unvaccinated and 3% in vaccinated individuals.

Hemorrhagic-Type Smallpox

This is the most virulent form of the disease. It occurs in 3% of the patients and is characterized by hemorrhages into the skin and/or the mucous membranes and toxemia. Death rate is 96% in unvaccinated and 94% in vaccinated individuals, usually before the occurrence of the lesions.

Other Types

The modified-type smallpox or milder-type, the flat-type smallpox, variola sine eruptione, and variola minor are other less virulent types of smallpox.

Diagnosis

Case definition of suspected or confirmed cases is described in Table 12.1. Differentiation between smallpox and other orthopoxes can be done by electron microscopy and by PCR assay and/or restriction fragment length polymorphism (RFLP).[27,36] Definitive characterization of the variola virus is made by culture in eggs and cell monolayers.

Treatment

Patients with smallpox must be isolated and managed, preferably if possible, in negative pressure rooms until death or for about 3 weeks until all scabs have been shed. There is no proof of any antiviral drug being effective in clinical cases. Antibiotics may be useful in secondary infections. The most effective measure of prevention is vaccination before exposure. Side effects due to vaccination are low but higher than with other vaccines. The more severe complications noted were postvaccinial encephalitis, progressive vaccinia, eczema vaccinatum, and generalized vaccinia.[35] However, vaccination can also modify the course of the disease and reduce mortality by 100% if given immediately after exposure, and by up to 50% if given within 4 days after exposure. Currently, a second generation of vaccine is being developed, and there is a need for developing a third-generation vaccine with an acceptable safety profile by attenuating or genetically engineering (disabling) vaccinia vaccine strains, while retaining their immunizing properties.

Plague

Plague is an acute bacterial infection caused by *Yersinia pestis*, a Gram-negative bacillus. Historically, three plague pandemics caused the death of more then 200 million people.[38] The disease, primarily the bubonic form, is still endemic in some parts of the world, mainly in Africa and in the former Soviet Union. Each year about 1,500 cases are reported. Plague is an enzootic infection of rodents, prairie dogs, and squirrels. Human transmission occurs via flea vectors from rodents and by respiratory droplets from animals to humans or humans to humans.

Clinical Features

The three clinical syndromes of plague are bubonic, secondary pneumonic, and primary pneumonic. The last one is the most likely in the event of a bioterror attack, being dispersed by aerosol.[39] Incubation period varies from 2 to 8 days. Bubonic plague is the most common naturally occurring form of the disease. Patients often present with a sudden onset of fever (38.5°C to 40°C) and fatigue and development of a bubo, an acutely tender lymph node. A small fraction of patients develop primary septicemic plague, which is remarkable for the absence of buboes. Secondary pneumonic plague develops via hematogeneous spread of the bacilli to the lungs and manifests as dyspnea, chest pain, hemoptysis, and/or severe bronchopneumonia. Primary pneumonic plague, plague meningitis, and plague pharyngitis are some of the other clinical syndromes associated with plague (Table 12.5).

In primary pneumonic plague, the patient presents with symptoms suggestive of pneumonia, with early onset of high fever, myalgia, malaise, headache, and hemoptysis, often progressing rapidly to sepsis and respiratory failure with signs of dyspnea, stridor, and cyanosis. Patients may also progress to shock and have extensive ecchymosis. Plague pneumonia is highly contagious to other humans by droplet transmission, and patients remain contagious up to 3 days after starting antibiotic treatment. But with prompt use of antibiotics the fatality rate decreases below 10%.

Diagnosis

Case definition of suspected cases or confirmed cases is described in Table 12.6. *Y. pestis* can be cultured from blood, sputum, bubo aspiration, and cerebrospinal fluid. Specimens should be taken before initiating antibiotic treatment. Smears can be stained with Gram, Giemsa, or Wayson's stains to demonstrate the bipolar coccobacilli. Serological tests and direct immunofluorescence for F1 antigen,

TABLE 12.5. Summary of clinical and biological characteristics of plague

Clinical description
– Incubation period: 1–6 days
Pneumonic plague
– Abrupt onset of intense headache and malaise, high fever, vomiting, abdominal pain, diarrhea and marked prostration, chest pain, cough, dyspnea, and hemoptysis
– Chest X-ray: multilobar consolidation, cavities, or bronchopneumonia
– Respiratory failure develops quickly with septicemic/shock
Bubonic plague
– Fever (38.5–40°C), chills, headache, weakness, and bubo
– Surrounding edema and the overlying skin is warm, erythematous, and adherent
Septicemic plague
– Septic shock, vasculitis, livid cyanotic petechiae, large ecchymoses, gangrene of acral regions, and multiorgan failure
– Meningitis occurs in 5% of cases
Presumptive diagnosis
– Staining of specimens
– ELISA, direct immunofluorescence, PCR
Diagnosis
– Isolation of *Yersinia pestis* from a clinical specimen
– Demonstration of a specific antibody response to *Y. pestis* fraction 1 (F1) antigen
– Elevated serum antibody titers to *Y. pestis* F1 antigen (without documented specific change) in a patient with no history of plague vaccination
– Detection of F1 antigen in a clinical specimen by fluorescent assay
Management of treatment
– If plague pneumonia, isolation in a negative pressure room (if possible)
– Gentamicin or streptomycin as first-line therapy with ciprofloxacin as an alternative (see also Table 12.7)
– Chloramphenicol should be used for the treatment of meningitis
– Persons in contact (<2 m) with pneumonic plague should receive antibiotic prophylaxis with doxycycline or ciprofloxacin for 7 days. Other antibiotics (chloramphenicol, sulfadiazine, trimethoprim-sulfamethoxazole, etc.) could also be used

Source: Data from: Bossi et al.[39]
PCR polymerase chain reaction, ELISA enzyme-linked immunosorbent assay

TABLE 12.6. Case definitions of possible, probable, and confirmed cases of plague

Possible case
– Sudden onset of severe, unexplained febrile respiratory illness
– Unexplained death following a short febrile illness
– Sepsis with Gram-negative coccobacilli identified from clinical specimens
Probable case
– A case that clinically fits the criteria for suspected plague, and in addition, positive results are obtained on one or more specimens
Confirmed case
– A clinically compatible case with confirmatory laboratory results
– Culture of *Yersinia pestis* from a clinical specimen and confirmation of identification by phage lysis
– A significant (fourfold) change in antibody titre to F1 antigen in paired serum samples
– A definitive diagnosis, by positive PCR or detection of F1 antigen on suspect isolates, will be available within one working day

Source: Data from the Official Journal of the European Communities[40,41]

Table 12.7. Criteria for suspecting deliberate release of plague

Deliberate release
– A single confirmed case in the European Union must be regarded with a high degree of suspicion of deliberate release[a]
– A confirmed case of plague in a person without history of being outdoors or having contact with animals
– ≥2 suspected cases of plague that are linked in time and place, especially if the suspected cases are geographically related according to a particular wind pattern

[a]Cases that occur in people who have returned from endemic areas should be investigated to ascertain that the illness did not occur with intent to deliberately release *Yersinia pestis*

specific phage lysis, and PCR for the plasminogen activator gene, are all available, preferably to be done at reference laboratories (Table 12.7).

Treatment

Treatment should be initiated as soon as the diagnosis is suspected; see Table 12.8. Many antibiotics are active against *Y. pestis*, and most guidelines suggest using Gentamycin or streptomycin as first-line therapy with ciprofloxacin as an alternative.[25,35,36,38,39,42] Chloramphenicol should be used for the treatment of meningitis. Persons who come in contact (<2 m) with patients with pneumonic plague should receive antibiotic prophylaxis with doxycycline or ciprofloxacin for 7 days. Prevention of human-to-human transmission from patients with pneumonic plague pneumonia can be achieved by implementing standard isolation precautions until at least 4 days of antibiotic treatment have been administered. For the other clinical types of the disease, patients should be isolated for the first 48 hours after the initiation of treatment. Health care workers should wear high-efficiency respirators.

Botulism

Aerosols of botulinum toxin could be used as a biological weapon.[37,43–45] Deliberate release may also involve contamination of food or water supplies with toxin or *Clostridium botulinum* bacteria. Botulinum toxin is extremely lethal and easy to produce.[8] The *C. botulinum* is a large, Gram-positive, strictly anaerobic bacillus that forms a subterminal spore. These spores can be found in soil and marine sediments throughout the world. Four groups of *C. botulinum* are shown in Fig. 12.1.

The toxins are ingested or inhaled and their effect is similar. Botulinum toxin does not penetrate intact skin. Toxins act by binding to the presynaptic nerve terminal at the neuromuscular junction and at cholinergic autonomic sites. This binding prevents release of acetylcholine and interrupts neurotransmission. Human botulism is almost always caused by toxin types A, B, E, and in rare cases F. By inhalation, the LD50 (dose that kills 50% of exposed persons) is 0.003 μg/kg of body weight. This toxin is 100,000 times more toxic than sarin gas.[37]

TABLE 12.8. Recommendations for treatment and postexposure prophylaxis of plague

Target	Population	Treatment of suspected or confirmed clinical cases (10 days)	Postexposure prophylaxis (7 days)
Adults (including pregnant women)	First-line treatment	– Gentamicin: 5 mg/kg IV in 1 or 2 doses daily or – Streptomycin: 1 g IM twice daily	
It is recommended, when possible, to cease breast-feeding	Second-line treatment; First-line prophylaxis	– Ciprofloxacin: 400 mg IV bid followed by 500 mg per os bid or – Ofloxacin: 400 mg IV bid followed by 400 mg per os bid or – Levofloxacin: 500 mg IV once a day, followed by 500 mg per os once a day	– Ciprofloxacin: 500 mg per os bid or – Ofloxacin: 400 mg per os bid or – Levofloxacin: 500 mg per os once a day
	Third-line treatment; Second-line prophylaxis	– Doxycycline: 100 mg IV bid followed by 100 mg bid per os	– Doxycycline: 100 mg bid per os
Children	First-line treatment	– Gentamicin: 2.5 mg/kg IV in 3 doses daily or – Streptomycin: 15 mg/kg IM twice daily (max, 2 g)	
	Second-line treatment; First-line prophylaxis	– Ciprofloxacin: 10–15 mg/kg IV bid followed by 15 mg/kg per os bid	– Ciprofloxacin: 10–15 mg/kg per os bid
	Third-line treatment; Second-line prophylaxis	– Doxycycline: >8 years and >45 kg: adult dose >8 years and <45 kg or >8 years: 2.2 mg/kg IV bid followed by 2.2 mg/kg per os bid (max 200 mg/d)	– Doxycycline: >8 years and >45 kg: adult dose >8 years and< 45 kg or <8 years: 2.2 mg/kg per os bid (max 200 mg/d)

Source: European Agency for the Evaluation of Medicinal Products[26] and Bossi et al.[39]
IV intravenous, *IM* intramuscular

Group I are proteolytic in culture and produce toxin types A, B or F.

Group II are non proteolytic and produce toxins types B, E or F.

Group III produce toxin types C or D.

Group IV toxins produce toxin type G.

FIG. 12.1. Four groups of *Clostridium botulinum.*

Clinical Features

Several forms of botulism are known: three natural forms—food or waterborne, wound, and intestinal (adult and infant)—and a fourth, inhalational botulism, which is a man-made form that results from aerosolized botulinum toxin. The incubation period can be brief, depending on the type and dose of toxin: 12–72 hours (range: 2 hours to 10 days).[46,47] Following aerosol exposure, onset of symptoms may be more rapid, possibly 1 hour after exposure. Person-to-person transmission has never been described.

Regardless of the route of contamination, illness is an acute, afebrile, symmetric, descending flaccid paralysis that begins in the head. Multiple cranial nerve palsies produce diplopia, ptosis, blurred vision, enlarged or sluggishly reactive pupils, photophobia, facial weakness, dysphonia, dysphagia, and dysarthria. This is followed by a symmetrical, descending skeletal muscle paralysis with hypotonia, weakness in the neck and arms, after which respiratory muscles and then distal muscles are affected.[37] There is no loss of sensation, and patients are well oriented. Autonomic signs like postural hypotension, dry mouth, cardiovascular, gastrointestinal, and urinary autonomic dysfunction may also be present. Gag reflex may not be lost. Deep tendon reflexes may be present or absent. Pupils are dilated and fixed. Respiratory paralysis may require mechanical ventilation. Laboratory test results, including analysis of cerebrospinal fluid, are unremarkable.

Diagnosis

Clinical diagnosis may be difficult without strong clinical suspicion. The first and early cases are commonly misdiagnosed. Case definitions of suspected or confirmed cases due to deliberate release are reported in Table 12.2. Laboratory diagnosis relies on isolation and identification of the neurotoxins from sera or other samples like stool, gastric specimen, vomitus, and suspected food. The aerosolized toxin may be detected by ELISA on nasal mucous membranes or bronchoalveolar lavage for 24 hours after inhalation.

Treatment

Without supportive treatment, death often occurs from respiratory failure. Patients with respiratory failure require long-term mechanical ventilation, from 60 days to 7 months.[44] Trivalent (A, B, E) equine antitoxins must be given to patients as soon as possible after clinical diagnosis by slow intravenous infusion.[47] Patients with botulism who survive may have asthenia and dyspnea for years. Muscle function returns after 3–6 months as the neuromuscular junction regenerates. In the United States, investigational pentavalent (A–E) botulinum toxoid vaccine is used for laboratory workers at high risk of exposure and by military personnel. Immunity is induced slowly by this vaccine, and frequent boosters are required.[45]

Tularemia

Francisella tularensis is a nonmotile, obligatory aerobic, facultative intracellular Gram-negative coccobacillus. One of the most infectious pathogenic bacteria known, ten organisms are sufficient to initiate human infection.[48] Inhalational tularemia following intentional release of a virulent strain of *F. tularensis* would have great impact and cause high morbidity and mortality. Another route of contamination in a deliberate release could be contamination of water.[49]

Clinical Features

The incubation period of tularemia is of 3–5 days (range 1–25 days). Seven clinical forms are known, according to route of inoculation: skin, mucous membranes, gastrointestinal tract, eyes, respiratory tract, glandular. Usually, whatever the clinical form, the onset of symptoms is abrupt with fever, chills, myalgias, arthralgias, headache, coryza, sore throat, and sometimes pulse–temperature dissociation, nausea, vomiting, and diarrhea. Inhalational exposure commonly presents as an acute flu-like illness without prominent signs of respiratory disease (Tables 12.9 and 12.10).

The diagnosis of tularemia due to a deliberate release would be suggested if large numbers of patients present with an atypical pneumonia (Tables 12.11, 12.12). Ulceroglandular tularemia is the most common (75–85%) reported form. Ulcers are usually single lesions of 0.4 to 3.0 cm in diameter. The lesion is associated with tender enlargement of one or more regional lymph nodes, which may become fluctuant and rupture releasing caseous material. Lymphadenopathy may persist for as long as 3 years. Neither severe diseases nor complications are usually noted with this form of tularemia. Tularemia sepsis is potentially severe and fatal. Any form of tularemia can be complicated by sepsis.

Diagnosis

Clinical diagnostic suspicion remains crucial. Case definitions of suspected or confirmed cases, and cases due to deliberate release, are shown in Table 12.11. *F. tularensis* may be identified by direct examination of secretions, exudates, or biopsy specimens using direct fluorescent antibody or immunohistochemical stains. Culture is possible but difficult and poses a significant risk of infection to laboratory workers.

Antigen detection assays, PCR, ELISA techniques may be used to identify *F. tularensis*. A fourfold change in titer between acute and convalescent serum specimens, a single titer of at least 1/160 to tube agglutination or 1/128 for microagglutination is diagnostic for *F. tularensis*.[42,48] Serum antibody titers do not attain diagnostic level until 10–14 days after onset of illness. Serologic testing is useful only retrospectively but confirms the diagnosis. For definitive laboratory confirmation, culture and an increase in specific antibodies in paired sera are required.

TABLE 12.9. Summary of clinical and biological description of tularemia

Clinical features

- Incubation period: 3–5 days
- Tularemia pneumonia (primary and secondary pneumonia)
- Inhalational exposure presents as an acute flu-like illness
- Progression to severe pneumonia with bloody sputum, respiratory failure, and death, if appropriate treatment is not started
- Chest radiography: peribronchial infiltrates, bronchopneumonia, pleura effusions, and hilar lymphadenopathy
- Ulceroglandular tularemia, most common form (75% to 85%)
- Local papule at the site of inoculation associated with fever and aches
- Papule pruritic ≥enlarges to pustule ≥ruptures to painful, indolent ulcer, which may be covered by an eschar
- Tender enlargement of ≥1 regional lymph nodes, which may become fluctuant and rupture releasing caseous material

Glandular tularemia

- Lymphadenopathy and fever
- No ulcer

Oculoglandular tularemia

- Purulent conjunctivitis, chemosis, conjunctival nodules, or ulceration
- Periorbital edema
- Tender preauricular or cervical lymphadenopathy

Oropharyngeal tularemia

- Stomatitis, exudative pharyngitis or tonsillitis + painful mucosal ulceration
- Retropharyngeal abscess or suppuration of regional lymph nodes

Typhoidal tularemia

- Acute flu-like illness
- Diarrhea, vomiting, headache, chills, rigors
- Myalgia, arthralgia, weight loss, prostration
- No indication of inoculation site
- No anatomic localization of infection

Tularemia sepsis

- Nonspecific signs confusion
- Septic shock, disseminated intravascular coagulation and hemorrhage, acute respiratory distress syndrome, organ failure, and coma

Diagnosis

Confirmatory tests for identification of *Francisella tularensis* [40,41]

- Isolation of *F. tularensis* from a clinical specimen
- Demonstration of a specific antibody response in serially obtained sera

For probable case

- A single high titer
- Detection of *F. tularensis* in a clinical specimen by fluorescent assay

Treatment [26,42,48,49]

- Private room placement for patients with pneumonia is NOT necessary
- Treatment of choice: Streptomycin and gentamicin (10 days)
- Quinolones effective alternative (10–14 days)
- Tetracyclines and chloramphenicol are associated with high relapse rate, therapy at least 14–21 days
- Combination of two (aminoglycosides and fluoroquinolones) in severe cases

Postexposure prophylaxis

- Streptomycin, gentamicin, doxycycline, or ciprofloxacin (14 days)
- Vaccination is NOT recommended for postexposure prophylaxis

Source: Data from Bossi et al.[49]

TABLE 12.10. Case definitions of tularemia

Possible case
– NA
Probable case
– A severe, unexplained febrile illness or febrile death in a previously healthy person
– Severe unexplained respiratory illness in otherwise healthy people
– Severe unexplained sepsis or respiratory failure not due to a predisposing illness
– Severe sepsis with unknown Gram-negative coccobacillary species that fails to grow on standard blood agar, identified in the blood or cerebrospinal fluid
– A clinically compatible case that fulfils the laboratory criteria for a probable case or has an epidemiological link
Confirmed case
– A clinically compatible case with positive confirmatory laboratory tests

Source: Data from the Official Journal of the European Communities[40,41]

TABLE 12.11. Definition of a deliberate release with *Francisella tularensis*

Suspected deliberate release
– Two or more suspected cases of tularemia that are linked in time and place, especially geographically related groups of illness following a wind direction pattern
Deliberate release
– Single confirmed case of indigenous tularemia NOT explained by occupational exposure

Source: Data from Bossi et al.[49]

Treatment

Guidelines have been published for treatment and prophylaxis of tularemia (13.12). Streptomycin and gentamicin are currently considered the treatment of choice for tularemia. Treatment with aminoglycosides should be continued for 10 days. Quinolone may be an effective alternative drug. Despite the absence of large data in patients with tularemia, ciprofloxacin principally, or ofloxacin should be prescribed for 10–14 days. In severe cases, combination of two antibiotics such as aminoglycosides and fluoroquinolones should be considered.[48,49] Use of macrolides in tularemia is not recommended. Usually, the beta-lactamase are considered ineffective. No isolation measures are necessary for patients with pneumonia.

Streptomycin, gentamicin, doxycycline, or ciprofloxacin are recommended for postexposure prophylaxis and must be taken for at least 14 days. An unlicensed live-attenuated vaccine is available. That vaccine appears to offer protection against ulceroglandular and pneumonic tularemia. In the absence of additional data, the vaccine is not recommended for postexposure prophylaxis.

Viral Hemorrhagic Fevers

Viral hemorrhagic fevers (VHFs) are a variety of diseases, associated with fever and bleeding disorders caused by RNA viruses (Table 12.13). These include Arenaviridae, which are composed of the Lassa, Argentine, Bolivian, and Brazilian

TABLE 12.12. Recommendations for treatment and postexposure prophylaxis of tularemia

Target population		Treatment of suspected or confirmed clinical cases (10–21 days)	Postexposure prophylaxis (14 days)
Adults (including pregnant women). It is recommended, when possible, to stop breastfeeding	First-line treatment (10 days)	– Gentamicin: 5 mg/kg IV in 1 or 2 doses daily or – Streptomycin: 1 g IM twice daily	
	Second-line treatment: first-line prophylaxis (14 days)	– Ciprofloxacin: 400 mg IV bid followed by 500 mg per os bid or – Ofloxacin: 400 mg IV bid followed by 400 mg per os bid or – Levofloxacin: 500 mg IV once a day, followed by 500 mg per os once a day	– Ciprofloxacin: 500 mg per os bid or – Ofloxacin: 400 mg per os bid or – Levofloxacin: 500 mg per os once a day
	Third-line treatment; second-line prophylaxis (21 days)	– Doxycycline: 100 mg IV bid followed by 100 mg bid per os	– Doxycycline: 100 mg bid per os
Children	First-line treatment (10 days)	– Gentamicin: 2.5 mg/kg IV 3 times daily or – Streptomycin: 15 mg/kg IM twice daily (max; 2 g)	
	Second-line treatment: first-line prophylaxis (14 days)	– Ciprofloxacin: 10–15 mg/kg IV bid followed by 10–15 mg/kg per os bid	– Ciprofloxacin: 10–15 mg/kg per os bid
	Third-line treatment; second-line prophylaxis (21 days)	– Doxycycline: >8 years and >45 kg: adult dose >8 years and <45 kg or <8 years: 2.2 mg/kg IV bid followed by 2.2 mg/kg per os bid (max 200 mg/d)	– Doxycycline: >8 years and >45 kg: adult dose >8 years and <45 kg or <8 years: 2.2 mg/kg per os bid (max 200 mg/d)

Source: Data from European Agency for the Evaluation of Medicinal Products[26] and Bossi, P et al.[49]
IV intravenous, IM intramuscular

([Junin, Machupo, Guanarito, Sabia] viruses; Bunyaviridae, which cause Rift Valley fever [RVF] and the Congo-Cremean hemorrhagic fever, [CCHF]); and Filoviridae, which are composed of Ebola, Marburg, and yellow fever viruses.[50,51]

Most of these viruses have zoonotic life cycles independent of humans (dengue and yellow fever partially excepted). These agents are usually transmitted to humans from animals or arthropod reservoirs via mosquitoes, ticks, or infected animal urine or feces. Except for RVF and the *flaviviruses*, person-to-person transmission can occur with close contact but it is not a usual route of transmission.

TABLE 12.13. Hemorrhagic fever viruses (HFVs) that could be involved in biological warfare

Family	Virus	Disease	Vector in nature
Filoviridae	Ebola	Ebola hemorrhagic fever	Unknown
	Marburg	Marburg hemorrhagic fever	Unknown
Arenaviridae	Lassa	Lassa fever	Rodent
	Machupo	Bolivian hemorrhagic fever	Rodent
	Junin	Argentine hemorrhagic fever	Rodent
	Guannarito	Venezuelan hemorrhagic fever	Rodent
	Sabia	Brazilian hemorrhagic fever	Rodent
Bunyaviridae	Rift Valley fever	Rift Valley fever	Mosquito
	Crimean-Congo hemorrhagic fever	Crimean-Congo hemorrhagic fever	Tick
Flaviviridae	Yellow fever	Yellow fever	Mosquito
	Omsk hemorrhagic fever	Omsk hemorrhagic fever	Tick
	Kyasanur Forest disease	Kyasanur Forest disease	Tick

Most of these viruses may be transmitted to humans through aerosolization. Biological weaponization has been proven successfully in nonhuman primates. Hemorrhagic fever viruses (HFVs) are associated with high morbidity, and in some cases high mortality. No specific treatment or vaccines exist for these viruses.

Diseases

Most of the HFVs induce a similar syndrome. The incubation period varies from 1 to 21 days (Table 12.14). Depending on the virus, the disease can progress with respiratory problems, severe bleeding, kidney failure, and shock. All HFVs can induce microvascular damage and capillary leak syndrome. Severity of illness can range from relatively mild to death. Most patients infected with these viruses experience a nonspecific febrile illness, without prominent involvement of a single organ system. A summary of clinical description of HFV is detailed in Table 12.13. Laboratory criteria for diagnosis and case definition are detailed in Table 12.15. Recommendations for treatment and postexposure prophylaxis of VHF are detailed in Table 12.16 and the status of vaccine development is detailed in Table 12.17.

Conclusion

Unlike most types of weapons, biological agents come in many forms ranging from bacteria and viruses to plants and toxins. Some agents cause contagious disease while others do not. Some are lethal while others are likely to cause debilitating illness but not death. Nevertheless, all select agents are recognized as potential weapons that could have serious and even devastating effects on victims. Although more than 70 biological agents have been designated by the CDC as possibly useful for hostile purposes, the six agents deemed especially attractive as terrorist weapons are those in Category A. They are responsible for smallpox, anthrax, plague,

TABLE 12.14. Summary of clinical description of hemorrhagic fever viruses (HFV)

Virus	Incubation (days)	Clinical feature	Mortality (%)
Ebola	2–21	Onset abrupt: high fever, chills, asthenia, headache, muscle aches, anorexia, conjunctivitis, abdominal pain, nausea, vomiting, diarrhea, pharyngitis, sore throat, chest pain, and erythematous macular rash. After 3 days, prostration, hemorrhagic manifestations, petechiae, ecchymosis, conjunctival hemorrhage, gingival bleeding, bleeding from injection site, frank bleeding from gastrointestinal tract with melena, vaginal bleeding, hematemesis, and bleeding from other sites such as internal organs. Patients may die of organ failure and shock.	72
Marburg	3–10	Idem Ebola	23
Lassa fever	10–14	Usually asymptomatic or mild illness. The onset of the disease is insidious with fever and general malaise over a 2 - 4 day period. In more severe cases; weakness, retroorbital pain, joint and lumbar pain, myalgia, headache, pharyngitis, cough and conjunctival injection. In the most severe form of the disease; prostration; abdominal pain, facial and neck edema, hemorrhages (conjunctival hemorrhages, mucosal bleeding, melena, hematochezia, hematuria, vaginal bleeding, hematemesis), encephalitis, capillary leak syndrome and shock. Hepatitis is frequent. Pulmonary manifestations can be significant with ARDS. Long-term sequelae of Lassa infection; sensorineural deafness.	15–20
New World Arenaviruses	7–14	Idem Lassa fever Hemorrhage, and neurological signs are more common; hemorrhage along the gingival margins is characteristic. Neurologic signs may include delirium, confusion, encephalopathy, convulsions and coma. Conjunctival injection, facial flushing, petechial and/or vesicular palatal enanthem and skin petechiae, generalized lymphadenopathy and orthostatic hypotension are common.	10–16

TABLE 12.14. (continued)

Virus	Incubation (days)	Clinical feature	Mortality (%)
Rift Valley fever	3–6	The initial clinical manifestations are a biphasic fever, the first bout lasting 4 days. After 1 or 2 days without fever the second fever spike occurs, lasting for 2 to 4 days. Usually the illness is mild and associated with fever and liver abnormalities. In severe cases hemorrhage (<1%), encephalitis (1%), and retinitis (10%).	1
Crimean-Congo hemorrhagic fever	3–6	Onset of symptoms is abrupt with fever, myalgia, dizziness, neck pain and stiffness, backache, headache, sore eyes and photophobia, nausea, vomiting, diarrhea and abdominal pain. The patient may experience sharp mood swing, and may become confused and aggressive. After 2 to 4 days, sleepiness, depression and lassitude may replace the agitation, and the abdominal pain may localize to the right upper quadrant, with hepatomegaly. Other clinical signs include tachycardia, lymphadenopathy, and a petechial rash or ecchymoses, both on mucosal surfaces and on the skin. Hemorrhagic symptoms include melena, hematuria, epistaxis and bleeding from the gums. A hepatitis is usually present. Multiorgan failure with hepatorenal and pulmonary failures may develop after the fifth day of illness.	30
Yellow fever	1–3	The onset of the illness is abrupt with fever, headache, generalized malaise, weakness, lumbosacral pain, bradycardia, nausea, and vomiting. This period lasts 3 days and is followed by a remission lasting 24h. Then intoxication, which can progress to death 7–10 days after presentation appears. Symptoms include jaundice, scleral icterus, albuminuria, oliguria, cardiovascular instability, and hemorrhagic manifestations.	25–50
Omsk Hemorrhagic fever	3–8	The onset is abrupt with fever, headache, severe myalgias, diarrhea, vomiting, severe prostration, conjunctival suffusion, photophobia, cervical and axillary adenopathy, and more rarely splenomegaly or hepatosplenomegaly. Papulovesicular lesions involving the soft palate are frequent. Pulmonary manifestations are also frequent during the first stage of the illness. The second stage of the illness is associated with neurological involvement. Hemorrhagic manifestations are those observed with other VHFs.	0.5–10
Kyasanur Forest fever	3–8	Idem Omsk hemorrhagic fever	3–10

Source: Bossi et al.[51]

TABLE 12.15. Laboratory criteria for diagnosis and case definition

Laboratory criteria for diagnosis
Positive virus isolation
Positive skin biopsy (immunohistochemistry for Ebola/Marburg viruses, Lassa fever virus)
Detection of specific viral nucleic acid sequences
Positive serology, which may appear late in the course of the disease
Case definition of suspected and confirmed cases of viral hemorrhagic fever (VHF)
Possible: Not applicable
Probable: A clinically compatible case with an epidemiological link
Confirmed: A clinically compatible case that is laboratory confirmed
Case definition of a suspected deliberate release of VHF
≤1 confirmed case in Europe which is not an imported case

Source: Data from the Official Journal of the European Communities[40,41]

TABLE 12.16. Recommendations for treatment and postexposure prophylaxis of viral hemorrhagic fever (VHF)

	Treatment of suspected or confirmed clinical cases of VHF (10 days)	Postexposure prophylaxis (7 days)
Adults (including pregnant women). It is recommended, when possible, to stop breastfeeding	*Ribavirin IV*: Initial dose of 2 g followed by 1 g every 6 h for 4 days, followed by 0.5 g every 8 h for 6 days or Initial dose of 20 mg/kg followed by 15 mg/kg every 6 h for 4 days, followed by 7.5 mg/kg every 8 h for 6 days or *Ribavirin per (os)*: 2 g orally (loading dose) followed by 4 g/day in 4 divided doses for 4 days followed by 2 g/day for 6 days	Ribavirin: 2 g/day orally in 4 divided doses
Children	No recommendations can be given	No recommendations can be given

Source: Data from: European Agency for the Evaluation of Medicinal Products[26]

botulinum toxin-caused illness, tularemia, and VHFs. As such, these agents and diseases should be of special interest to members of the medical community, who may be called upon to treat victims of their effects.

The threat of bioterrorism poses a challenge for many sectors of society including public health, primary care, hospitals, first responders, as well as agencies beyond the health community. Coping successfully with bioterrorism will depend upon awareness of the threat, a high level of pre-event preparedness, coordination, and practiced performance at both national and local levels.

TABLE 12.17. Status of vaccine development against hemorrhagic fever virus (HFV) in 2002

Virus	Vaccine candidate	Development stage
Ebola	Recombinant subunit	Preclinical
	Replicons	Preclinical
Marburg	Not mentioned	
Lassa fever	Not mentioned	
New World arenaviruses	Not mentioned	
Rift Valley fever	Inactivated Live, attenuated	Phase II
		Phase I
Yellow fever	Live attenuated (17D strain)	Licensed
	Infectious clone	Preclinical
Omsk hemorrhagic fever	Not mentioned	
Kyasanur Forest fever	Not mentioned	

Source: US Department of Health and Human Services[52]

References

1. HHS Public Health Emergency Medical Countermeasure Enterprise. Implementation Plan for Chemical, Biological, Radiological and Nuclear Threats. US Department of Health and Human Services, Office of The Assistant Secretary For Preparedness and Response, Office of Public Health Emergency Medical Countermeasures, April 2007.
2. Inglesby T, Grossman R, O'Toole T. A plague on your city: observations from TOPOFF. Biodefense Quarterly 2000;2:1–10.
3. DARK WINTER, Bioterrorism Exercise Andrews Air Force Base June 22–23, 2001. http://www.upmc-biosecurity.org/website/events /2001_darkwinter/dark_winter.pdf.
4. Comments and Recommendations by Members of New Jersey Universities Consortium for Homeland Security Research. Lioy PL, Roberts FS, McCluskey B, et al. J Emerg Manag. 2006;4:41–51.
5. Centers for Disease Control and Prevention Web site: Bioterrorism Overview. Available at: http://www.bt.cdc.gov/bioterrorism/overview.asp#intro/. Accessed September 30, 2008.
6. Noah DL. The history and threat of biological warfare and terrorism. Emerg Med Clin N Am. 2002;20:255–271.
7. Petro JB, Plasse TR, McNulty JA. Biosecurity and bioterrorism: biodefense strategy, practice, and science. *Biosecur Bioterror*. 2003;1(3):161–168.
8. Bossi P, Garin D, Gay F, et al. Bioterrorism: management of major biological agents. Cell Mol Life Sci. 2006;63:2196–2212.
9. Khandori N, Kanchanapoom T. Overview of biological terrorism: potential agents and preparedness. Clin Microbiol News. 2005;27:1–8.
10. Stewart C. Toxins and biowarfare in biological warfare: preparing for the unthinkable emergency. In: Topics in Emergency Medicine, Vol II. Atlanta: American Health Consults, 2001.
11. Hawley RJ, Eitzen EM Jr. Biological weapons—a primer for microbiologists. Annu Rev Microbiol. 2001;55:235–53.

12. Khandary N. Bioterrorism and bioterrorism preparedness: historical perspective and overview. Infect Dis Clin North Am. 2006;20:179–211.

13. Cole LA. *The Anthrax Letters: A Medical Detective Story*. Washington DC: Joseph Henry Press/National Academies Press, 2003.

14. Rotz LD, Khan AS, Lillibridge SR, et al. Public health assessment of potential biological terrorism agents. Emerg Infect Dis. 2002;8:225–230.

15. Leissner KB, Holzman RS, McCann ME. Bioterrorism and children: unique concerns with infection control and vaccination. Anesthesiol Clin N Am. 2004;22:563–577.

16. Bravata DM, Holty JC, Wang E, et al. Inhalational, gastrointestinal, and cutaneous anthrax in children. A systematic review of cases: 1990–2005. Arch Pediatr Adolesc Med. 2007;161(9):896–905.

17. American Academy of Pediatrics: Chemical-biological terrorism and its impact on children: a subject review. Pediatrics. March 2000;105(3):662–670.

18. Mackay B. SARS poses challenges for MDs treating pediatric patients. CMAJ. 2003; 168:1457.

19. Inglesby TV, Henderson DA, Bartlett JG, et al. Working group on civilian biodefense, anthrax as a biological weapon: medical and public health management. JAMA. 1999;281: 1735–1745.

20. Inglesby TV, O'Toole T, Henderson DA, et al. Anthrax as a biological weapon. 2002: updated recommendations for management. JAMA. 2002;287:2236–2252.

21. Advisory Committee on Immunization Practices. Use of anthrax vaccine in the United States. MMWR Recom Rep. 2000;49(RR-15):1–20.

22. Verkey P, Poland GA, Cokerill FR, et al. Confronting bioterrorism: physicians on the front line. Mayo Clin Proc. July 2002;77:661–672.

23. Centers for Disease Control and Prevention (2001) Update: investigation of bioterrorism-related anthrax—Connecticut. MMWR. 2001;50:1077–1079.

24. Jernigan JA, Stephens DS, Ashford, DA, et al. Bioterrorism-related inhalational anthrax: the first 10 cases reported in the United States. Emerg Infect Dis. 2001;7:933–944.

25. Bossi P, Tegnell A, Baka A, et al. Task Force on Biological and Chemical Agent Threats, Public Health Directorate, European Commission, Luxembourg (2004) Bichat guidelines for the clinical management of anthrax and bioterrorism-related anthrax. EuroSurveill.9,E3-http://www.eurosurveillance.org./em/v09n12/0912–231.asp.

26. European Agency for the Evaluation of Medicinal Products (2002) Guidance document on use of medicinal products for treatment and prophylaxis of biological agents that might be used as weapons of bioterrorism. 25 July 2002: www.emea.eu.int.

27. Center for Disease Control and Prevention (2001) Update: investigation of bioterrorism-related anthrax and interim guidelines for clinical evaluation of persons with possible anthrax. MMWR. 2001;50:941–948.

28. Meselson M, Guillemin J, Hugh-Jones M, et al. The Sverdlovsk anthrax outbreak of 1979. Science. 1994;266:1202–1208.

29. Swartz M. Current concepts: recognition and management of anthrax—an update. N Engl J Med. 2001;345:1621–1626.

30. Bell D, Kozarsky P, Stephens D. Clinical issues in the prophylaxis, diagnosis, and treatment of anthrax. Emerg Infect Dis. 2002;8:222–225.

31. Health Protection Agency Web Site. http:/www.camr.org.uk/. Accessed September 30, 2008.

32. Freidlander A, Pittman P, Parker G. Anthrax vaccine: evidence for safety and efficacy against inhalational anthrax. JAMA. 1999;282:2104–2106.

33. National Institute of Allergy and Infectious Diseases of the National Institutes of Health Web Site, Anthrax Vaccine. Availbale at: http:/www3.niaid.nih.gov/newsnews releases/2002/anthraxvacc.htm. Accessed September 30, 2008

34. Breman J, Henderson D. Diagnosis and management of smallpox. N Engl J Med. 2002;346:1300–1308.

35. Bossi P, Tegnell A, Baka A, et al. Task Force on Biological and Chemical Agent Threats, Public Health Directorate, European Commission, Luxembourg (2004) Bichat guidelines for the clinical management of smallpox and bioterrorism-related smallpox. Euro Surveill. 2004;9(12). http://www.eurosurveillance.org/em/v09n12/0912-233.asp.

36. Henderson DA, Ingelsby TV, Bartlett JG, et al. Smallpox as a biological weapon. Concensus statement. JAMA. 1999;281:2127–2137.

37. Franz DR, Jahrling PB, Freidlender AM, et al. Clinical recognition and management of patients exposed to biological warfare agents. JAMA. 1997;278:399–411.

38. Inglesby TV, Dennis DT, Bartlett JG, et al. Plague as a biological weapon. Medical and public health management. JAMA. 2000;283:2281–2290.

39. Bossi P, Tegnell A, Baka A, et al. Task Force on Biological and Chemical Agent Threats, Public Health Directorate, European Commission, Luxembourg (2004) Bichat guidelines for the clinical management of plague and bioterrorism-related plague. Euro Surveill 2004;9(12). http://www.eurosurveillance.org/em/v09n12/0912-232.asp.

40. Commission of 19 March 2002. Case definitions for reporting communicable diseases to the community network under decision N° 2119/98/EC of European Parliament and the Council. Official Journal of the European Communities. OJL. 2002;86:44.

41. Amending Decision N° 2119/98/EC of the European Parliament and Council and Decision 2000/EC as regards communicable diseases listed in those decisions and amending decision 2002/253/EC as regards to case definitions for communicable diseases. Official Journal of the European Union. OJL 2003;184:35–39.

42. Scientific Institute of Public Health, France, Epidemiology Unit Web site. Available at: http://www.iph.fgov.be/epidemio/epien/index.htm and http://afssaps.sante.fr/. Accessed September 30, 2008.

43. Lecour H, Ramos H, Almeida B, et al. Botulism. A review of 13 outbreaks. Arch Intern Med. 1998;148:578–580.

44. Centers for Diseases Control and Prevention (1998) Botulism in the United States, 1899–1996. Handbook for epidemiologists, clinicians, and laboratory workers. Centers for Diseases Control and Prevention, Atlanta, GA.

45. Siegel, L. Human immune response to botulinum pentavalent (ABCDE) toxoid determined by a neutralization test and by an enzyme linked immunosorbent assay. J Clin Microbiol. 1998;26:2351–2356.

46. Bossi P, Tegnell A, Baka A, et al. Task Force on Biological and Chemical Agent Threats, Public Health Directorate, European Commission, Luxembourg (2004) Bichat guidelines for the clinical management of botulism and bioterrorism-related botulism. Euro Surveill 2004;9E:13–14: http://www.eurosurveillance.org/em/v09n12/0912-236.asp

47. Arnon S, Schechter R, Inglesby TV, et al. Botulinum toxin as a biological weapon. JAMA. 2001;285:1059–1070.

48. Dennis DT, Inglesby TV, Henderson DA, et al. Tularemia as a biological weapon. Medical and Public Health Management. JAMA. 2001;285:2763–73.

49. Bossi P, Tegnell A, Baka A, et al. Task Force on Biological and Chemical Agent Threats, Public Health Directorate, European commission, Luxembourg (2004) Bichat guidelines for the clinical management of Tularemia and bioterrorism-related Tularemia. Euro Surveill 2004;9E(12). http://www.eurosurveillance.org/em/v09n12/0912-234.asp

50. Borio L, Inglesby T, Schmaljohn A, et al. Hemorrhagic fever viruses as a biological weapon: medical and public health management JAMA. 2002;287:2391–2405.
51. Bossi P, Tegnell A, Baka A, et al. Task Force on Biological and Chemical Agent Threats, Public Health Directorate, European commission Luxembourg (2004) Bichat guidelines for the clinical management of Hemorrhagic Fever viruses and bioterrorism-related Hemorrhagic Fever viruses. Euro Surveill 2004;9E(12):1–6.
52. The Jordan report. 20th Anniversary. Accelerated Development of Vaccines 2002. US Department of Health and Human Services, National Institute of Allergy and Infectious Diseases. 156pp.

13
Chemical Agents and Terror Medicine

Kristan Staudenmayer and William P. Schecter

A toxic chemical is the most likely nonconventional weapon to be employed in a terrorist attack because of the availability and simplicity of production, storage, and deployment.[1] Several chemical-based acts of terrorism have occurred during the last three decades. Cyanide-laced Tylenol® capsules resulted in the deaths of seven people in the United States in 1984.[2] The Aum Shinrikyo terrorist organization released sarin nerve agent in a residential area of Matsumoto, Japan, in June 1994 resulting in seven deaths and ~600 injuries.[3] The same organization released sarin again in March 1995 into a Tokyo subway.[4] This attack resulted in 12 deaths and over 1,000 injuries. United States (US) intelligence analysts believe that the al Qaeda Terrorist Network has attempted to develop a chemical weapons capability.[5,6] In September 2003, the Department of Homeland Security issued an "Information Bulletin" informing law enforcement agencies of a suspected al Qaeda attempt to disseminate hydrogen cyanide.[7] In fact, the 1993 attack on the World Trade Center in New York did indeed have a cyanide component to it that failed. Government and law enforcement officials and health care personnel must be prepared to identify, manage, and treat victims of a chemical weapon attack.

Epidemiology

Toxic chemicals that may be used as chemical weapons are classified in three groups. This classification was devised by the Organization for the Prohibition of Chemical Weapons and is based on the quantities of the substances produced commercially for legitimate purposes.[8] The classification scheme follows:

Schedule 1: Chemicals solely employed as weapons such as mustard agents and nerve agents.
Schedule 2: Toxic chemicals which have small-scale industrial uses such as dimethyl methylphosphonate (a precursor of sarin) used as a flame retardant and thiodiglycol (a precursor of mustard agent) used as a solvent in ink.[5] This extensive category is growing as hundreds of new chemicals are introduced each month.[9]
Schedule 3: Toxic chemicals used in large quantities for multiple applications in industry. Examples include phosgene (used to manufacture plastics) and chloropicrin (used as a fumigant).

S.C. Shapira et al. (eds.), *Essentials of Terror Medicine*,
DOI: 10.1007/978-0-387-09412-0_13, Springer Science+Business Media, LLC 2009

A list of both traditional chemical weapons and improvised weapons are listed in Table 13.1. Chemical agents may exist in gaseous, aerosol, solid, or liquid states. The state of the chemical and its dissemination method determine the route of entry, which in turn affects both the clinical presentation and the time to onset of symptoms.[10] Symptoms are also dependent on the dose and potency of each chemical. The type of weapon deployed and the method of chemical dispersion have a critical impact on the severity of the attack.[7] For example, cyanide vapor released in an open space may be diluted rapidly and result in minimal impact. The same amount of vapor released in an enclosed space may be lethal.

A chemical terror attack may present either as an overt or covert release of a chemical agent.[9,11,12] Terrorist chemical acts are likely to be overt because the effects of most chemical agents are immediate and obvious.[9] There are three possible types of overt chemical attacks. The first is the release of a traditional chemical weapon (such as sarin nerve gas) against a civilian or military target.[5] Alternatively, terrorists could employ improvised chemical weapons, such as an insecticide.[5] Finally, terrorists could attack or sabotage an industrial chemical facility or chemical transport vehicle causing the release of toxic material. Industrial facilities are frequently located near residential areas in the United States. One-hundred-twenty-three US chemical facilities located near population centers have the potential to affect more than 1 million people in the case of an accident or terrorist attack. An additional 700 facilities could each threaten at least 100,000 people in the surrounding areas. Approximately 3,000 other industrial facilities could threaten at least 10,000 people if attacked.[13] For example, an accident at the Union Carbide industrial plant in Bhopal, India, in 1984 resulted in the release of methyl isocyanate (a precursor of the pulmonary agent phosgene) resulting in 3,800 deaths and 2,700 injuries.[14]

Depending on the agent and means of dissemination, a covert chemical attack is also possible. In either case, health care workers risk secondary exposure.[9,15] A covert attack presents a particular risk to health care workers and rescue teams because unidentified secondary exposure can lead to spread of the agent.

Most toxic gases are colorless. Liquids can range from colorless to brown.[16] The odor of a chemical residue may on occasion provide a clue, but many chemicals are odorless.

There are several epidemiologic clues that might suggest the covert release of a chemical agent including (1) an increase in the number of patients seeking care for symptoms potentially caused by a chemical weapon, (2) unexplained deaths in otherwise healthy individuals, (3) emission of unexplained odors from patients, (4) clusters of similar illnesses, (5) the rapid-onset of symptoms after exposure to a potentially contaminated source, or (6) unexplained death of plants or animals.[12,17]

Victims of a covert attack will likely present first to local area hospitals. The hospital staff must be trained to recognize these epidemiologic clues to mobilize appropriate resources and prevent secondary exposure. Identification of an overt chemical release or suspicion of a covert attack should result in activation of local area disaster management protocols and immediate initiation of decontamination procedures.

TABLE 13.1. Chemical agents which may be used for terrorist attacks

Categories	Agents	Signs/symptoms
Nerve Agents: Agents which directly incapacitate the nervous system	G agents→ Sarin (GB) Soman (GD) Tabun (GA) GF V agents→ VX	Time to onset of symptoms: Vapor—seconds to minutes. Liquid—minutes to hours Signs/Symptoms: *Muscarinic*: "SLUDGE": salivation, lacrimation, urination, defecation, GI symptoms (diarrhea, abdominal cramps) emesis; diaphoresis, miosis, blurred vision, bradycardia, bronchorrhea, dypsnea, chest tightness. *Nicotinic*: fasciculations, muscular weakness, muscle paralysis, hypertension, tachycardia. *CNS*: confusion, restlessness, stlessness, anxiety, ataxia , headaches, fatigue, loss of consciousness, respiratory depression, seizures, coma. *Note*: children may exhibit different symptoms (CNS, stupor, flaccidity, dypsnea).
Blood Agents: Agents which affect the body by being absorbed into the blood	Arsine (SA) Carbon monoxide Cyanides→ Cyanogen chloride (CK) Hydrogen cyanide (AC) Potassium cyanide (KCN) Sodium cyanide (NaCN) Sodium monofluoroacetate (compound 1080)	Time to onset of symptoms: seconds Signs/Symptoms: Headaches, dizziness, nausea, vomiting, drowsiness, hallucinations, gasping for air, loss of consciousness, brady/tachycardia, seizures, respiratory/cardiac arrest. Liquid cyanogen chloride may cause eye and respiratory tract irritation and chemical burns on exposed skin.

Traditional chemical warfare agents

(continued)

TABLE 13.1. (continued)

Categories	Agents	Signs/symptoms

Blister Agents/ Vesicants: Chemicals that induce blistering of the eyes, respiratory tract, and skin	Mustards→ Distilled mustard (HD)
	Sulfur mustard gas (H)
	Mustard/lewisite (HL)
	Mustard/T
	Nitrogen mustards (HN-1,2,3)
	Sesqui mustard
	Lewisites/chloroarsine agentsà
	Lewisite (L, L-1, L-2, L-3)
	Mustard/lewisite (HL)
	Phosgene oxime (CX)
		Time to onset of symptoms:
		  Onset: Lewisite—immediate
		  Mustard—effects may be delayed 2–24 hours.
		  Phosgene oxime—immediate
		
		Signs/Symptoms:
		Pain initially, followed by erythema, blisters, necrosis.
		Mustards produce groups of small blisters over erythematous areas.
		Lewisite blisters expand, taking up to 4 days to cover entire erythematous areas.
		Conjunctivitis, corneal opacity, blepharitis. Dry cough, nose, throat, lung irritation to marked airway damage. Epistaxis. Nausea, vomiting, diarrhea, abdominal pain, hyperexcitabilty, convulsions.

Choking/Pulmonary Agents: Chemicals that cause severe irritation or edema of the respiratory tract	Ammonia
	Bromine (CA)
	Chlorine (CL)
	Hydrogen chloride
	Methyl bromide
	Methyl isocyanate
	Osmium tetroxide
	Phosgene→ Diphosgene (DP)
	Phosgene (CG)
	Phosphine
	Phosphorus
	Sulfuryl fluoride
		Time to onset of symptoms:
		  Immediate.
		  Phosgene can be delayed 24 hours
		
		Signs/Symptoms:
		Eye and airway irritation, dypsnea, chest tightness, rapid breathing, coughing, wheezing, rales, hemoptysis, stridor, frothy secretions (2–24 hrs), cyanosis, upper airway swelling, pulmonary edema, lung collapse; tachycardia, initial hypertension, hypotension, possible cardiovascular collapse; nausea, vomiting; skin burns, blisters.

Traditional chemical warfare agents

Improvised chemical agents			
Incapacitating Agents: Agents that induce altered sensorium or decrease in consciousness	Opioids (fentanyl) BZ (an anticholinergic)	Time of onset of symptoms: Opioids: Dependent on route. Aerosolized may be immediate, ingested minutes to hours. BZ: The onset of incapacitation is dose-dependent and ranges from 1 to 48 hours. Signs/Symptoms: Opioids: CNS and respiratory system depression (lethargy, coma, decreased respiratory rate, miosis, and apnea) BZ: hallucinations; agitation; mydriasis; blurred vision; dry, flushed skin; urinary retention; ileus; tachycardia; hypertension; and elevated temperature (>101°F).
Riot Control Agents/Tear Gas: Highly irritating agents used to disable	Bromobenzylcyanide (CA) Chloroacetophenone (CN) Chlorobenzylidenemalononitrile (CS) Chloropicrin (PS) Dibenzoxazepine (CR) Capsaicin	Time to onset of symptoms: Immediate. Signs/Symptoms: Respiratory: cough, hoarseness, dyspnea, tachypnea, wheezing, hypoxemia, cyanosis, pulmonary edema Skin and mucous membranes: erythema, pain, blistering. Eye: lacrimation, redness, blurred vision, corneal burns Oropharynx: oral burns, sore throat, dysphagia, salivation Nose: rhinorrhea, burning, irritation, edema
Insecticide agents: Used in large quanitities can become weapons	Organophosphates	Time of onset to symptoms: variable and depends on agent Signs/Symptoms: See nerve agents.

Data from: Website Emergency Preparedness & Response: Chemical Agents: Department of Health and Human Services: Centers for Disease Control and Prevention (CDC); An Epidemiology Publication of the Orgeon Department of Human Services: Preparing for a Chemical Terrorist Event--A Primer. In: Services ODoH, ed. CD Summary. Vol 52: 2003; and Biological and Chemical Terrorism: Strategic Plan for Preparedness and Response. Recommendations of the CDC Strategic Planning Workgroup. In: (CDC) DoHaHScfDCaP, ed. Vol 49: Morbidity and Mortality Weekly Report (MMWR); 2000.

Pre-Hospital Issues

Individuals exposed to a hazardous material (HAZMAT) have a greater chance of recovery when emergency treatment is provided by appropriately trained medical personnel at both the scene and the receiving hospital as part of an integrated emergency medical response.[14] Prearranged plans should be used because the timing and nature of a terrorist attack cannot be predicted.

Although preplanning should occur at the national, state, and local levels, local governments and hospitals will most likely bear the initial brunt of the attack.[18–21] Unfortunately, many local governments, businesses, and hospitals do not have a coordinated response plan in place.[22] Furthermore, many hospitals currently are not prepared to manage chemical threats.[20,23,24]

A detailed discussion of general disaster preparedness at the state and local levels is beyond the scope of this chapter. However, a review of several fundamental principles of disaster management is important. Local emergency medical systems must develop a written disaster response plan. This plan should be coordinated with local hospitals and emergency medical services. This plan should include policies governing on-scene rescue procedures, communication, transportation, and the incident command system. Plans should be reviewed regularly and appropriately revised. Regularly scheduled training drills are essential. Specific plans for management of a chemical attack should be developed.

The key objectives of the pre-hospital management of a chemical attack include (1) reduction in the number and severity of injuries caused by the toxic chemical, (2) prevention of additional injuries during the first aid and decontamination process, (3) control of the spread of the chemical agent, and (4) evacuation to definitive medical care.[25] Table 13.2 shows the steps necessary to achieve the goals of pre-hospital care.[17,18,26]

The plan for decontamination after a chemical attack is based on prior experience with HAZMATs. HAZMAT guidelines have been adopted and further developed to apply to a chemical terrorist event. HAZMAT procedures should be initiated at the scene of a chemical terrorist attack. HAZMAT equipment, however, is expensive and not readily accessible to all potential responders to a chemical event.[27] For this reason, hospitals should be prepared for their own decontamination procedures in case there is difficulty with on-site decontamination.

The goals of decontamination are isolation and containment of the threat during transport of patients from the affected area to safety. If a chemical event is identified, these procedures should be initiated at the scene of attack because the most effective decontamination occurs within the first few minutes following exposure.[25] In addition, on-site decontamination prevents possible contamination of the receiving hospital which would effectively incapacitate an important medical asset.

The "hot line" concept is employed to isolate the area. One side of the line is considered to be in the "hot zone," while the other side is considered "clean."[17,25,28] (Fig. 13.1). The hot line is best delineated with the assistance of a chemical detector, if possible. The hot zone is placed downwind of the decontamination zone. Wind

TABLE 13.2. Steps to achieve the goals of pre-hospital care

1. Recognition of the chemical attack
2. Isolation and security at the scene of attack
3. Implementation of the Incident Command System
4. Provision of personal protective equipment (PPE) for rescue personnel
5. Decontamination of casualties
6. Identification of the chemical agent
7. Communication and coordination of security, rescue, and medical personnel
8. Triage of victims
9. Initiation of treatment
10. Transportation to hospital
11. Psychological management of the "worried well"
12. Fatality management

Data from Kenar and Karayilanoglu,[17] Waeckerle,[18] and Staten[26]

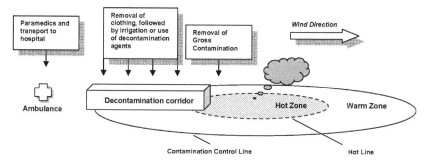

FIG. 13.1. Hot Zone

direction should be monitored during the incident. Any rescue worker who enters the hot zone must wear appropriate personal protective equipment (PPE). PPE is classified according to the level of protection provided. Level A, the maximal level, consists of a full chemical suit, positive pressure breathing apparatus, double layers of chemical-resistant gloves, and boots. Airtight seals prevent chemical exposure at the junctions between the suit and the breathing apparatus, gloves, and boots. Level A suits are protective against all chemicals, including those in the gas or vapor state. Level B PPE consists of a positive pressure breathing apparatus and suits, which provide complete protection against chemicals in the liquid but not the vapor state. Level C equipment consists of a face cartridge mask, splash-protective suit, gloves, and boots. Level C protection should provide adequate respiratory and contact protection.[27] Level D protection employs only latex gloves and eye splash protection.[29] Specific data to guide the appropriate level of protection is lacking.

Rescuers should be trained and appropriately attired before entering the hot zone. If the proper equipment is not available, or if rescuers have not been trained in its use, assistance from a local or regional HAZMAT team or other properly equipped response organization should be sought.

Before leaving the hot zone, patients and properly gowned workers must pass through a decontamination zone. The decontamination zone serves to neutralize or remove the toxic chemical before entry to the clean area. Physical removal of the chemical agent is the most important step in decontamination. Simple removal of clothing eliminates up to 85% of toxic agent.[17,30] Once the bulk of the toxic chemical has been physically removed, the remaining substance should be removed by chemical methods. Chemical methods of decontamination include soap and water, oxidation, and acid/base hydrolysis. Decontamination studies have shown that water, soap and water, or flour followed by tissue wipes are as effective as some decontamination agents depending on the specific toxic chemical.[25] Furthermore, water has the additional benefit of assisting with physical decontamination. Oxidative and acid/base hydrolytic agents were specifically developed to neutralize traditional chemical warfare agents but may not be readily available. Dilute (0.5%) hypochlorite solutions may be used to oxidize chemical agents located on the skin and superficial wounds.[25] If the chemical weapon is known and an antidote is available, treatment with the antidote should begin immediately. First aid also can be administered as needed after safety measures have been instituted.

After decontamination and first aid, the patient can be triaged to local area hospitals. Hospitals should have their own decontamination area in the likely event that patients arrive by private transportation before decontamination. The principles of hospital decontamination are the same as field decontamination. Hospital workers must strictly follow decontamination procedures to prevent the spread of the agent and avoid the temptation to circumvent this process if a patient is having difficulty. If a patient requires an immediate life-saving intervention, the caregiver should be appropriately protected by PPE. The performance of endotracheal intubation and other resuscitative maneuvers while wearing PPE is difficult.[31] After passing through effective decontamination, patients do not pose a risk to hospital workers. Hospital personnel should be safe in standard universal precautions.

Hospital Issues

The management of the patient following decontamination depends on the specific chemical weapon and the nature of any associated injuries. Traditional chemical weapons include nerve agents, blood agents, vesicants, and pulmonary agents. Nerve agents are organophosphate compounds that incapacitate the nervous system by inducing a cholinergic crisis. Blood agents include chemicals that are absorbed into the vascular system ultimately poisoning cellular metabolism. Vesicants, also known as blister agents, induce cutaneous and mucous burns and bone marrow suppression. Pulmonary agents, also known as choking agents, injure the respiratory tract causing pulmonary edema and hypoxia. In addition to the traditional classes of chemical weapons, two newer categories have been added: incapacitating agents (e.g., fentanyl, BZ) and riot control agents (e.g., tear gas).

Nerve Agents and Insecticides

Nerve agents are organophosphate compounds that are inhibitors of cholinesterase. Acetylcholine is a neurotransmitter which, after release from the presynaptic vesicles, binds to postsynaptic receptors. Acetylcholine is broken down by cholinesterase, resulting in termination of the presynaptic signal. Inhibition of cholinesterase results in excess acetylcholine binding to the postsynaptic receptor causing a cholinergic crisis. There are two receptors for acetylcholine: the muscarinic and the nicotinic receptors. Depolarization of the muscarinic receptors stimulates smooth muscle and the secretory glands. Depolarization of the nicotinic receptors stimulates skeletal muscle contraction and the sympathetic ganglia.

The symptoms caused by overstimulation of the muscarinic receptors are bronchospasm, decreased pulmonary compliance, nausea, vomiting, miosis, blurring of vision, bradycardia, and hypersecretions. An acronym for these symptoms is *SLUDGE* (salivation, lacrimation, urination, defecation, GI symptoms, and emesis). Overstimulation of the nicotinic receptors results in fasciculations, flaccid paralysis, pallor, hypertension, and tachycardia.[32,33] The effects on blood pressure and heart rate can be variable due to the opposing effects of the muscarinic and nicotinic receptors. The initial effect of organophosphate poisoning is usually tachycardia followed by bradycardia as the severity of the cholinergic crisis increases.[30]

The severity of the symptoms depends on the dose. At moderate doses, patients may experience respiratory distress, incontinence, and fasciculations. A large dose results in coma, seizures, apnea, and death.

The time from exposure to symptoms depends on the physical state and route of entry of the organophosphate. When in the gaseous state, nerve agents have an immediate effect. Deposition on the skin results in a time-release effect which may be delayed for hours.[25] Laboratory studies demonstrated a delayed but lethal response after deposition of nerve agent residue on skin in a pig model.[34]

There are five types of nerve agents which have been developed by state-sponsored weapon development programs. The North Atlantic Treaty Organization (NATO) designates two classes of nerve agents: G and V. Within these two classes, agents are given a NATO designation and may also have a common name. The G agents include Tabun (GA), Sarin (GB), Soman (GD), and GF, while the V agent is VX. VX is the most potent nerve agent.[25,30]

Two antidotes must be given to counteract the adverse effects of organophosphates. The first, atropine, is a competitive inhibitor of acetylcholine at the postsynaptic *muscarinic* receptor. Atropine has no effect at the *nicotinic* receptor. Atropine is given in incremental doses until the clinical signs of bronchorrhea, wheezing, decreased pulmonary compliance, miosis, and diarrhea resolve. The second antidote is an oxime compound. The oximes function as "molecular crowbars" which separate the organophosphate from the cholinesterase molecule, thereby permitting metabolism of acetylcholine. Pradiloxime chloride (PAM) is the oxime antidote used in the United States.[31] Unfortunately, the chemical bond between the organophosphate and cholinesterase becomes very difficult to separate over time. This phenomenon is called "aging." Different nerve agents age at different rates. For example, the aging half-life of soman is only 2 minutes, which means that oximes are not helpful for treatment unless given immediately after exposure.[25]

Patients exposed to a nerve agent should be removed to an area free of the chemical, receive the antidote, and undergo decontamination. For mild symptoms, patients should receive 2 mg of atropine intramuscular (IM) followed immediately by 600 mg (1 ampule) of PAM IM. Further doses of atropine may be required. IM atropine should be given every 5–10 minutes for symptoms of hypersecretion, wheezing, or shortness of breath. If there has been a severe exposure, the military recommends 6 mg atropine IM, 1,200–1,800 mg PAM IM, and 10 mg diazepam IM (for seizure control).[30] A repeat dose of 600 mg of PAM may be given after 1 hour if fasciculations persist. The maximum dose of PAM is 2,000 mg. Additional PAM may cause hypertension.

Many hospitals have an inadequate supply of nerve agent antidote because the pharmaceuticals have variable shelf lives and replacement is costly.[10] For this reason, the US Centers for Disease Control and Prevention (CDC) implemented the CHEMPACK project (program's mission is to provide state and local governments a sustainable nerve agent antidote cache that increases their capability to respond quickly to a nerve agent event such as a terrorist attack). In the case of a nerve agent attack, a stockpile of antidote will be deployed to the area of exposure. However, this supply is likely to arrive too late to significantly affect the outcome of the attack.

The US military has developed a controversial program to protect soldiers at risk for exposure to nerve agents. Pretreatment with the carbamate pyridostigmine to reversibly bind the cholinesterase enzyme in theory should block potential binding sites for organophosphates. In animal studies, pretreatment with pyridostigmine and posttreatment with an oxime reduced the toxicity of soman.[30]

Pretreatment with carbamates, however, produces cholinergic symptoms. During the Gulf War, many soldiers were pretreated with pyridostigmine. Despite the cholinergic symptoms, these soldiers continued to demonstrate an ability to perform their duties.[35-37] The efficacy of this pretreatment could not be assessed because fortunately no nerve agents were employed during the Gulf War.

The organophosphate insecticides are similar to nerve agents in inhibiting cholinesterase. However, the cholinergic crisis is generally much longer after exposure to an insecticide. Much larger doses of atropine are usually required to control the muscarinic symptoms after massive insecticide exposure.

Blood Agents

Blood agents are absorbed into the circulation and act by either blocking oxygen transport to the tissues (arsine, carbon monoxide) or oxidative metabolism [cyanide, sodium monoflouroacetate (compound 1080)]. Cyanide is the only blood agent for which an antidote is available.

Cyanides exist as highly volatile liquids or gases and can be absorbed by inhalation, percutaneous absorption, or ingestion. There are several different cyanides including cyanogen chloride (CK), hydrogen cyanide (AC), potassium cyanide (KCN), and sodium cyanide (NaCN). The cyanide ion has an affinity for transitional metals and binds to the ferrous iron in the mitochondrial cytochrome system. The binding of the cyanide ion to cytochrome a_3 interrupts mitochondrial oxidative metabolism resulting in lactic acidosis. The initial signs of cyanide poisoning include tachypnea and tachycardia. The skin is pink and the blood is bright red due to high oxygen saturation. Cyanide vapor may have the odor of bitter almonds. In the presence of a severe exposure, patients rapidly lose consciousness, develop apnea and cardiac arrest. The antidote for cyanide poisoning is treatment with a nitrite compound followed by sodium thiosulfate.[38]The nitrite oxidizes the ferrous ion in hemoglobin to the ferric ion creating methemoglobin. The ferric ion in methemoglobin has a much stronger affinity for the cyanide ion than the ferrous ion in cytochrome a_3. As a result, the cyanide ion binds to methemoglobin creating cyanomethemoglobin. Intravenous (IV) sodium thiosulfate then converts cyanomethemoglobin to thiocyanate and sulfite, two metabolically inert compounds which are excreted in the urine.[34] In adults, the nitrites may be administered by sniffing an ampule of 0.3 cc of amyl nitrite or by administration of 10 cc of a 3% solution of sodium nitrite IV followed by 50 cc of a 35% solution of sodium thiosulfate IV over 1 min.

If a patient has also been in a fire or explosion, both carbon monoxide and cyanide poisoning may be present. Nitrite therapy should be initiated with caution under these circumstances. If the carboxyhemoglobin level is elevated due to smoke inhalation, the addition of methemoglobin may further reduce oxygen delivery to the tissues. A delay in nitrite therapy may be necessary until the carboxyhemoglobin level is reduced.

Vesicants/Blister Agents

Vesicants, also known as blister agents or mustards, are viscous liquids at room temperature which induce blistering of the eyes, respiratory tract, mucous membranes, and skin. They also cause bone marrow suppression.[30] The time of onset and specific symptoms depend on the type of vesicant. The onset of symptoms may be delayed for as long as 24 hours. Massive exposure to aerosolized vesicants causes death due to respiratory tract burns and bone marrow suppression. After decontamination, the wounds are treated as burns.[35,36]

Vesicants were first used in battle in 1917 near Ypres in Belgium and were most recently used by the Iraqis against Iranian soldiers during the Iran–Iraq War in the 1980s. Although vesicants remain potential military weapons, their use in a terrorist attack is less likely because of difficulty with storage and delivery of the weapon to the site of the attack.

Pulmonary/Choking Agents

Pulmonary or choking agents cause severe irritation to the respiratory tract. Chlorine and phosgene are the classic pulmonary agents, but other gases such as bromine, hydrogen bromide, and sulfuryl fluoride produce a similar clinical syndrome. The clinical picture resembles an inhalation burn injury.

Patients exposed to pulmonary agents present initially with chest tightness and shortness of breath. Both the initial physical examination and chest X-ray may be normal. The development of pulmonary edema may be delayed by several hours. Bacterial pneumonia commonly occurs several days after exposure. Severe exposure leads to acute pulmonary edema, upper airway obstruction, and death. There is no antidote. Treatment consists of intubation and mechanical ventilation in the event of respiratory insufficiency.

Incapacitating Agents

This category includes agents used to tranquilize or incapacitate a population. In 2002, Russian Special Forces probably used aerosolized fentanyl to subdue Chechen terrorists holding hostages in a Moscow theater.[39] Unfortunately, the dose was lethal and caused the death of 129 (16%) of the 800 hostages and 41 of the 50 terrorists. All but two of the hostages' deaths were due to fentanyl.[40]

BZ, an incapacitating agent developed by the military, is an anticholinergic agent with effects similar to atropine. Individuals exposed to BZ manifest the classic symptoms of anticholinergic toxicity (see Table 13.3).

The treatment for BZ is carbamate cholinesterase inhibitors. These drugs increase the amount of acetylcholine in the synapse and competitively inhibit BZ at the muscarinic receptor. Physostigmine is the preferred carbamate because it crosses the blood–brain barrier to reverse the effects of BZ on the central nervous system.[25] Treatment consists of 2 mg of physostigmine diluted in 10 mL saline and administered IV over 5 minutes.

TABLE 13.3. Cholinergic versus anticholinergic symptoms

Anticholinergic toxicity (from BZ):
Dry as a bone (decreased secretions)
Red as a beet (skin flushing)
Blind as a bat (loss of visual accommodation)
Hot as a hare (heat retention)
Mad as a hatter (confusion, hallucinations, slurred speech)
Cholinergic toxicity (from nerve gas or oganophosphates) Muscarinic effects
S→Salivation
L→Lacrimation
U→Urination
D→Defecation
G→GI symptoms
E→Emesis
Nictoinic effects
Muscular: Fasciculations, flaccid paralysis
Cardiovascular: Variable (initial effect may be tachycardia followed by bradycardia as the severity of the cholinergic crisis increases)

Riot Control Agents/Tear Gas

Riot control agents are chemicals used by the police and the military to disperse large crowds. The term "tear gas" is actually a misnomer as the agents in this category are in the solid state at standard temperature and pressure. Delivery is accomplished by aerosolization. These chemicals irritate the skin and mucous membranes. The agents in this class include bromobenzylcyanide (CA), chloroacetophenone (CN, also known as "mace"), chlorobenzylidenemalononitrile (CS), chloropicrin (PS), dibenzoxazepine (CR), capsaicin (pepper spray), and diphenylaminearsine (DM). Management consists of decontamination and exposure to fresh air. Dilute hypochlorite solution should not be used as it may exacerbate dermatitis. It is also important to note that while these chemicals are not generally lethal, if persons with preexisting pulmonary disease (e.g., asthma) are exposed they may trigger a secondary lethal event.

Management of Patients Before the Identification of the Chemical Weapon

The agent responsible for a mass poisoning may not be identified in the immediate aftermath of the attack. A large number of people may arrive at local hospitals with similar symptoms after exposure before the identification of the chemical weapon as occurred in Bhopal, India, in 1984,[14] and Tokyo in 1995.[4,15]

A symptom-based algorithm for managing victims of chemical weapons during the first few minutes to hours after the attack is important. An example of such an algorithm is shown in Fig. 13.2. We developed this algorithm based on known chemical weapon symptoms, CDC recommendations, as well as a symptom-based protocol.[41]

Outcomes

The outcome of the attack will depend on both the potency and the quantity of the specific nerve agent released, the location (closed verses open space), and the ability of the exposed population to flee the area. Victims with severe exposure are at greater risk of dying at the scene. A relatively small number of moderately exposed victims can be salvaged by decontamination and timely administration of the antidote if one is available. Most of the patients presenting to the hospital will be the "worried well," as occurred after the sarin attack in the Tokyo subway in 1995. Identification of the small number of sick patients in the midst of the large number of worried well patients will be a major challenge.

Many survivors may experience long-term effects from chemical exposure. Persons who experienced one or more episodes of symptomatic organophosphate poisoning have reported neuropsychiatric changes for 1 year or longer after the initial exposure.[25] The duration of the neuropsychiatric effects after nerve agent attack is less well documented, but available information suggests that these effects persist for several weeks or possibly several months.[25]

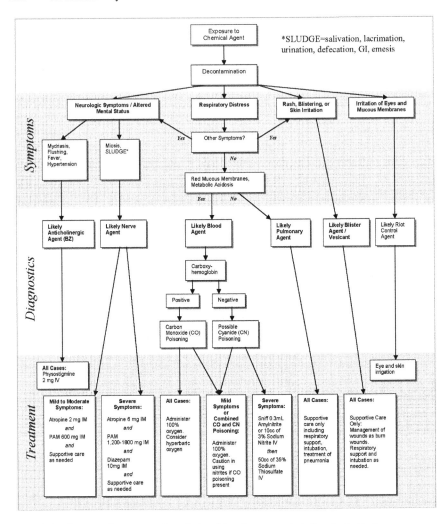

FIG. 13.2. Suggested symptom-based algorithm for suspected chemical attack.

Life-threatening delayed cardiotoxicity resulting from exposure to organophosphate compounds has also been described. The first report[42] documented an 18% mortality rate due to arrhythmias caused by organophosphate poisoning. One characteristic common to the patients who died was a prolonged QT interval. These findings have been confirmed in animal models of organophosphate toxicity.[43]

English, German, and Japanese mustard factory workers with repeated exposure to vesicants experience an increased incidence of airway cancer.[44-46] Mustard agent has been classified as a mutagen for its ability to cause chromosomal breaks. Mustard agents have also been shown to produce nonairway cancers in animals.

The effect of a single exposure to mustard agent on the future risk of cancer in humans is unknown.[25]

Conclusion

A terrorist chemical attack is a significant potential threat. Pre-hospital and hospital workers are likely to be directly involved in the care of the victims. The principles of management include event recognition, implementation of the Incident Command System, on-site and/or hospital decontamination, and protocolized medical management based on symptoms and signs until the toxic chemical is identified with certainty. Antidotes are available only for nerve agents, cyanide, and BZ. Decontamination and supportive medical care for victims of most chemical weapons is the only treatment. In the absence of an overt attack, pre-hospital and hospital workers must be prepared to recognize a chemical event and initiate decontamination procedures to minimize secondary exposure. A prearranged plan for response to a chemical weapon attack is essential for an organized, coordinated, and effective response.

References

1. Silberman LH, Robb CS, Levin RC, et al. Commission on the Intelligence Capabilities of the United States Regarding Weapons of Mass Destruction: Report to the President of the United States; 2005.
2. Beck M, Monroe S. The Tylenol scare: the death of seven people who took the drug triggers a nationwide alert—and a hunt for a madman. *Newsweek*. Oct 11 1982;100(15):32–36.
3. Morita H, Yanagisawa N, Nakajima T, et al. Sarin poisoning in Matsumoto, Japan. *Lancet*. Jul 29 1995;346(8970):290–293.
4. Nozaki H, Aikawa N, Shinozawa Y, et al. Sarin poisoning in Tokyo subway. *Lancet*. Apr 15 1995;345(8955):980–981.
5. Kosal ME. Near-Term Threats of Chemical Weapons Terrorism. *Strateg Insights*. July 2006;V(6):1–4.
6. Commission on the Intelligence Capabilities of the United States Regarding Weapons of Mass Destruction: Report to the President of the United States March 31, 2005.
7. Terrorist Chemical Device (Update). In: Security DoH, Investigation FBO, eds; 2004.
8. Convention on the Prohibition of the Development, Production, Stockpiling, and Use of Chemical Weapons and on their Destruction: The Organization for the Prohibition of Chemical Weapons; 1997.
9. Khan AS, Levitt AM, Sage MJ. Biological and Chemical Terrorism: Strategic Plan for Preparedness and Response. Recommendations of the CDC Strategic Planning Workgroup. *Morbidity and Mortality Weekly Report (MMWR)*. 2000;49:1–14.
10. Lawrence DT, Kirk MA. Chemical terrorism attacks: update on antidotes. *Emerg Med Clin North Am*. May 2007;25(2):567–595; abstract xi.
11. Noeller TP. Biological and chemical terrorism: recognition and management. *Cleve Clin J Med*. Dec 2001;68(12):1001–1002, 1004–1009, 1013–1006.
12. Patel M, Schier J, Belson M, Rubin C, Garbe P, Osterloh J. Recognition of illness associated with exposure to chemical agents — United States, 2003. *MMWR Weekly*. 2003;52:938–940.

13. Homeland security: Voluntary initiatives are under way at chemical facilities, but the extent of security preparedness is unknown. In: Office USGA, ed. U.S. General Accounting Office; 2003.

14. Bhopal Information Center Web site. http://www.bhopal.com/index.htm?404;http://www.bhopal.com/review.htm. Accessed July 11, 2007.

15. Okumura S, Okumura T, Ishimatsu S, Miura K, Maekawa H, Naito T. Clinical review: Tokyo—protecting the health care worker during a chemical mass casualty event: an important issue of continuing relevance. *Crit Care*. Aug 2005;9(4):397–400.

16. An Epidemiology Publication of the Oregon Department of Human Services: Preparing for a Chemical Terrorist Event–A Primer. *CD Summary*. 2003;52.

17. Kenar L, Karayilanoglu T. Prehospital management and medical intervention after a chemical attack. *Emerg Med J*. Jan 2004;21(1):84–88.

18. Waeckerle JF, Seamans S, Whiteside M, et al. Executive summary: developing objectives, content, and competencies for the training of emergency medical technicians, emergency physicians, and emergency nurses to care for casualties resulting from nuclear, biological, or chemical incidents. *Ann Emerg Med*. Jun 2001;37(6):587–601.

19. *Health Aspects of Biological and Chemical Weapons*. Geneva: World Health Organization; 2001.

20. Bennett RL. Chemical or biological terrorist attacks: an analysis of the preparedness of hospitals for managing victims affected by chemical or biological weapons of mass destruction. *Int J Environ Res Public Health*. Mar 2006;3(1):67–75.

21. Simon R, Teperman S. The World Trade Center attack. Lessons for disaster management. *Crit Care*. Dec 2001;5(6):318–320.

22. Managing Hazardous Materials Incidents (MHMI). Volumes 1, 2, and 3. Agency for Toxic Substances and Disease Registry (ATSDR). 2001. Atlanta, GA: U.S. Department of Health and Human Services, Public Health Service.

23. Keim ME, Pesik N, Twum-Danso NA. Lack of hospital preparedness for chemical terrorism in a major US city: 1996–2000. *Prehospital Disaster Med*. Jul–Sep 2003;18(3):193–199.

24. Treat KN, Williams JM, Furbee PM, Manley WG, Russell FK, Stamper CD, Jr. Hospital preparedness for weapons of mass destruction incidents: an initial assessment. *Ann Emerg Med*. Nov 2001;38(5):562–565.

25. *Medical Aspects of Chemical and Biologic Warfare*. Washington, DC: Office of the Surgeon General at TMM Publications; 1997.

26. Staten C. EMS Management for Hazardous Materials Incidents. *Emergency Response & Research Institute*; 1992.

27. Macintyre AG, Christopher GW, Eitzen E, Jr., et al. Weapons of mass destruction events with contaminated casualties: effective planning for health care facilities. *JAMA*. Jan 12 2000;283(2):242–249.

28. Sidell FR. What to do in case of an unthinkable chemical warfare attack or accident. *Postgrad Med*. Nov 15 1990;88(7):70–76, 81–74.

29. OSHA Technical Manual. *Section VIII: Chapter 1 Chemical Protective Clothing* [http://www.osha.gov/dts/osta/otm/otm_viii/otm_viii_1.html. Accessed July 11, 2007.

30. Schecter WP, Fry DE. The surgeon and acts of civilian terrorism: chemical agents. *J Am Coll Surg*. Jan 2005;200(1):128–135.

31. Ben Abraham R, Rudick V, Weinbroum AA. Practical guidelines for acute care of victims of bioterrorism: conventional injuries and concomitant nerve agent intoxication. *Anesthesiology*. Oct 2002;97(4):989–1004.

32. Sidell FR. Clinical effects of organophosphorus cholinesterase inhibitors. *J Appl Toxicol.* Mar–Apr 1994;14(2):111–113.
33. Taylor P. Anticholinesterase agents. In: Hardman JG, Limbird LE, eds. *Goodman and Gilman's the Pharmacological Basis of Therapeutics.* 9th ed. New York: McGraw-Hill; 1996:161–170.
34. Field Management of Chemical Casualties Handbook. July 2000. 2nd ed; 2000.
35. Arad M, Varssano D, Moran D, Arnon R, Vazina A, Epstein Y. Effects of heat-exercise stress, NBC clothing, and pyridostigmine treatment on psychomotor and subjective measures of performance. *Mil Med.* Apr 1992;157(4):210–214.
36. Gawron VJ, Schiflett SG, Miller JC, Slater T, Ball JF. Effects of pyridostigmine bromide on in-flight aircrew performance. *Hum Factors.* Feb 1990;32(1):79–94.
37. Keeler JR, Hurst CG, Dunn MA. Pyridostigmine used as a nerve agent pretreatment under wartime conditions. *JAMA.* Aug 7 1991;266(5):693–695.
38. Marrs TC. Antidotal treatment of acute cyanide poisoning. *Adverse Drug React Acute Poisoning Rev.* Winter 1988;7(4):179–206.
39. Coupland RM. Incapacitating chemical weapons: a year after the Moscow theatre siege. *Lancet.* Oct 25 2003;362(9393):1346.
40. Donahoe JJ. The Moscow Hostage Crisis: An Analysis of Chechen Terrorist Goals. *Strateg Insights.* 2003;II(5):1–4.
41. Subbarao I, Johnson C, Bond WF, et al. Symptom-based, algorithmic approach for handling the initial encounter with victims of a potential terrorist attack. *Prehospital Disaster Med.* Sep–Oct 2005;20(5):301–308.
42. Luzhnikov EA, Aleksandrovskii VN, Tsunikov AI, Kosarev VA, Pavlov AS. [Neurological and electrophysiological changes after acute peroral poisoning with organophosphate insecticides]. *Voen Med Zh.* Nov 1975(11):41–44.
43. Allon N, Rabinovitz I, Manistersky E, Weissman BA, Grauer E. Acute and long-lasting cardiac changes following a single whole-body exposure to sarin vapor in rats. *Toxicol Sci.* Oct 2005;87(2):385–390.
44. Easton DF, Peto J, Doll R. Cancers of the respiratory tract in mustard gas workers. *Br J Ind Med.* Oct 1988;45(10):652–659.
45. Wada S, Miyanishi M, Nishimoto Y, Kambe S, Miller RW. Mustard gas as a cause of respiratory neoplasia in man. *Lancet.* Jun 1 1968;1(7553):1161–1163.
46. Weiss A, Weiss B. [Carcinogenesis due to mustard gas exposure in man, important sign for therapy with alkylating agents]. *Dtsch Med Wochenschr.* Apr 25 1975;100(17):919–923.

14
Radiological Agents and Terror Medicine

JEFFREY S. HAMMOND and JILL LIPOTI

Few words can elicit more fear and misunderstanding than "radiation." A terrorist's chief aim is psychological, to instill fear. This fear is compounded if radioactivity is involved because it is invisible and undetectable without specialized equipment, it may be perceived to be untreatable and associated with cancer, the long-term impact is unknown and it evokes historical mental images of Hiroshima and Chernobyl.

The attacks of 9/11 focused attention on unconventional terrorist events, including those potentially involving radioactive materials. Consequently, greater attention has been paid to increased security at nuclear power plants. Prudence dictates that we consider and plan for all types of radiological emergencies, however.

A terrorist event involving radioactive material would likely take the form of one of four scenarios: detonation of a small tactical nuclear device ("suitcase bombs"), sabotage of a nuclear reactor, nonexplosive dispersal, or placement of an unshielded high-energy source of radioactive material via a radiological exposure device (RED), or dispersal of radioactive material in association with a conventional explosive, a so-called radiological dispersal device (RDD) or "dirty bomb."[1]

In September 2005, the International Atomic Energy Agency (IAEA) documented the inadequate security of radioactive materials in 100 countries, especially in those of the former Soviet Union. The smuggling of radioactive sources rose from 8 incidents in 1996 to 77 in 2003, including at least one case of weapons grade material.[2] Since 1993, the IAEA has confirmed 18 incidents involving highly enriched uranium or plutonium. Smuggling of nuclear material in the form of spent fuel rods and by-products of civilian nuclear power plants, or radioactive sources from medicine, mining, and industrial sources such as cesium-137 or cobalt-60, further increases the risk of use to construct an RDD.

Indeed, with the exception of the detonation of a nuclear device, such events have already occurred. The episodes of nuclear reactor meltdown at Chernobyl, and near-meltdown at Three Mile Island, are constant reminders of the risk reactors pose, in an urban environment. A minute amount of Polonium 210 placed in a drink at a restaurant was used to kill a former Soviet agent in London in 2006. In 1995, Chechen separatists buried a source of cesium-137 in a Moscow public park and then alerted the news media. While there were no injuries, the aim of the terrorist is to disrupt the social fabric of his or her target, and the message in this case was quite clearly made.

S.C. Shapira et al. (eds.), *Essentials of Terror Medicine*,
DOI: 10.1007/978-0-387-09412-0_14, Springer Science+Business Media, LLC 2009

In 2002, a United States citizen was arrested, and later convicted, on charges that he conspired to deploy an RDD, or "dirty bomb," in the United States.

Planning, responding, management, and recovery would be more challenging than after a conventional explosive device. Treatment of casualties is complicated by contamination.

The decontamination effort is compounded by the necessity to include the area of the event and associated debris. Hence, the affected area may be much larger than the immediate area of the attack. Unlike a bombing or conventional blast, the size and nature of the event will not be known for an indeterminate time. Consequently, the opportunity to induce hysteria among both uniformed public and health professionals may lead to panic. The potential for social disorder and panic has lead to RDDs being considered a "weapon of mass disruption." The need for specialized mental health services and debriefing, as well as medical follow-up for those exposed, those potentially exposed, or those fearing exposure will be significant.

Moreover, the consequences of the radiological event will be uncertain in terms of long-term health impacts. This may contribute to both public panic and health care worker distress. In addition to the immediate threats to public health, social issues, including potential stigmatization of victims as being unclean or contaminated, and the need for environmental remediation, may result in economic disruption of markets and essential services. This may be mitigated by a communication strategy that includes pre-event education, intra-event communication, and post-event counseling and debriefing.

Radiation Basics

Radiation is a form of energy. It is naturally occurring, invisible, and ubiquitous. Radioactivity is the mechanism by which an unstable nucleus rearranges itself to achieve a more stable configuration, ejecting charged particles to do so. There are 92 naturally occurring elements that make up the periodic table, and each undergoes some form of decay over time. It is this process of natural decay that creates emission of radiation.

Radiation energy can be in the form of either particles or electromagnetic waves. Alpha particles represent emission of a helium nucleus, two protons and two neutrons. They are heavy, slow moving particles with limited potential for penetration, and are readily blocked by paper or skin. However, if an alpha-emitting material causes internal contamination through inhalation, ingestion, or via a wound it can cause ionization resulting in damage to tissue.

Beta particles represent emission of either a positron or electron. Smaller and faster than alpha particles, they have the potential for moderate penetration, but are blocked by plaster, glass, or foil. Some beta radiation can penetrate human skin to the basement membrane layer where new skin cells are produced, and, in the event of prolonged contact, may cause skin injury.

Neutron radiation is a third form of particle, and requires water, concrete, or lead shielding to block. Gamma radiation is electromagnetic wave activity in the form of high-energy photons. Gamma waves penetrate well but may be blocked by less than 1 inch of lead.

Ionizing radiation is measured in either the English unit, the *rad*, or the international scientific unit, the *gray* (Gy). The rad denotes the deposition of 0.01 joules of energy per kilogram of tissue. Both rads and Gy measure the amount of energy absorbed per unit mass, and 1 Gy equals 100 rads. However, rads of differing types of ionizing radiation produce different tissue damage potentials. Therefore, the *rem* was introduced to account for this variation is tissue damage potential. Rems measure the absorbed dose weighted by type of radiation, or the biological dose conferring tissue damage. This distinction is important since victims may be exposed to multiple types of radiation emitters.

For one-time flash exposures, 1 rad effectively equals1 rem. The corresponding international unit for the biological risk of exposure is designated the seivert (Sv). One seivert equals 100 rem and may be thought of as a cumulative dose. For beta particles and gamma rays, Gy and Sv are numerically equivalent. Seivert is commonly used when referring to internal contamination.[3]

Radiation is a natural process, to which we are subjected on a daily basis. The average annual dose from all sources of ionizing radiation in the United States is 360 mRem. A barium enema examination may expose a patient to 870 mrem, while a cardiac catheterization may deliver a skin dose of up to 26,000 mrem. Prodromal signs of acute radiation sickness may appear with exposure to 100 rem (1.0 Sv). The LD50, or the lethal dose for 50% of the population at 60 days, is 400–500 rems (4–5 Gy or 4–5 Sv).[4]

The physical half-life of an isotope is the time (in minutes, hours, days, or years) required for the activity of a radioactive material to decrease by one half due to radioactive decay. Half-lives range from fractions of seconds to millions of years (Fig. 14.1). The biological half-life, on the contrary, is the time required for the body to eliminate half of the radioactive material, and depends on the chemical form.

Radioactive Contamination

Exposure reduction techniques are based on the three principles of time, distance, and shielding. Distance is related to the area of a sphere ($4\Pi r^2$). Since intensity (I) is related to source strength (S) divided by the surface area of the sphere, energy levels at twice the distance from the source spread over four times the area, and is therefore one-quarter of the intensity. At three times the distance, the intensity is reduced to one-ninth.

It is important to remember that casualties that have been irradiated are not radioactive themselves. In this regard, the victim of a radiological incident differs from the victim of a biological or chemical exposure. While basic hazardous material (HAZMAT) response guidelines were originally derived from radiation response documents,[5] they have evolved separately since radiation does not pose the same potential degree of hazard.

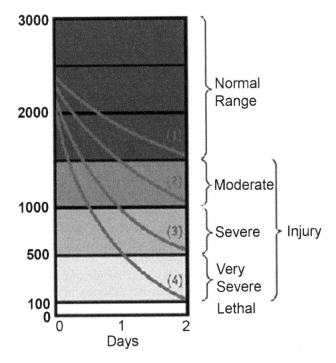

F<small>IG</small>. 14.1. Patterns of early lymphocyte response in relation to dose.

Health care workers must understand the essential difference and ramifications between exposure and contamination. Irradiation is exposure to penetrating radiation. Irradiation occurs when all or part of the body is exposed to radiation from an unshielded source. However, exposure does not necessarily connote contamination. For example, a person receiving medical X-rays is exposed but not contaminated. External irradiation *does not* make a person radioactive. Such a patient can receive care from doctors and nurses utilizing basic universal precautions without risk.

Contamination occurs when material that contains radioactive atoms is deposited on skin, clothing, in wounds, or is ingested. It is important to remember that radiation per se does not spread or get "on" or "in" people; rather it is radioactive contamination that can spread. A person contaminated with radioactive materials will be irradiated until the source of radiation (the radioactive material) is removed.

A person is *externally* contaminated if radioactive material is on skin or clothing. External contamination may come as a result of dust, powder, or liquid. External radiation contamination has been likened to dirt as an analogy, both for the relative ease of removal and the limited risk to health care workers. The victim is *internally* contaminated if radioactive material is inhaled, swallowed, or absorbed through wounds. Such radioactive material may or may not be eliminated from the body in urine, feces, or sweat. Various drugs are available that can be used to block uptake (e.g., KI, potassium iodide) or enhance elimination (e.g., Prussian blue).

The US Department of Energy maintains a 24-h hotline [(865) 576–1005] for questions about radiation exposure and management at the Radiation Emergency Assistance Center/Training Site (REAC/TS) in Oak Ridge, Tennessee (www.orise.orau.gov/reac).

Response to a Terrorist Event Involving Radioactivity

Planning

The planning for, and response to, a radiological terrorist event presents unique requirements for assessment, treatment, personal protection, public health, and mental health.

In the event of a radiation-related event, a planned course of action should include verification and notification. Key data include ascertaining, if possible, the number of victims, mechanism of injury, on-site efforts at surveillance for contamination, the victims' radiological status, and identity of the contaminant.

Each member of the response team should be familiar with the hospital's written plan. This mandates active participation in scheduled hospital-based drills and regional exercises. The Joint Commission (formerly the Joint Commission for Accreditation of Health Care Organizations), a regulatory and certifying body in the United States, requires at least two disaster drills annually. More frequent drills should be scheduled for specific subgroups directly involving HAZMAT-related activities such as decontamination.

The general principles of emergency preparedness and hospital disaster planning are described elsewhere in this text, and will not be repeated here. However, while a disaster plan should adhere to an "all-hazards" approach, there should be an annex or appendix specific to radiation events. This addendum would address specific needs such as notification of a radiation safety or health physics officer, establishment of receptacles for contaminated material and waste, distribution of radiation survey meters, and radiation-specific decontamination and physical plant maneuvers, such as floor covering.

This annex would also delineate specific roles for other members of the health care team that would be unique to the situation. For example, the pharmacist would assume a HAZMAT role, would deploy a nuclear antidote cart, monitor inventory, and report the exposure to the appropriate regulatory agencies.[6] A radiological incident may be associated with cutaneous burns, and each facility should have a formalized transfer and support relationship with a regional burn center.

A special consideration to basic disaster triage is the phenomenon of the worried well. This will likely be compounded by the hysteria associated with a radiological event. For this reason, radiological devices and radiation have been described as "weapons of mass hysteria," in contradistinction to weapons of mass destruction. An incident caused by nuclear terrorism may create large numbers of contaminated people who are not injured and worried people who may not be injured or contaminated. Measures, including triage outside the emergency department (ED) and a lockdown of the ED, must be taken to prevent these people from overwhelming the facility.

Since the sine qua non of radiation decontamination is removal of clothing and showering ("wet decon"), which will remove over 85–90% of the contamination, facility disaster planning should include provisions for multiple showers in a temperature-controlled area, including a decon area for those people contaminated but otherwise uninjured. In addition, plans must include provisions for management of children separated from parents, assistance for the elderly, bagging and identification of clothing for later forensic investigation and disposal, and replacement clothing.

Members of the radiological emergency response team do not need high-level personal protective equipment (PPE). Universal precautions will suffice. Pregnant staff should be excluded from decontamination teams. Organize staff into decon teams with set rotation schedules to minimize exposure. Emergency staff should dress in surgical clothing (scrub suit, gown, mask, cap, eye protection, and gloves) and don waterproof shoe covers. A radiation dosimeter should be assigned to each team member and attached to the outside of the surgical gown or PPE where it can be easily removed and read. These dosimeters are different from routine radiology department monitors, in that they can be read in real time on-site by the radiation safety officer (RSO). Dosimeters come with and without alarms. Finger ring dosimeters are preferred; however, the RSO can estimate the radiation dose to the hands based on total body dosimetry.[7]

To prepare a treatment area, remove or cover equipment that will not be needed during emergency care of the radiation accident victim. Multiple large plastic-lined waste containers will be needed. If possible, survey instruments should be checked and ready for use before the patients arrive. Background radiation levels should be documented.

Rolls of brown wrapping paper or butcher paper 3 to 4-feet wide can be unrolled to make a path from the ambulance entrance to the decontamination room. This will facilitate cleanup after the event. Chux can also be used if paper is not available. This route should then be roped off and marked to prevent unauthorized entry.

The floor of the decontamination room or treatment area should be covered in a similar way if time allows.

While it may be desirable that the treatment area have either a ventilation system that is separate from the rest of the hospital or can be isolated to prevent the unfiltered exhaust air from the radiation emergency area from mixing with the air that is distributed to the rest of the hospital, there is little likelihood that contaminants will become suspended in air and enter the ventilation system. Therefore, separate ventilation systems are not recommended.

Patient Care

Triage is an iterative process. Some patients may be triaged and decontaminated in the field, but the majority will bypass the emergency medical services (EMS) system and self-refer or self-transport. Therefore, a triage station should be set up outside the ED. No patient should be admitted to the ED or facility without passing through the hospital triage station. Instruct EMS personnel to stay with their vehicle until they, their vehicle, and equipment are surveyed and released by a RSO.

The most common type of radiation detector is a Geiger-Mueller tube, also called a Geiger counter. The operator should first survey, and record, background readings over a 60-second span. The probe should be held approximately ½–1 inch from the skin and moved slowly in a sequential fashion over the entire body, paying particular attention to the palms of the hands and soles of the feet.

When in doubt, a critically injured patient may be taken immediately into the treatment area. If the victim's condition allows, an initial, brief radiation survey can be performed to determine if the victim is contaminated. Any radiation survey meter reading above background radiation levels indicates the possibility of contamination. A more thorough survey will be performed once life-threatening problems are addressed.

During triage, serious medical problems have priority over radiological concerns, and immediate attention is directed to life-threatening problems. Radiation injury rarely causes unconsciousness or immediate visible signs of injury and is not immediately life threatening unless severe and fatal acute radiation sickness is present; therefore, other causes of injury or illness must be considered. Life-saving maneuvers, such as hemorrhage control or airway management, should not be withheld pending wet decon. In such cases, removal of clothing, followed by immediate patient care, should precede wet decon. Medical stabilization of the patient is the first priority, and full decontamination can follow.[8]

Risk to health care staff is an obvious concern. Computer modeling of a hypothetical RDD employing a cobalt-60 fragment indicated that surgical staff might receive a does that could exceed the LD_{50} over a 2-hour period.[9] However, this was an extreme simulation example, as the dose received by the patient was a lethal one, and the patient would likely have been considered expectant. The occupational dose limit of 5 rem per year does not apply in life-saving operations, and is extended to 25 rem per event by the US Environmental Protection Agency, and 150 rem by NATO.[10] The National Council on Radiation Protection and Measurements (NCRP) advises that emergency exposure may exceed that limit and even approach 500 rem, but in the context that this is considered an once-in-a-lifetime event.[11] The International Committee on Radiation Protection estimates, based on Japanese data from WWII, that the lifetime risk of excess fatal cancer is 5% per Gy of whole body irradiation.[12] The doses received by ED staff after the Chernobyl accident were less than 1 rem.[13]

Time to first emesis is an important biological marker that may guide triage. The time to onset of prodromal symptoms is the most important factor in determining whether significant exposure has occurred. Initial symptoms include nausea, vomiting, diarrhea, and skin tingling. Early emesis, 1–4 hours from the time of exposure, indicates a dose likely to be at least 3.5 Gy, and indicates the need for urgent treatment.[14] These patients may warrant cytokine therapy with colony-stimulating factors.[15] Emesis less than 1 hour from exposure is associated with doses exceeding 6.5 Gy and uniformly fatal outcomes. These patients can be considered "expectant" during triage. Patients with emesis occurring more than 4 hours from exposure may be deferred for delayed evaluation after management of the more urgent cohort.

Use care to avoid spread of any contaminants embedded in or on the clothing. Clothing, and any accompanying linens should be placed in a marked, red plastic bag. If practicable, washing fluid should be collected for later analysis by the health physicist, to determine the dose received and for forensic analysis. If not practical, washwater can simply be directed to the domestic sewerage system. Caregivers should change gloves after handling clothing or other potentially contaminated items. Once the patient is decontaminated, he or she is given a bracelet or tag to designate that the procedure has been completed for later caregivers.

Noncontaminated individuals can be cared for as in any other emergency case. The victim of exposure without contamination poses no radiological hazard to others. If exposure is known or suspected, a stat complete blood count (CBC) should be ordered with particular attention given to determining the total lymphocyte count (TLC). After the baseline test, repeat every 4–6 hours to detect decreases in TLC. Be sure to document the time the blood sample is obtained. Findings may be plotted against an Andrews lymphocyte curve (see Fig. 14.2) to predict the clinical course.[16] While the TLC is less reliable in patients with combined injuries, such as trauma and burns, a decrease of 50% to less than 1000/mm^3 in the first 24–48 hours is indicative of at least a moderate radiation dose. An absolute neutrophil count of less than 500 at 48 hours is prognostic for a lethal injury.[17]

Contaminated wounds should be gently irrigated and washed, not scrubbed, with soft sponges and lukewarm water. Since intact skin forms a barrier, care must be taken to avoid creating abrasions or open wounds which increase morbidity and mortality. Debride surgically only as needed. Avoid overly aggressive decontamination. A dosimeter can monitor the process, which should continue until radiation levels are less than two times the background radiation.

In cases where open wounds are present, consider all such wounds as contaminated until proven otherwise. Swab wounds with a cotton-tip applicator and survey the cotton tip for levels of radioactivity. Remove visible radioactive material and place it into a lead pig for proper evaluation and disposal by the RSO. Remove foreign bodies with forceps or pick-ups or a water-pik; never handle directly without instruments.

To assess for internal contamination, swab body orifices including the nostrils, mouth, ears, and rectum and survey the swabs. The most common site of injury is

Technetium-99m	6 hours
Thallium-201	73 hours
Cobalt-60	5 years
Cesium-137	30 years
Americium-247	432 years
Uranium-238	4.5 billion years

FIG. 14.2. Half-life of representative nuclear isotopes.

the lungs, resulting from inhalation of contaminated air. Nasal swabs within 1.5 hours of the event will give an indication of isotope size and lung burden.[18]

Gastric lavage and laxatives may reduce the gut load after ingestion. In a mass casualty event, the volume of patients may preclude collection of urine and stool for evaluation. Medical countermeasures in the event of internal contamination include radiation mitigators and eliminators (see Table 14.1). It is essential that appropriate drugs and supplies be readily available. As such, hospitals or other local facilities should have on hand or know where to obtain ample quantities of antidotes and neutralizers. These include, for example, potassium iodide to protect against thyroid deposition of radioactive iodine, sodium bicarbonate to mitigate the effects of uranium exposures, and Prussian blue to help negate the effects of radioactive poisoning from cesium, rubidium, or thalium.

There is no evidence to support the use of steroids for neurological symptoms.[19]

In addition to routine medical records, note survey readings, type and time of samples obtained, time of first emesis if any, and completion of decontamination.

Take care to note preexisting conditions such as rashes, healing wounds, or scars. This information may assist in reconstructing the event, or making a prognosis.

A threshold dose of 0.5 Gy is required to induce most substantial adverse fetal effects.[20] The risk of major malformations is primarily between gestational days 18

TABLE 14.1. Drugs to mitigate effects of internal contamination

Radionuclide	Medication	Ingestion/Inhalation dose	Principle of action
Iodine	KI (potassium iodide)	130 mg (tablet) stat, followed by 130 mg q.d. × 7–14 d (if indicated); 65 mg/d for children aged 3–18 years	Blocks thyroid deposition
Rare earths Plutonium Transplutonics Yttrium	Zn-DPTA Ca-DTPA	1 gm Ca-DTPA (Zn-DTPA) in 150–250 ml 5% D/W IV over 60 min for up to 5 d	Chelation
Uranium	Bicarbonate	2 ampules sodium bicarbonate (44.3 mEq each; 7.5%) in 1000 cc normal saline at 125 cc/h; alternately, oral administration of two bicarbonate tablets every 4 h until the urine reaches a pH of 8–9	Alkalinization of urine; reduces chance of acute tubular necrosis
Cesium Rubidium Thallium	Prussian Blue [Ferrihexacyano-Ferrate (II)]	1 g with 100–200 ml water p.o. t.i.d. up to 10 g/d for 3 weeks (titrate by fecal and urine assay)	Blocks absorption from GI tract and prevents recycling.
Tritium	Water	Force fluids, approximately >3–4 L/d	Isotopic dilution

Adapted from Radiation Event Medical Manager. www.remm.nlm.gov

and 40, although the specific window for fetal harm leading to embryonic death is 4–11 days.[17] Termination of pregnancy is not justified based on radiation-related risk for fetal doses less than 10 rem. Exposure to 5 rem increases the risk of severe heredity effects by approximately 0.02%.[21] Fetal doses greater than 50 rem can cause significant damage however, depending on the dose and stage of gestation, leading to difficult care decisions for the mother and treatment team.

When surgery is required, it is preferable to do so within the first 48–72 hours. Beyond that window of opportunity, bone marrow suppression and derangements in wound healing, bleeding diathesis and infection risk make operative management complicated and risky.[22] Examples of the practical considerations of this restriction include a decision for early wound closure rather than management of the abdomen with temporary abdominal closure, and limited use of external fixation in preference to definitive open reduction and fixation.

If no symptoms appear within 24 hours, and there is no aberration in the peripheral blood count, especially the TLC, the patient can be discharged home.[23] Mental health considerations will pose a large public health burden. In keeping with other terrorist events, an RDD will likely produce four psychological casualties for every physical victim.[1] It is imperative that following initial care and treatment, someone with knowledge of radiation effects spend adequate time answering the patient's questions and addressing concerns of the staff.

Aftermath and Recovery

The first 24–48 hours are the worst; after that, you will likely have many additional resources. Over time, the event will evolve from a response to a recovery phase. Early symptoms and their intensity are an indication of the severity of the radiation injury.

However, because of the prolonged time frame associated with radiation sickness, which extends into months, and potential long-term appearance of malignancies, this will likely be spread over a longer time frame than other types of disasters.

Survey the facility for contamination and decontaminate as necessary. Normal cleaning routines (mop, strip waxed floors) are typically very effective and generally adequate.

Replace cloth furniture, floor and ceiling tiles, and other physical plant items that cannot be adequately decontaminated. The decontamination goal is less than twice normal background levels. Consult the health physics officer or staff for instructions for proper disposal of radioactively contaminated debris.

Management of the deceased requires coordination with the medical examiner or coroner's office. The US Centers for Disease Control and Prevention has published guidelines for handling decedents contaminated with radioactive materials.[24] Worker monitoring, debriefing, and counseling as needed is an essential part of a successful response. The most important take-home message is train and drill to ensure competence and confidence. Despite this need, a 2004 study of 10 Philadelphia area hospitals reported that less than half were observed using Geiger counters, dosimeters, lead pigs, or antidotes/chelating agents during a full-scale regional exercise.[25]

The key planning and treatment axioms are outlined in Table 14.2.

TABLE 14.2. Key points in planning for and managing of radiation injuries

- This is a weapon of mass *hysteria*, not a weapon of mass destruction. Given proper precautions, the *risk* to health care workers is negligible.
- Externally exposed patients do not become radioactive and therefore do not pose a significant risk to emergency medical services (EMS) or other responders. *Do not delay* medical treatment.
- The major hazard to health and safety is the *explosion* itself and/or injury from shrapnel or fragments.
- *Contact* your *radiation safety officer* or health physics specialist early.
- *Universal precautions* will help delay or prevent the spread of contamination. This includes *double gloving*. Lead shields are not necessary and give a false sense of security.
- A high gamma source may be present at the emergency site. Perform a *radiological assessment*. The incident commander should limit access to the "hot zone" to what is necessary to assist victims.
- Assess and treat life-threatening injuries immediately, treatment of such takes *priority* over decontamination. Do not delay advanced life support.
- *Removal* of patient's clothing will *reduce contamination by 85–90%*. Place clothing in a plastic bag and label with name and location. Washing of skin with water and a mild soap is effective for initial decontamination after clothing removal. It is not necessary to collect the water used for decontamination.
- *Decontamination* is successful when radiation counts are <2× background. Document contamination pattern on a body diagram.
- *Gently wash* the skin during decon. *Do not* use scrub bushed or *abrade* the skin during washing, as this may create a wound and lead to internal contamination.
- In the medical facility, set up a *controlled area* for victims. Use a *buffer zone* for added security. *Cover floor areas* (butcher block paper, Chux, etc.) to prevent tracking of contaminants.
- All staff should wear a *dosimeter*. These are different from routine X-ray film badges. They should be worn outside any surgical gown at the neck to be easily read and removed. *Monitor* anyone and everything leaving the controlled area.
- *Assess for internal contamination*. Swab body orifices (nose, ears, mouth, rectum) and evaluate for isotope. Evaluate for radioactive fragments. This should be removed with instruments. Avoid touching with ungloved hands.
- If surgery is required, there may be a *36 to 48-hour window* before the onset of cytopenias and acute radiation syndrome. Wound closure should be accomplished in this time frame or may be delayed 2–3 months.
- Patients who exhibit *vomiting* less than 1 hour after exposure have overwhelming acute radiation syndrome and should be treated expectantly.
- After the event, *survey* the facility for contamination. Mop and strip waxed floors if readings twice background are encountered. Remove ceiling tiles or cloth furniture that cannot be cleaned.
- *Debrief* staff and provide psychological support postevent.

Conclusion

The use of radioactive materials as a terrorist weapon is both plausible and potentially highly disruptive and destructive. In the context of terror medicine, the challenges include not only treatment of affected patients and contaminated surfaces but also the special precautions that health care workers must take and knowledge they must have to ensure their personal safety.

While only one of many possible terrorist threats, the nature of a radiological attack requires unique preparedness and response procedures. Optimal medical management of such an attack can only be achieved with proper education, planning, training, and drills on the part of the responders, physicians, nurses, and other personnel likely to become engaged.

References

1. Barnett DJ, Parker CL, Blodgett DW et al. Understanding radiologic and nuclear terrorism as public health threats: Preparedness and response perspectives. J Nucl Med 2006; 47: 1653–1661.
2. Averting radiation terrorism, December 9, 2005. http://www.janes.com/security/international_security/news/rus1/rjhm051209_1_n.shtml
3. Burnham JW, Franco J. Radiation. Crit Care Clin 2005; 21: 785–813
4. Goans RE, Waselenko JK. Medical management of radiologic casualties. Health Phys 2005; 89: 505–511.
5. Fong FH. Medical Management of Radiation Accidents, in Hogan D and Burstein J (eds.), *Disaster Medicine*. Lippincott, Williams & Wilkins, Philadelphia, 2002.
6. Cohan V. Organization of a health system pharmacy team to respond to episodes of terrorism. Am J Health Syst Pharm 2003; 60: 1257–1263.
7. Centers for Disease Control and Prevention. Protecting responding personnel. Available at: http://www.remm.nlm.gov/ext_contamination.html. Accessed September 30, 2008.
8. Cone DC, Koenig K. Mass casualty triage in the chemical, biological, radiological or nuclear environment. Eur J Emerg med 2005; 12: 287–302.
9. Smith JA, Ansari A, Harper FT. Hospital management of mass radiological casualties: Reassessing exposures from contaminated victims of an exploded radiological dispersal device. Health Phys 2005; 89: 513–520.
10. Mettler FA, Voelz GL. Major radiation exposure—what to expect and how to respond. NEJM 2002; 346: 1554–1561.
11. National Council on Radiation Protection and Measurement, NCRP report #116, "Limitations of exposure to ionizing radiation." Bethesda, MD, 1993.
12. Fry RJ, Fry SA. Health effects of ionizing radiation. Med Clin NA 1990; 74: 475–488.
13. Bushberg JT, Kroger LA, Hartman MB, et al. Nuclear/Radiological terrorism: Emergency department management of radiation injuries. J Emerg Med 2007; 32: 71–85.
14. Koenig K, Goans RE, Hatchett RJ, et al. Medical treatment of radiological casualties: Current concepts. Ann Emerg Med 2005; 45: 643–652.
15. Waselenko JK, MacVittie TJ, Blakely WF, et al. Medical management of acute radiation syndrome: Recommendations of the Strategic National Stockpile Working Group. Ann Intern Med 2004; 140: 1037–1051.
16. Andrews GA. Medical management of accidental total body irradiation, in Hubner KF, Fry Sa (eds.), *The medical basis for radiation accident preparedness*. Elsevier, North Holland, 1980.
17. Chambers JA, Purdue GF. Radiation injury and the surgeon. J Am Coll Surg 2007; 204: 128–139.
18. Edsall K, Keyes DC. Treatment of radiation exposure and contamination, in Keyes DC (ed.), *Medical Response to Terrorism*. Lippincott, Williams & Wilkins, Philadelphia, 2005.
19. Fry DE, Schecter WP, Hartshorne MF. The surgeons and acts of civilian terrorism: Radiation exposure and injury. J Am Coll Surg 2006; 202: 146–154.
20. US Nuclear regulatory Commission. Regulatory Guide 8.13: Instruction Concerning Prenatal Radiation Exposure, revision 2, December 1987.

21. Mossman KL, Hill LT. Radiation risks in pregnancy. Obst Gynecol 1982; 60: 237–242.
22. Hirsch EF, Bowers GJ. Irradiated trauma victims: The impact of ionizing radiation on surgical considerations following a nuclear mishap. World J Surg 1992; 16: 919–923.
23. Radiation Emergencies. Centers for Disease Control and Prevention, Atlanta, Georgia, 2008. www.bt.cdc.gov/radiation.
24. Guidelines for handling decedents contaminated with radioactive materials. Centers for Disease Control and Prevention, Atlanta, Georgia, 2007. http://www.bt/cdc.gove/radiation/pdf/radiation-decedent-guidelines.pdf
25. Jasper E, Miller M, Sweeney B, et al. Preparedness of hospitals to respond to a radiological terrorism event as assessed by a full-scale exercise. J Pub Health Management Prac 2005; November (suppl): S11–S16.

15
Cyber-Terrorism: Preparation and Response

Abraham R. Wagner and Zvi Fisch

Cyber-terrorism represents the intersection of two distinct historical phenomena – cyberspace and terrorism. Cyberspace may be understood as the "virtual world" of symbolic or binary representations of information – a place where computer programs function and data move. In other terms, it is the world of computers and networks. Terrorism has been described as premeditated, politically motivated violence perpetrated against noncombatant targets by subnational groups or clandestine agents. Combining these characterizations, the result is what is now commonly known as "cyber-terrorism."

Cyber-Attacks Really Do Matter

The past three decades have seen the world become one where possible cyber-attacks are a serious concern. There has been movement at an astonishing pace from an analog world to a digital one dominated by interconnected systems, for communications, information, medical services, finance, and national security. This has been not only a technological revolution but a social and cultural one as well. While these systems provide great efficiencies and capabilities, they also create significant vulnerabilities. The real questions are just what vulnerabilities they create; what can be done about them; and by whom.

Cyber-attacks differ from other forms of hostile actions in that both the weapons and the targets are highly dynamic in nature. Other forms of terrorist activity are largely static, in that the weapons and the targets do not change very much from year to year. Consider some "classic" terrorist targets and weapons:

- Crowded markets have been around for millennia; crowded buses for almost a century.
- Tall buildings have been with us for over a century (New York's original "skyscraper" – the Flatiron Building, was constructed in 1902, and even the World Trade Center lost in the 9/11 tragedy was some 30 years old).

S.C. Shapira et al. (eds.), *Essentials of Terror Medicine*,
DOI: 10.1007/978-0-387-09412-0_15, Springer Science+Business Media, LLC 2009

- Airports have not changed a great deal, in technical terms in over 50 years, and train stations in over 100. The addition of guards and metal detectors is the only recent advancement.
- Tunnels and bridges have been around for centuries, and even the "new" technology here is decades old.
- Military camps date back to biblical times, even though tents are now more modern and air-conditioned.
- Bombs and explosives date back centuries and the "recent" invention of such things as plastic explosives is decades old.
- Rifles and automatic weapons also date back a century or more.

In the cyber-world, the story is much different, with the technology changing to a "new generation" about every 18 months. The target environment is also highly dynamic and "weapons" must be constantly upgraded or replaced to work at all. Being an effective cyber-terrorist requires a serious, ongoing development program. Countermeasures also require an appreciation for the dynamics of the situation and the need for ongoing development as well.

The Enabling Technology

Cybernetics and modern information technology, including the digital world and the Internet, are a very recent phenomenon. What began as a Massachusetts Institute of Technology (MIT) doctoral dissertation in 1962, and a US Defense Department experiment in communications in 1968, rapidly evolved into a technological revolution going far beyond simple communications.* Criminals and terrorists have become increasing users of the Internet for many functions. As in years past, when they relied on other technologies such as the telephone, radio, and mail, they cannot effectively be barred from net access and will continue to use net resources for their criminal purposes.

True revolutions in information and communications do not come along very often. Possibly, the only thing that comes close in comparison to the Internet was Morse's invention of the telegraph in the early nineteenth century.† Cyberspace and the Internet began at the Defense Department's Advanced

---

*In terms of making information available, it is likely the most significant advance since printing and Gutenberg's invention of moveable type in the sixteenth century. Internet use has exploded from a handful of scientists to a world where "net" access is almost universal and has become a medium for all – criminals and terrorists are no exception.

†In May 1844, Samuel Morse sent his famous message "What hath God wrought" over a 37-mile telegraph line from Washington to Baltimore, funded by a $50,000 grant from the US Army. Although ignored in the first few years, by 1851 there were 50 competing telegraph companies, and by 1866 Western Union (formed by a merger of several of these) had over 4,000 offices and had become the first communications giant in history.

Research Projects Agency (ARPA) and a research group around MIT.‡ The project did not lead immediately to the ARPAnet or the Internet, and the concepts of privacy and security were not central to the program.

At the outset, the "net" did not expand rapidly and received little notice outside the scientific community. Electronic mail (e-mail) was not even part of the initial ARPAnet concept, and the "web" was not a part of the original vision either. It was several years before these features that revolutionized information operations, communications, and the media were developed. As Table 15.1 illustrates, the early years of the net were characterized by relatively few "nodes" and users, largely ARPA (later DARPA) contractors.

By the late 1980s, millions of PCs were being sold, and the means to connect this growing number of computers to the net were developed. Commercial Internet service providers (ISPs) gave the public a means to access the net, previously limited to ARPA researchers, and in 1988 the ARPAnet transitioned to the Internet for all to use.§ The global Internet infrastructure is now made up of many root routers that manage the millions of domains and countless net users. Strategically placed around the world, the routers serve an estimated 1.173 billion Internet users.

---

‡ Formed during the Cold War, in an effort to fund a wide range of defense technologies of possible importance to the Unied States, ARPA has been at the forefront of technical developments in a host of critical areas. Over the years, the word "Defense" has been added, then subtracted, and then added again to its name, and it is currently known as DARPA. In the early days of the net, the "D" was not there, so the net was known as the ARPAnet. DARPA itself does no work internally. Its relatively small staff of technical experts is responsible for the direction of research funds to universities, contractors, national laboratories, and others who perform the actual research tasks. The results have been nothing less than astounding. This approach has given rise to an entire information technology industry, and several others. For a good historical account, see Segaller.[1] This novel concept proposed "packet switching" as a more efficient use of a network than "line switching" that had been used since the time of Morse in 1848. In simple terms, "line switching" means that the sender and recipient are somehow "connected" for the duration of their communication, and tie up the line for that period. Alternatively, the "packet switching" concept breaks all communications into uniform digital "packets" which are sent over available network resources, and then reassembled by the recipient. No single line is tied up, and the network routs the packets in the most efficient way possible. In the analog world of the 1960s, it was an interesting concept, but of limited practical use. In the digital world of the 1990s, it became a multibillion dollar revolution. It has changed both the technology and economics of communications as nothing else in history.

§ The principal sponsor of this law in the US Senate was Senator Albert Gore, Jr. While Gore later misstated in his unsuccessful 2000 Presidential Campaign that he had "invented" the Internet, he was indeed largely responsible for its successful evolution, and the world is indebted to Gore for this. The final results of this revolution in the economics of telecommunications have still not been seen. Most carriers evolved on the basis of being able to charge individual users for service. International telex, telephone, FAX, and so on were a major revenue base for these carriers. Since Internet users were now paying nothing to the carriers to send the same (or much more!) data, a significant problem has evolved.

TABLE 15.1. Nodes on the net

Year	Nodes	Events
1969	4	UCLA, Stanford, UCSB, Utah; net 56kb
1970	5	BBN technologies added; net spans United States
1971	15	MIT, Rand, Harvard, others added
1974	62	Transmission control protocol (TCP) developed
1977	111	Apple II launched as PC
1981	213	Microsoft has 40 employees
1983	562	TCP/IP protocols developed; Internet is born
1984	1,024	Domain names invented (.com)
1986	5,000	First bulletin board with GUI
1987	10,000	25-million PCs sold in United States; net is T1 (1.54 mb)
1989	100,000	ARPAnet deinstalled; now Internet
1992	1,000,000	Mosaic browser developed
2008	Unknown	Internet is a global resource

The following decades saw order of magnitude changes in the base technologies and the capability they provided. The original "net" has grown from a test bed with four nodes to millions of Internet servers and countless users worldwide. This has become a communications and information technology environment never dreamed of even a few short years ago, and is largely due to the convergence of four key technology developments:

Moore's Law – Cheap Computers for Everybody: The world is full of increasingly cheap and powerful integrated circuits making possible low-cost computers and other electronic devices.

Packet Switching: Switched packet communications has enabled the Internet and worldwide communications networks.

Digital Everything: In the information age, the world moved from analog to digital, where data, voice, video, images, and other media are all digital.

Infinite/cheap Bandwidth: New technologies such as fiber optic cable, advanced radio-frequency (RF) systems, and others enabled major increases in high-quality, low-cost bandwidth worldwide, resulting in virtually free worldwide communications.[¶]

The world has moved from an analog one with paper files to a digital one where information operations are dominated by networked digital systems, used for all

---

[¶] The final results of this revolution in the economics of telecommunications have still not been seen. Most centers evolved on the basis of being able to charge individual users for service. International telex, telephone, fax, and so on were a major revenue base for these carriers. Since Internet users were now paying nothing to the carriers to send the same (or much more) data, this has evolved into a significant problem.

aspects of commerce, government, and personal matters. People around the globe have adopted these technologies and now consider them indispensable. Besides efficient and low-cost communications, they offer a revolutionary ability to deal with information important to every facet of life. Internet use has spread across the globe and is found not only in the developed world but even the most desolate areas of the Third World, with users from all ages and walks of life – including criminals and terrorists.

In terms of actual threats to these technologies and systems, it is possible to bind the problem quickly. At one end, the little chips that run your watch or permit your auto to start will escape even the best-laid plans of the *Hezbollah* and *al Qaeda*. At the other end, the penultimate apocalypse of cyber-terrorism depicted in films such as "War Games," "Terminator 3" and "the Net" is equally unlikely.‖

Internet Security and Privacy

In the early days of the net, security and privacy were not major concerns. In retrospect this seems difficult to understand, but it is in fact the case. The "net" began as a communications experiment involving only a few ARPA contractors connected to the ARPAnet. The ARPAnet was a technology development effort, not seen as a "military" system. Most ARPA contractors were universities and technology firms – not weapons contractors.** ARPA and Department of Defense regulations prohibited use of the ARPAnet for any classified data while the original users were largely scientists whose desire was to share data with other scientists.

With substantial government support in the late 1980s and early 1990s, the ARPAnet transitioned into the modern Internet, bringing this revolutionary technology to a far greater set of users, organizations, and individuals throughout the world. Almost overnight, commercial ISPs emerged to provide connectivity and accounts to new users, offering connections with "dial up" telephone modems as well as more costly direct, higher-bandwidth connections. Using the Internet as the communications backbone, modern information operations quickly developed to provide

---

‖ Although produced some 20 years apart, these films involved plots where computers controlling the release of US nuclear weapons were taken over by terrorists, or terrorist software, causing an end to the planet. A similar plot is used in "The Net" (1997) that inspired President Clinton to issue Presidential Directive PD-63, focused on protection of national infrastructure.

** Stories about the ARPAnet being developed as a communications system to survive a nuclear war are incorrect. As a practical matter, the net's switched-packet architecture has a large degree of inherent survivability, and can withstand many crises, but the driving concept was one of efficiency of network resources.

- *Communications:* Asynchronous, networked communications and e-mail, later including telephones (voice over IP) and hybrid devices such as personal digital assistants (PDAs).
- *Electronic data and other record systems:* Record systems, such as medical records which for years had been moving to computers from paper files, were now on systems connected to larger networks and accessible via the Internet.
- *Information and other media:* Books, journals, and all forms of information previously available only in printed hardcopy were rapidly becoming available "on-line" in digital form.

No one at ARPA envisioned this scenario at the outset. Use of these new technologies presented special problems for those with sensitive data, whether classified information or sensitive medical records. These users rapidly began to move from specialized systems to common commercial technologies and the Internet, and developed their own means to protect their data. Requirements here include the following:

Reliability of service and data storage: Users want systems that are essentially 100% reliable and always available with 24/7 access becoming the baseline. Users do not want to hear about systems that are "down" or broken, even for "routine maintenance." They will not accept loss of data from systems that have failed or are broken, even in the case of a major national disaster.[††]

Security and privacy: While early net users were not concerned about data privacy and security, users now demand them. The net is now used for personal and private communications, as well as for the transfer of medical records and financial data.[‡‡]

Net users do not necessarily need the level of security that the military requires, but still want a high level of assurance that their communications will not be seen by unintended readers. They also want systems that are safe from invasion. The same network that has enabled legitimate users to get "out" to the world has also enabled illegitimate users to get "into" many computers to steal data or cause problems. Using malicious software, or "malware" such as viruses, worms, and Trojans, they have given rise to an entire new category of computer crimes and annoyances.

[††] It is worth noting the problems encountered by banks in New Orleans as a result of Hurricane Katrina. Several local banks and electronic records were destroyed. Users could not gain access to their accounts, and transfers to alternate sites and servers were significantly delayed.

[‡‡] Just a few years ago, some 70% of VISA card users believed that it was not safe to use their credit cards for Internet purchases. Major changes in the systems and procedures have made such use a great deal safer, and now the vast majority of cardholders do believe that such use is safe.

Implications for Health and Hospital Services

The medical world increasingly depends on advanced computer systems. Initially used to replace manual, paper billing systems use has proliferated to virtually all aspects of medical practice and public health services. Current systems enable the connection of electronic medical records (EMR), or electronic patient records (EPR), with other medical digital equipment, such as imaging and archiving systems that contains findings of X-rays, magnetic resonance imaging (MRI), computerized tomography (CT), as well as echo and ultrasound images of a particular patient. Other systems contain laboratory test results and a host of other medical applications.

Modern medical technology allows the implementation of complicated procedures by experts who are not physically present, using online instant communication technology (telemedicine), advanced apparatus including miniaturized robotics to treat orthopedic problems, and even miniature cameras that are swallowed like pills and broadcast online transmission of the state of the patient's intestines.[§§] Medical teams exchange information through relevant forums set up to allow interaction on specific subjects utilizing websites, medical forums, online chats groups, and other conferencing systems.

Various publications have stated that terrorist attacks in general and cyber-attacks in particular would not be aimed at hospitals, public health, or other medical services.[2] Unfortunately, it is important to consider the possibility that terrorists do not think likewise, and to prepare for scenarios including

- *Data corruption:* Alteration or deletion of vital data (blood type, medical test results, images, allergy information, and medicine doses) could cause patients to die. Infiltration of computers in medical centers by computer viruses and alteration or deletion of information on databases, mainly EPR records, would delay treatment of patients, and prevent doctors from receiving vital information which could enable life-saving procedures.
- *Theft:* There is also the possibility of monetary loss where medical information stored on a hospital's computer could have a high value if it concerns a well-know celebrity or a politician.[¶] Cyber-thieves would also have great interest in personal data of patients and staff in a hospital, including their bank and credit card details.
- *Denial of service:* A coordinated attack on a medical center's computers could cause the system to temporarily crash, thereby affecting computerized medical equipment, preventing certain procedures (nonaccess to computerized patients

---

[§§] The systems to support telemedicine were also developed at DARPA in the late 1980s and early 1990s as a specialized application of the network technology developed earlier.
[¶] At Hadassah University Hospital in Jerusalem, attempts were made to gain illegal access to Israeli former Prime Minister Ariel Sharon's medical records while he was hospitalized there in January 2006.

records, and to laboratory, operation rooms, and blood bank control systems). It could also neutralize the administrative apparatus that controls day-to-day operation of a hospital such as staff transportation schedules, food and drink management, and billing procedures.

Sources of Threats to Health and Hospital Services

With the rapid growth of the Internet has come a wave of threats to the legitimate and secure use of these systems. Hospitals and health systems might be less likely targets than some other enterprises, but the threat to them could still come from the same pools of likely perpetrators. Criminal and terrorist abuses include the potential for attacking individual computers as well as the Internet itself, or "cyberterrorism." These threats include the following categories:

Hackers: Most cyber-attacks come from "hackers" who commonly are bored high school youngsters who are malicious, but not serious criminals or terrorists. Their goal is neither money nor destruction but perverse pleasure from annoying others. A smaller number of sophisticated hackers bridge into the criminal category, seeking to invade computers to access files or personal data, using such software "tools" including viruses, worms, and Trojans to defeat security software.

Criminals: As commerce has moved to networked systems, criminals have moved there as well. Cyber-attacks have caused commercial users to protect their systems from sophisticated hacking and criminal penetration. Unlike the misguided school youngsters, criminals are seeking to steal from unwitting net users, either cash or goods from fraudulent transactions. Net-based crime is a growth industry.

Disgruntled employees: Many cyber-attacks come from former employees (e.g., system administrators) still angry with their employers – not the nation. Cases often involve current or former "insiders" with at least some technical skills, and more importantly still have active passwords and system access.

Firms seeking data: The exponential increase in Web sites has brought a myriad of sites that seek to extract data users, then resold or used for commercial purposes. Employing tools such as "cookies" and backweb applications, they collect data that many people would prefer kept private, and which is then used to bombard the users with "spam" communications.

Police and intelligence services: As data that were once in paper files have moved to databases and computer servers, investigations by police and intelligence agencies have increasingly focused on these systems. Even though "legal" in most cases, they are nonetheless a threat to the security and privacy of the users.

Given the worldwide reach of the Internet, and the ability to access the net from almost any place on earth, these threats have taken on an international aspect. Often attackers are in a nation far from their target, operating from locations that either difficult to locate or hard to prosecute.

Means of Protection

All net users want protection from the disruptions discussed above, and seek to maintain the security and privacy of their data. The basic means of maintaining security, privacy, and data protection fall into three categories:

1. *Physical security:* The easiest and surest way to maintain the security of data is to physically protect the computer and not connect it to a network. Computers not connected to an "outside world" are simply not subject to invasion. For many years, classified data was maintained in this manner, with host computers locked in secure facilities with no external connections. Increasingly, even these systems have been connected to secure networks as their users have demanded remote access. Modern operations place a high priority on connecting computers to both local and wide area networks, as well as the Internet.

2. *Technical solutions – hardware and software*: Many threats exist because the computers and software evolved very quickly and contain a wide range of security vulnerabilities. Most of these vulnerabilities are software-related, and often are cases where developers have rushed to market systems not fully debugged. Currently, most major software developers recognize user demands for security and have made major efforts to fix these vulnerabilities when identified, making "patches" or software upgrades available to users. Other software firms market security tools that protect computers from attacks by viruses, worms, and Trojans. Virtually, all of these tools provide online updates as new spyware and malware are found. An additional technical solution lies in the use of encryption software that enables users to protect important data.

3. *Legal protection:* Many nations have sought to protect the security and privacy of information through legal means. Increasingly, laws in the United States and elsewhere place severe criminal penalties on cyber-crimes. Prosecution of cyber-criminals has acted as a deterrent in some cases. Further, international cooperation in the prosecution of cyber-criminals, such as that between the United States and Germany, and the United States and Russia, has had a deterrent effect here as well. Clearly, such cooperation is to be valued, but cyber-criminals are working to improve their skills and avoid capture wherever they operate.

Organizational Information Protection System

Every entity with a computer network must be obliged to set up an organizational information protection system with security standards and regulations. These should include physical security of the computer environment (the building, the room, and the actual computer), awareness by employees of potential dangers and how to prevent them, work rules that explicitly state who is allowed to do what, prevention of unlimited access by users to potentially dangerous applications.

As part of organizational threat containment activity, a survey of potential threats should be carried out by specialists in this field who can advise on the threat level and recommend appropriate protective measures for stored information, applications, workstations, networks, and also physical measures and worker discipline. The survey should cover three main areas:

- *Dangers* facing the organization from virus infection, loss of information through fire, flooding, and so on, information theft by employees and transfer to competitors or public disclosure, and collapse of computer infrastructure/servers/communications.
- *Probability* of each occurrence (stated in percentages).
- *Recommendations* for preventing the dangers and minimizing the probability of such occurrences, while laying out blueprints for relevant actions in a document defined as information protection policy.

After completing the threat survey, the organization should establish an information protection policy based on the threat, probability, and cost considerations. IT information security should include the following:

- Implementation of strict supervision at key work points and servers to prevent workers from installing (accidentally or otherwise) unauthorized software or introducing outside material on portable media (disk-on-key, CD);
- Using spam blockers and e-mail filters to weed out unwanted and potentially dangerous communications;
- Periodic password changes using passwords with a minimum of eight digits including letters and numbers in a nonlogical format (i.e., not using birthday dates, telephone numbers, etc.);
- Using a strict access-as-needed system without granting administrator rights to users (which would enable unlimited viewing, editing and deletion of data);
- Maintaining a number of backup copies of data in different places, preferably secure and distant from the organization's location;
- Immediate cancellation of all computer access rights of workers who leave the organization, whether they are leaving voluntarily or not;
- Keeping detailed logs of computer activity reporting "who did what and when" for audit and trail purposes;
- Selecting appropriate security devices or software, such as a firewall, which is designed to prevent outside penetration into a company's computers, or access by workers in the organization to outside sources that could be potential threats;
- Encryption of sensitive data so that even in hostile hands, it cannot be used; secured data transmission technology between users;
- Biometric identification (fingerprints, eye or ear identification, voice recognition, electronic signature) of the user to verify that he is actually the person requesting access and not someone using a stolen identity.

Current Trends

In this highly dynamic world, computers and related hardware continue to grow cheaper and more powerful almost daily while hybrid devices "connected" to the world are proliferating at an even greater rate. The only real questions are the extent to which medicine, business, government, and national security depend on systems that are vulnerable, and can these vulnerabilities be addressed? The reality is that there is no stopping this technical revolution. It is simply too cost-effective and brings about great capabilities – private citizens, as well as business and the military are all "hooked."

But there is good news for at least two reasons. First, the technology is fundamentally asymmetrical.[3] Technology and economics ultimately favor the defense, and over time it will become increasingly difficult and costly to attack networks, computers, and other critical infrastructure elements. Hardware and software "fixes" to various vulnerabilities are being developed and implemented on an ongoing basis. Hacking is simply really getting much harder.

Second, and equally important, this is a technology we understand, and we are in a position to provide relatively cost-effective technical solutions. The technology came from an American agency, DARPA, and not a foreign agency. Initially, the United States (and other nations) failed to provide better security solutions, with both the government and industry at fault. In the pre-9/11 era, these problems were addressed in Presidential Directive PD-63, but the incentive to "cure" the problems was not there. In the post-9/11 world, the incentives have been far stronger. Preventing cyber-terrorism is much less of a technological problem than one of economics and national will. This is an area where the problems can actually be solved.

There is no stopping the technical revolution – none of the current technical trends is likely to abate in the foreseeable future. Computers and related hardware will continue to grow cheaper and more powerful. Hybrid devices "connected" to the world will continue to proliferate at an escalating rate. These technologies are cost-effective and popular, introducing all sorts of new capabilities. Individuals as well as public and private institutions including the health services are all addicted. The essential challenge is to protect our commerce, government, and national security by addressing the vulnerabilities in the cyber-systems.

The convenience of remote access to information led the commercial world to rush headlong into reliance on networked systems. Growing information systems and databases were grafted onto a network that was not designed for wide access. The decentralized nature of the Internet and existing network protocols provided network reliability and scalability, but little in the way of security.

What Can Be Done?

In the past, the United States government had more technical resources and investment in communications and computer security than did the private sector. The balance has shifted to the point that, aside from some unique government needs and concerns, the commercial sector will be dominant in the development of information technologies and services. Thus, the increasing government reliance on commercial services means that the government activities in information protection will build on an increasingly sophisticated commercial infrastructure. The issue of defense against cyber-attack can thus be simplified by understanding where commercial and government concerns and capabilities may diverge. From this, one can focus government efforts on areas where the market is unlikely to provide an adequate solution. Efforts undertaken by the United States government and others in this area include

NIPC: The Federal Bureau of Investigation's (FBI) National Infrastructure Protection Center (NIPC) was an effort at an early warning and analytic capability, but it still lacks most of the reporting and monitoring mechanisms, the intelligence support, and the federal interagency integration that a fully effective capability would require.

ISAD: The International Standard Archival Description (ISAD) Information Sharing and Analysis Center (ISAC) offers a national-level monitoring capability integrating government agencies and the private sector. This center exists largely on paper, however, and would not provide a reactive or real-time monitoring capability for effective early warning.

International cooperation: Cooperation is mandatory between organizations engaged in the same purpose nationally and worldwide, such as the FBI or its NIPC. These organizations provide national critical infrastructure threat assessment; early warnings regarding vulnerability; and law enforcement investigation and response. Together with security and intelligence units that analyze terror threats, effective protection can be coordinated.

At the organizational and personal level, there are a number of things that can be done to improve the security posture:

Separation and disconnection: Separation of the personal and organizational workplace from the Internet can provide a level of protection from the outside. Many organizations that require a high level of information security now use a separate operational network that is secured and separated from any Internet connection.

Threat survey: As part of organizational threat containment activity, a survey of potential threats should be undertaken to assess the threat level and to recommend protective measures for stored information, applications, workstations, and networks. After completing the threat survey, the organization should make a decision on implementation of an information protection policy based on threat, probability, and cost considerations.

Data protection management standards: Organizations should comply with recognized standards such as provided for in the Gramm-Leach-Bliley Act to protect consumers' personal financial information held by financial institutions.[4] International standards can provide a model for establishing, implementing, operating, monitoring, reviewing, maintaining, and improving an information security management system.[5]

Good practices at the level of the individual computer or network need to be supplemented by a synoptic view of the overall system. Every addition to the infrastructure can increase the level of threat to the existing nodes. Thus, in recognizing that infrastructures are dynamic systems, probing must be ongoing to assess real-world security. Network design should also incorporate redundancy and reconstitution mechanisms, to assure continuity of operations in the event of attack. Such mechanisms would minimize the impact of local failure on the larger infrastructure.

Conclusion

On balance, the response of the United States to evolving cyber-threats has been very little, very late. Some aspects of US policy even seem senseless, such as efforts to place export controls on software and data that are already available on the worldwide web. Such action is unlikely to impede a terrorist.

Even at DARPA, cradle of the cybernetics revolution, with an annual budget of $2.7 billion, the investment in cyber-defense has been minimal. In fact, cyber-defense would not require the level of funding that went into defense against nuclear weapons in the 1950s. But the problems of providing an effective warning and response capability are nevertheless similar. The United States has invested great sums toward nuclear defense – strategic intelligence and contemporaneous warning capabilities, attack assessment, maintenance of essential services. Moreover, a government priority is the ability to attribute the source of an attack. Although deterrence of a cyber-attack is a less critical requirement, it should receive more attention and support than is now the case.

The passive defenses of network security and information assurance are the crucial platform on which to build an information warfare defense capability. However, the appearance of sophisticated cyber-threats will require an active, consolidated system that integrates capabilities for warning, attack assessment, response, and reconstitution across the government/commercial divide.

In the final analysis, do the terrorists really care? Will a cyber-attack give them the sort of visibility and destruction they are looking for? Are they willing to invest in the technical capability to pull it off? It is a different technology than wrapping a terrorist in explosives who self-destructs on a bus or in a crowded marketplace.

On the other hand, will the commercial sector preempt government action and make such cyber-attacks increasingly difficult? Network operators and communications providers continue to added security features and layers of protection. The net itself is inherently survivable, and is a characteristic of packet switching. The infrastructure is one without a single point of failure.

There are no magic wands to deal with these problems. As the industry matures, security will increasingly be a selling point for hardware, software, and service providers. As medical service providers and commerce in general rely increasingly on secure information flows, the private stakes associated with computer security will rise. At the same time, with the emergence of the next-generation Internet, there is the potential to replace the current, jury-rigged, system with one that has security designed in from the start.

References

1. Segaller S. *Nerds 2.0.1: A Brief History of the Internet*, New York: TV Books, 1998.
2. Clem A, Galwankar S, Buck G. Health implications of cyber-terrorism. http://pdm.medicine.wisc.edu/18-3pdfs/272Clem.pdf. Accessed 27 June 2007.
3. Berinato S. The truth about cyber-terrorism (2002). www.cio.com/archive/031502/truth.html. Accessed June 24, 2007.
4. U.S. Federal Trade Commission. The Gramm-Leach Bliley Act. http://www.ftc.gov/privacy/privacyinitiatives/glbact.html. Accessed June 25, 2007.
5. ISO/IEC 27001. http://www.standardsdirect.org/iso17799.htm. Accessed June 25, 2007.

Part IV
TYPES OF INJURY

16
Penetrating Injury in Terror Attacks

GIDON ALMOGY and AVRAHAM I. RIVKIND

The US Department of Defense defines terrorism as "the calculated use of unlawful violence or threat of unlawful violence to inculcate fear; intended to coerce or to intimidate governments or societies in the pursuit of goals that are generally political, religious, or ideological."[1] The method used by the attacker will depend on various factors and include conventional as well as nonconventional weapons.

Penetrating injuries may result from stabbing, high- and low-velocity firearms, objects that impale, and shrapnel. Injuries caused by these means have been extensively described in surgical and medical literature. This chapter covers penetrating injuries caused by methods and weapons used commonly by terrorists. Among them, stabbings and suicide bombings result in distinctive patterns of injury that are of particular relevance to terror medicine.

Terror-Related Stab Wounds

The knife has long served as an instrument of attack, especially in the Middle East. During the Middle Ages, the Hashashin in their struggle with other Islamic groups, targeted high-ranking political or military leaders whom they regarded as the source of evil. The knife, usually the *shabari'ya*, a curved Arab dagger, was thrust into the victim's body in the name of Allah (God).[2]

Despite the availability of firearms, sharp penetrating instruments such as the knife, spear, dagger, sword, machete, and bayonet are popular to this day in causing civilian trauma. The attacker is most commonly male, between the ages of 25 and 31.[3] The majority of attacks occur over weekend evenings and nights and the motive is usually criminal or social in nature.[4] The associated mortality rate has been reported to range from 0% to 15%.[5,6]

In an innovative publication, Hanoch et al. have described the unique pattern of injury following terrorist-associated knife stabbings.[7] The attackers were almost uniformly males between the ages of 18 and 30.[8] Almost two-thirds of victims were between the ages of 18 and 35. Over 70% of attacks occurred in the morning hours, between 7 a.m. and 11 a.m. and a fourth between 7 a.m. and 8 a.m. The most common site of injury was to the right posterior thorax, via the back (46.1% of stab wounds). The median number of stab wounds per victim was 2 (range 1–28). The

S.C. Shapira et al. (eds.), *Essentials of Terror Medicine*,
DOI: 10.1007/978-0-387-09412-0_16, Springer Science+Business Media, LLC 2009

authors demonstrated that none of the victims who sustained 6 or more stab wounds survived. Mortality following terrorist stabbing was more than 25%.

The authors performed a multivariant analysis to identify predictors of mortality from stab wounds. The victim's age, the number of stab wounds, and injury to the left anterior chest were found to be significant predictors of death from stab wounds.

The authors also reported on the consequences of untimely removal of the assault weapon. In four cases, the knife was removed by a bystander (1), paramedic (1), victim (1), and in the operating room (1). The outcome of removing the knife was abrupt hemodynamic collapse. In fact, when the implement was removed by the bystander and the paramedic, the victims died. The authors concluded that removal of the knife should be performed only under the controlled conditions in the operating room, while the patient is anesthetized. Well-trained personnel must be available and the necessary surgical equipment must be easily accessible to control bleeding. In hemodynamically stable victims, the authors advocated identification of the depth of penetration by simple anterior and lateral X-rays.

Injury by Penetrating Missiles

Factors determining the type and extent of injury from a penetrating missile include the region of the body injured, the organs in proximity to the path of the penetrating object, and the velocity of the missile. The laws of energy offer a better understanding of the injury caused by a penetrating missile.[9] First, energy (or mass) is neither created nor destroyed; however, it can change its form. Thus, penetrating missiles slow considerably after hitting the body and transfer their kinetic energy to body tissues in the form of heat. Second, the kinetic energy of a missile is proportional to its mass multiplied by the square of its velocity. Therefore, in general, injury caused by high-velocity firearms is more extensive than injury caused by stab wounds and low-velocity firearms. Third, injury is dependent on the amount and speed of energy transmission, the surface area over which the energy is applied, and the elastic properties of the tissues to which the energy transfer is applied.

Energy transfer to the tissues can be considered as a shock wave that moves at various speeds through different media. Stress imparted to the human tissue is dependent on the velocity of the missiles initiating the wave, the velocity of the waves in the tissue, and the mass density of the material.[10] The stress level in the tissue at impact is controlled by the velocity of the material particles of the tissue and is directly proportional to it. Once the velocity exceeds the tolerance level of the tissue, tissue disruption occurs, and in this manner produces injury.[11]

According to the laws of physics, for a moving object to lose speed, its energy of motion must be transmitted to another object or transferred to another form. Direct energy transfer occurs when tissue cells are placed in the direction of motion away from the site of impact. The rapid movement of tissue particles away from the point of impact produces damage by tissue compression, and as the shock wave progresses an expanding cavity is created at a distance from the point of initial impact. This temporary phenomenon is known as cavitation and is proportional to the kinetic energy of the missile, or in other words, to the magnitude of energy exchanged.

Factors such as a missile's velocity and mass determine the amount of injury the missile will cause. Most civilian gunshot wounds result from low-velocity missiles (<1000 ft/s; 305 m/s). High-velocity missiles (>3000 ft/s; 915 m/s), usually a result of military type firearms, produce much more tissue damage than low-velocity firearms.[12] Tissue damage also depends on the missile's mass (see above) and configuration. Sharp missiles with small cross-sectional fronts slow with tissue impact, resulting in little injury or cavitation. Missiles with large cross-sectional fronts, especially those with serrated fronts, cause more injury.

Other factors that determine tissue damage are ballistic properties of the missile such as yaw, tumble, and cavitation. When a missile travels through tissue, the differential resistance it encounters causes its path to become unsteady. This instability results in yawing or deviation from the missile's longitudinal axis, and fragmentation.[13] Tumbling of a missile is associated with high-velocity firearms. These properties increase tissue damage by considerably slowing down the missile inside the tissue and enlarging the cavitation effect.

Penetrating Injury and Bombing Attacks

Suicide Terrorism

Undoubtedly, the most efficient conventional weapon in the hands of terrorists has been the suicide bomber. The "Tamil Tigers" (Liberation Tigers of Tamil Eelam or LTTE), a nationalistic terror organization operating in Sri Lanka, began perpetrating suicide attacks in 1987. By February 2001, the LTTE had carried out 168 suicide terror attacks in Sri Lanka and India, the largest number of suicide attacks until surpassed by Palestinian groups in 2003. It was probably the Tamils who "invented" the infamous suicide belt (Fig. 16.1).[15] Since then, this method has become perhaps the most serious threat to civilian lives and livelihood.

In the Middle East, suicide bombing was first used in Lebanon by a small (and until then unknown) group by the name of Hezbollah. In October 1983, two suicide bombings by Hezbollah militants killed 241 American servicemen and 58 French paratroopers, which prompted the Americans and the French to leave Lebanon.[16] The political success of those attacks undoubtedly encouraged the Hezbollah and other terror groups to propagate this tactic. As part of their successful campaign to drive Israeli forces from southern Lebanon, Hezbollah carried out 51 suicide attacks in Lebanon over a 17-year period. This new and devastating modus operandi gained wide publicity and helped inspire Palestinian suicide bombing attacks (SBAs), which began in April 1993.[17]

Attacks in Sri Lanka, Lebanon, Israel, Iraq, Great Britain, and elsewhere, have caused tens of thousands of deaths and disrupted daily life.[18] Global terrorist groups have identified and capitalized on the potential of suicide bombers both in terms

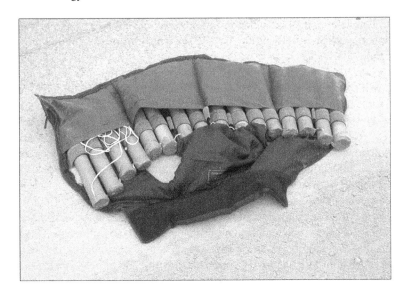

Fig. 16.1. Explosive belt armed and ready to use, found by the Israel Defense Forces during operation "Defensive Shield" in Nablus, West Bank (April 2002). From Almogy and Rivkind.[14] Reprinted with permission from Elsevier.

of lethality and psychological effect. Because of global political changes, terrorist groups have been able to acquire high-grade explosive material, which has enabled them to add large amounts of fragments to a bomb, thus intensifying the effects of penetrating trauma (Fig. 16.2).

The explosive device is detonated at the discretion of the attacker at the appropriate time to cause maximum bodily damage. Since the device is worn at chest height, it spreads the explosive fragments especially to the head and torso of the victims. Compared to explosive devices placed under bus seats in Israel, the introduction of the suicide attacker has increased the number of fatalities aboard buses from a median of 3 per year in the 1980s to a median of 9 in the recent intifada (2000–2006).[19,20]

Thus, an inexpensive explosive device, generally carried by a devout young man or woman, has emerged as a highly effective weapon. As a result, the suicide bomber has become a mainstay of Palestinian terrorist groups.

Management of Victims

Trauma after explosions has traditionally been categorized into primary (direct effect of pressure), secondary (effects of projectiles), tertiary (effect due to wind or motion of air propelling the victim against a stationary object), and quaternary injury (burns, asphyxia, and exposure to toxic inhalants),[21] (see Chap. 11 and Table 19.1).

Civilian trauma victims of events unrelated to terrorism may suffer multiple wounds, usually caused by a single mechanism. Blunt trauma can cause injuries of varying severity to several organs and several body regions. Penetrating firearm wounds can cause injury to multiple organs, but injury is usually limited to a

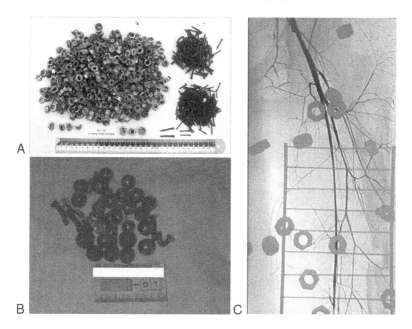

FIG. 16.2. a. Fragments found by the Israel Defense Forces during operation "Defensive Shield"; b. Fragments found at the site of a suicide bombing attack; and c. Angiography of the thigh of a 14-year-old girl showing multiple shrapnel. From Almogy and Rivkind.[14] Reprinted with permission from Elsevier.

single body region. Civilian victims of trauma are most often injured in random violence and are therefore brought into nearby hospitals in small numbers or as individuals.

This familiar scenario changes greatly following an attack by a suicide bomber. The attacker's aim is to target as many victims and cause as much bodily damage as possible. The attacker becomes a designated killing machine, detonating his device at the most effective place and time. Consequently, the number of simultaneous casualties can be very high. Furthermore, detonation of an explosive device within a short distance of a crowd causes injuries similar to those in war. The extent of injury is wide-ranging, with several casualties at the extremity of life while others may have only minor superficial injuries. The mechanism of injury can be a combination of blast injuries, blunt trauma, penetrating wounds and burns, usually to multiple body regions. The diagnostic and therapeutic approaches need to be adjusted to this type of multidimensional injury.

Scope of Injury

As noted, the range of injuries sustained by victims of terrorist attacks, especially suicide bombings, is often more complex than among victims of other forms of

TABLE 16.1. Demographic and clinical characteristics of terrorist bombing attacks compared to all other forms of trauma

	Terrorist bombing attacks	Other trauma
Age 15–44 (years)	71	36.1
ISS ≥ 16 (%)	28.7	10
Injury to ≥3 body regions (%)	28.3	6.2
Abdominal, thoracic, and/or vascular surgery (%)	22.9	4.5
Median ICU LOS (days)	5	3
Mortality (%)	6.1	2

From Kluger et al.[22] Reprinted with permission from Elsevier
ISS injury severity score, *ICU* intensive care unit, *LOS* length of stay

trauma. The degree of severity is of special concern. Severe injuries (injury severity score, ISS ≥ 16) were reported in 28.7% of victims of terrorist explosions compared to 10% of victims of other forms of trauma (Table 16.1). More victims of terrorist bombing attacks undergo abdominal, vascular, and neurosurgical procedures compared to victims of other types of trauma.[22] They are also significantly younger compared to victims of other forms of trauma.

The majority of victims of penetrating trauma sustain injuries to distinctive parts of the body such as the head, chest, abdomen, and limbs. Blunt trauma is more commonly a multisite injury, the severity of which depends on the mechanism of injury. The injuries sustained by victims of a SBA share "the worst of both worlds." The hallmark of injuries that follow an SBA is a combination of penetrating injury, blast wave effect, and effects of the heat wave, predominantly, burns. The multitude of heavy missiles causes damage to a large surface area, much like blunt trauma. Each particle causes extensive tissue damage at the site of entry, much like penetrating trauma. Survivors typically suffer a combination of wounds of varying severity and location (Fig. 16.3). This phenomenon, when different classes of injury occur simultaneously in the same patient, has been termed "multidimensional injury pattern."[23] The extent and severity of injury will depend on factors such as the explosive power of the device, distance of the victim from the site of detonation, quantity and mass of fragments, and attack setting.

Attack Setting

The physical characteristics of the setting have implications on the type (primary, secondary, tertiary, and quaternary) of blast injury. In Israel, three attack settings have been identified: buses, semiconfined spaces (SCS) such as covered open markets, restaurants and indoor cafés, and open spaces (OS) such as outdoor cafés and bus stops.[24] There is a trend, albeit not statistically significant, of an increasing number of casualties admitted to hospital per attack and an increasing number of severely injured casualties (ISS ≥ 16) per attack as the setting changes from OS to SCS to buses.

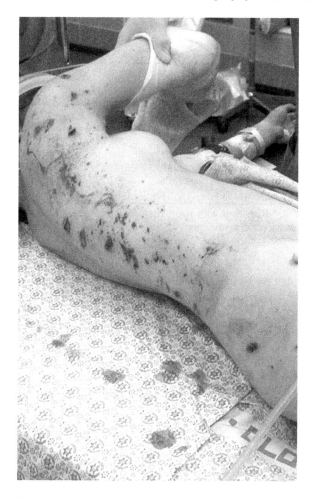

FIG. 16.3. A 15-year-old girl injured in the Sbarro pizzeria attack (August 9, 2001, Jerusalem) sustained multiple penetrating wounds to her right side and back. Shrapnel caused penetrating rectal injury which required a temporary colostomy. From Almogy and Rivkind.[14] Reprinted with permission from Elsevier.

The pattern of penetrating injury changes with the attack setting. The head typically sustains a higher percentage of penetrating wounds than its relative body surface area in all settings.[25] Penetrating head injury is more common among victims aboard buses (68.15%), and penetrating torso injury is more common in SCS (58.7%). Victims injured in OS are more likely to suffer from penetrating extremity and soft-tissue injury (66.7%) and less likely to suffer from the effects of the blast wave [burns and tympanic membrane (TM) rupture] compared to patients injured in SCS and buses (Table 16.2). A meta-analysis of 29 worldwide terrorist bombing

TABLE 16.2. The incidence of the various injuries according to attack setting

	All attacks (n = 154)	Bus (n = 72)	SCS (n = 46)	OS (n = 36)	p value
Penetrating injury (all)	135 (87.7)	64 (88.9)	40 (86.9)	31 (86.1)	0.90
Penetrating head injury	84 (54.5)	49 (68.1)	18 (39.1)	17 (47.2)	0.005
Penetrating torso injury	61 (39.6)	19 (26.4)	27 (58.7)	15 (41.7)	0.002
Penetrating extremity injury	76 (49.4)	26 (36.1)	26 (56.5)	24 (66.7)	0.005
Burns	42 (27.3)	27 (37.5)	13 (28.3)	2 (5.6)	0.002
Skull fractures	19 (12.3)	8 (11.1)	4 (8.7)	6 (16.7)	0.525
Open fractures	34 (22.1)	9 (12.5)	15 (32.6)	10 (27.8)	0.024
Tympanic membrane rupture	34 (22.1)	28 (38.9)	4 (8.7)	2 (5.6)	<0.0001
Blast lung injury	28 (18.2)	17 (23.6)	5 (10.9)	6 (16.7)	0.208
Intra-abdominal injury	13 (8.4)	4 (5.6)	7 (15.2)	2 (5.6)	0.143

From Almogy et al.[20] Reprinted with permission from Lipponcott, Williams & Wilkins
SCS semiconfined space, OS open space

attacks showed that the incidence of burns and TM rupture inside a confined space was 22% and 35%, respectively, compared to 1% and 5%, respectively, in OS.[26]

Gastrointestinal Tract Injury

Penetrating torso injury and primary blast injury to hollow viscera are the two main mechanisms that account for intra-abdominal injury sustained by victims of terrorist bombing attacks. Nearly 40% of victims of SBA suffer from penetrating injuries to the torso caused by missiles such as shrapnel and debris. Reviewing their more recent experience with terrorist bombing attacks (2000–2005), Almogy et al. reexamined the incidence and factors associated with intra-abdominal injury. Their data, based on 154 hospitalized victims of 17 SBAs in Jerusalem, showed that intra-abdominal injury was caused in all cases by penetrating shrapnel and not by the blast wave. The results also demonstrated that intra-abdominal injury can be suspected based on the presence of penetrating torso wounds and the presence of injuries to four or more body areas. Furthermore, the authors have shown that the presence of penetrating torso wounds and injuries to four or more areas serve as predictors of significant intra-abdominal injury with an odds ratio of 22.3, and 4.9, respectively.

Previous reports have highlighted the importance of the blast wave in causing bowel injury, often associated with delayed diagnosis and a high morbidity rate. Reports by Katz et al.[19] and Paran et al.[27] of terrorist bombings aboard a bus described five cases of blast wave-induced perforation of the bowel.[27] Hematomas and perforations of the bowel, mesenteric tears, and rupture of hollow viscera have been reported following isolated blast injury.[28]

The disparity between recent and previous reports in Israel can be explained by changes that have taken place in the type and mass of explosive material and the location of the explosive device. The explosive material has changed from low-grade to military-grade, fragmentation has changed from low- to high-mass and the location of the explosive device, which was previously concealed under seats, is now carried at chest height. Thus, victims in proximity to the explosive device absorb higher levels of energy and develop bowel perforation, and are less likely to survive; and, correspondingly, the severity of penetrating injuries among survivors is intensified.

Management of Abdominal Injury

Similar to other injuries caused by a blast, the management of intra-abdominal injury is based on Advanced Trauma Life Support (ATLS) guidelines. Victims with obvious signs of peritonitis are taken to the operating room without further work up. These constitute a small minority, following terrorist bombing attacks. Hypotensive victims with intra-abdominal fluid on focused abdominal sonogram for trauma (FAST) are also taken immediately to the operating room.

The majority of victims, however, undergo extensive imaging evaluation. FAST has been shown to be an effective screening tool for abdominal injury in mass-casualty incidents.[29,30] At Hadassah University Hospital, FAST is performed routinely on all victims admitted to the trauma unit, and on any victim with penetrating torso wounds or injuries to four or more body regions. Proximity to the epicenter evidenced by the presence of blast lung injury (BLI), TM rupture, burns and multiple penetrating injuries, mechanism of injury and abnormal sonographic findings warrant abdominal and pelvic CT scans. Data from Hadassah show that diagnosis can be established within 6 hours of injury based on FAST and CT. By utilizing this approach, only 2 (13.3%) nontherapeutic laparotomies were performed over a 5-year period, and there were no missed or delayed abdominal injuries. As is commonly accepted in trauma management, the authors found no use for diagnostic or therapeutic laparoscopy for the respiratory-compromised, multiple-injured victims.

The use of diagnostic peritoneal lavage (DPL) is selective. DPL is limited either to hemodynamically unstable victims who are taken for urgent nonabdominal surgery or to septic victims in the ICU to rule out delayed and/or missed injuries. Only four DPL's were performed at Hadassah following terrorist bombing attacks (2.6% of hospitalized victims). The procedures were performed in the operating room to rule out injury to hollow viscera in victims undergoing other surgical procedures. Because of the possibility of late onset abdominal crisis, in several cases catheters were left in situ for 48–72 hours for continued abdominal monitoring (Rivkind, personal communication).[31]

Auditory Injury

The ear has been consistently shown to be the most sensitive organ to blast injury. Penetrating ear injury is very uncommon and was not reported at Hadassah (Almogy, personal communication). Auditory injury has been reported in 35–41% of survivors of terrorist bombing attacks.[32] Peak overpressures as low as 5 psi can rupture the TM and overpressures of 15 psi will cause TM rupture in 50% of victims. The most common finding is rupture at the pars tensa region.[33] Blast overpressure tears sensory cells from the basilar membrane, which eventually heals with scars, leading to continued symptoms.[34] The setting in which the terrorist attack is perpetrated will determine the number of auditory injuries. The frequency of TM rupture ranges from 8% in OSs and can reach up to 50% in confined spaces (e.g., bus, restaurant).

Hearing loss may be conductive due to TM rupture, ossicular damage, or serous otitis. It may also be sensorineural due to cochlear damage. Inner ear injury is uncommon though it may manifest as a stunning of receptor organs, usually without long-term sequela.[35]

Management of Tympanic Membrane Rupture

To document the presence of TM rupture and initiate early treatment, the Hadassah University Hospital protocol calls for an otolaryngologist to evaluate and perform an otoscopic examination on all victims of an SBA. Treatment consists of avoiding additional auditory injury, removal of debris from the external canal by suction under a microscope, and keeping the ears dry. Some doctors recommend debridement of TM margins and insertion of a patch over the perforation under local anesthesia.[36] This approach may allow a higher percentage of eardrum closure compared to conservative management and prevent the formation of cholesteatoma.[37]

Cohen et al. reported on 17 survivors of an attack aboard a bus. Symptoms and signs immediately following the attack included aural fullness (88.2%), tinnitus (88.2%), otalgia (52.9%), ear discharge (52.9%), and dizziness (41.2%).[38] Of the 17 survivors, 16 (94.1%) had rupture of at least one TM and in 59.3% of affected ears the perforations were large. Spontaneous resolution of TM rupture was gradual and incomplete and by the end of a 6-month follow-up, 12 perforations (44.4%) were still present. These 12 perforations were repaired by surgery.

Of the 34 ears examined following the attack, only one had normal hearing. The remaining ears had sensorineural (26.5%), conductive (8.8%), or mixed hearing loss (61.8%). At 6-month follow-up some form of hearing loss, chiefly sensorineural, persisted in 81.8% of victims. Resolution of auditory symptoms varied. Ear ache and discharge were almost completely resolved at 6-month follow-up. Complaints of aural fullness and dizziness persisted for 11 of the 15 victims (73.3%) and 5 of 7 victims (71.4%), respectively.

Auditory Injury as a Predictor of Blast Injury

Controversy exists regarding the significance of TM rupture as a predictor of occult blast injury. In a recent review, the authors of this chapter advocated the value of routine otoscopy in triaging victims of terror bombing attacks to identify those suffering from severe blast injury in general, and BLI in particular.[39] We and others do not find such a significant role for the ear. Leibovici et al. reported on 647 victims of 11 terrorist bombing attacks.[40] Of the 49 victims who suffered from BLI, 18 (36.7%) did not have TM rupture at all. Similar experience from Hadassah has shown that of the 154 victims who were admitted for over 24 h, 34 (22.1%) had TM rupture. Univariate analysis showed that TM rupture is not associated with BLI (7/28 victims with TM rupture had BLI compared to 27/126 victims with TM rupture and without BLI, $p = 0.8$). TM rupture appears to be associated with blast injury in confined spaces such as buses.

Ocular Injury

The ocular surface is only 0.10% of the body surface area but can account for 2–16% of bombing injuries.[41] Penetrating eye injuries were present in 16% of victims following the 2004 Madrid bombings and 8.5% of victims at Hadassah University Hospital.[42] Penetrating injury from shrapnel and debris such as glass is the cause of an overwhelming number of eye injuries following explosions. Corneal abrasion (21%) and lid and eyebrow laceration (20%) were the most common types of injuries following the Oklahoma City bombing. Blast ocular injury is very rare and has rarely been reported following terrorist bombing attacks.

Management of Ocular Injury

Symptoms include eye irritation and pain, sensation of a foreign body, and periorbital swelling. Victims with suspected globe injuries, corneal abrasions and burns, and intraocular foreign bodies should be evaluated by an ophthalmologist.[43] Victims of terror attacks were more likely to require a surgical procedure and were more likely to suffer from a worse outcome of visual acuity compared to other causes of ocular injury. Treatment includes irrigation and ophthalmic ointment for superficial burns and topical antibiotics, cycloplegics and topical nonsteroidal anti-inflammatories for corneal abrasions. Surgical procedures include sutures (22.5%), vitrectomy (20%), and repair of retinal detachment (20%).

Vascular Injury

Vascular injury requiring surgical intervention was reported in 4.0% of victims of all types of terrorist attacks in Israel. Data from Hadassah for two periods of intensive terrorist bombing attacks in Jerusalem (1994–1997 and 2000–2005) show that following bombing attacks 10 victims (11%) and 14 victims (9.1%), respectively, suffered from vascular injury which required surgical intervention.[44]

Victims with vascular injury were more severely injured compared to other victims of terrorist bombing attacks (median ISS = 17, vs 11.5, respectively, p = non significant) (Almogy, personal communication). The most commonly injured vessel was the superficial femoral artery (5/14 victims, 35.7%), followed by the anterior tibial and radial arteries (3 victims each, 21.4%). In all cases, the vascular repair was performed immediately. In five cases (35.7%), there was injury to two or more vessels. These were repaired simultaneously by two or more teams of vascular surgeons (Fig. 16.4). Although very uncommon, blunt vascular injury to the descending aorta has also been described following severe blast injury.

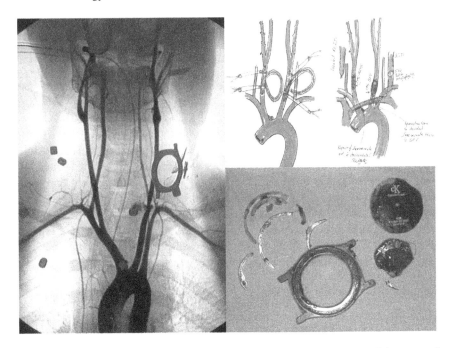

Fig. 16.4. The case of a 23-year-old female serves an astonishing example of the approach to penetrating vascular injury following a suicide bombing attack (SBA). She was injured aboard a bus and sustained a combination of penetrating and blast injuries, and burns. Angiography revealed bilateral carotid artery injury caused by multiple missiles. The injuries were repaired using autologous tissue. From Almogy and Rivkind.[14] Reprinted with permission from Elsevier. Photograph at bottom right courtesy of Dr. Y. Berlatzky, Hadassah University Hospital.

The rather large disparity between victims of all types of terrorist attacks and victims of terrorist SBAs can be explained by the fact that detonation of a heavy explosive device in an urban setting and within a crowd generates a large amount of flying debris, which causes multiple penetrating injuries to several body regions.

Management of Vascular Injury

Wolf and Rivkind summarized the experience accumulated with vascular trauma at Hadassah University Hospital following terror attacks.[45] The authors concluded that the most severe vascular injuries were extremity injury with skeletal fracture and extensive soft-tissue damage. The authors formulated a 5-step approach toward the treatment of such complex injuries. A biplanar arteriography is routinely performed before surgery. The first step is isolation of blood vessels and insertion of arterial shunts. Skeletal fixation is then established and followed with definitive vascular repair. Arterial reconstruction is preferably performed with the use of contralateral saphenous veins. Extensive soft-tissue damage may cause injury to collateral veins.

Therefore, the authors recommend reconstruction of major veins to prevent venous engorgement and stasis. To minimize the rate of infection, the authors recommend performing reconstruction using autologous tissue. The fourth step is four-compartment fasciotomy, performed in cases of severe soft-tissue damage. This is followed by soft-tissue coverage with split-thickness skin grafts or muscle flaps.

Assessing proximity of penetrating fragments and debris to vascular structures is often difficult. Bomb fragments are irregularly shaped and their path within the body is unpredictable. The authors therefore advocate a liberal approach to surgical exploration and removal of foreign bodies, or exclusion arteriography, especially in the neck.

Conclusion

The increased level of terrorism against the Israeli population between 2000 and 2006 resulted in thousands of casualties. Some assaults were conducted with knives, though most with car bombs, packages containing explosives, and suicide bombers whose explosive belts were packed with nails, screws, and other metallic pieces. The intensity and frequency of terror attacks have challenged the health care system, though the experience has also enabled responders and caregivers to develop optimal means of care.

This chapter has reviewed the medical management of victims of penetrating injuries particularly from stabbings or explosive-driven particles. Especially in the case of suicide bombings, as noted, injuries are more severe and complex than in accidents or other nonterrorist events. Unlike in other traumatic incidents, penetrating injuries from a terror attack commonly affect numerous organs and tissues in a single patient, from the head and neck down to the chest, abdomen, and beyond. Moreover, during the intifada, Palestinian terrorists launched assaults on buses, cafés, and outdoor places, including malls and shopping centers. As a result, medical caregivers gained a better understanding of the relationship of different environments – closed, semiconfined, and open – to the variety of injuries, including penetrating wounds.

Many parts of the world have experienced attacks by terrorists, intended to attain maximum publicity by inflicting injury and death. But the unusual number of assaults deliberately launched against Israeli citizens during the intifada also enabled the country's medical system to refine the response procedures. This information could be of great value to responders in other countries as well.

References

1. Modeling and Simulation Information Analysis Center Web site. Available at http://www. msiac.dmso.mil/ootw_documents/sscdictionary/body_t.htm. Accessed April 8, 2006.
2. Hanoch J, Feigin E, Pikarsky A, Kugel C, Rivkind A. Stab wounds associated with terrorist activity in Israel. JAMA 1996; 276: 388–90.
3. Goodman RA, Merci JA, Loya F, et al. Alcohol use and interpersonal violence: Alcohol detected in homicide victims. Am J Public Health 1986; 76: 144–9.

4. Lambrianides AL, Rosin RD. Penetrating stab injuries of the chest and abdomen. Injury 1984; 15: 300–3.

5. Walton CB, Blaisdell FW, Jordan RG, Bodai BI. The injury potential and lethality of stab wounds: A Folsom prison study. J Trauma 1989; 29: 99–101.

6. Wong K, Petchell J. Severe trauma caused by stabbing and firearms in metropolitan Sydney, New South Wales, Australia. ANZ J Surg 2005; 75: 225–30.

7. Hanoch J, Feigin E, Pikarsky A, Kugel C, Rivkind A. Stab wounds associated with terrorist activities in Israel. JAMA 1996; 276: 388–90.

8. Israel Ministry of Foreign Affairs Web site. Available at http://www.mfa.gov.il/mfa/terrorism. Last accessed June 11, 2007.

9. Stuhmiller JH, Phillips YY, Richmond DR. The physics and mechanics of primary blast injury. In: Bellamy RF, Zajtchuk R, eds. Conventional Warfare: Ballistic last and Burn Injuries. Washington, DC: Office of the Surgeon General of the US Army; 1991: 241–70.

10. Mellor SG. The pathogenesis of blast injury and its management. Br J Hosp Med 1988; 39: 536–9.

11. Stapczynski JS. Blast injuries. Ann Emerg Med 1982; 11: 687–94.

12. O'Connell KJ, Clark M, Lewis RH, Christenson PJ. Comparison of low- and high-velocity ballistic trauma to genitourinary organs. J Trauma 1988; 28: S139–44.

13. Fackler ML: Physics of missile injuries. In: McSwain NE Jr, Kerstein MD, eds. Evaluation and Management of Trauma. East Norwalk, Connecticut: Appleton-Century-Crofts; 1987: 25–53.

14. Almogy G, Rivkind AI. Terror in the 21st Century: Milestones and Prospects—Part II. Curr Probs Surg 2007; 44(9): 54.

15. Rohan Gunaratna. Lecture at ICT Conference: Countering Suicide Terrorism, worldpress, February 2000: 97–104.

16. Diego Gambetta (ed.). *Making Sense of Suicide Missions*. New York: Oxford University Press; 2005: 81.

17. Available at http://en.wikipedia.org/wiki/Hezbolla, accessed April 8, 2006.

18. Available at http://www.spur.asn.au/chronology_of_suicide_bomb_attacks_by_Tamil_Tigers_in_sri_Lanka.htm, accessed June 13, 2007.

19. Katz E, Ofek B, Adler J, et al. Primary blast injury after a bomb explosion in a civilian bus. Ann Surg 1989; 209: 484–8.

20. Almogy G, Mintz Y, Zamir G, et al. Suicide bombing attacks: Can external signs of trauma predict internal injuries? Ann Surg 2006; 243(4): 541–6.

21. Philips YY. Primary blast injuries. Ann Emerg Med. 1986; 15:1446–50.

22. Kluger Y, Peleg K, Daniel-Aharonson L, Mayo A; Israeli Trauma Group. The special injury pattern in terrorist bombings. J Am Coll Surg 2004; 199: 875–9.

23. Kluger Y, Kashuk J, Mayo A. Terror bombing-mechanisms, consequences and implications. Scand J Surg 2004; 93: 11–4.

24. Almogy G, Belzberg H, Mintz Y, Pikarsky AJ, Zamir G, Rivkind AI. Suicide bombing attacks: Update and modifications to the protocol. Ann Surg. 2004; 239(3): 295–303.

25. Rignault DP, Deligny MC. The 1986 terrorist bombing experience in Paris. Ann Surg 1989; 209: 368–73.

26. Arnold JL, Halpern P, Tsai M-C, Smithline H. Mass casualty terrorist bombings: A comparison of outcomes by bombing type. Ann Emerg Med 2004; 43: 263–73.

27. Paran H, Neufeld D, Shwartz I, et al. Perforation of the terminal ileum induced by blast injury: Delayed diagnosis or delayed perforation. J Trauma 1996; 40: 472–5.

28. Phillips YY, Zajtchuk R. Management of primary blast injury. In: Bellamy RF, Zajtchuk R, eds. Conventional Warfare: Ballistic last and Burn Injuries. Washington, DC: Office of the Surgeon General of the US Army; 1991: 295–335.

29. Sarkisian AE, Khondkarian RA, Amirbekian NM, Bagdasarian NB, Khojayan RL, Oganesian YT. Sonographic screening of mass casualties for abdominal and renal injuries following the 1988 Armenian earthquake. J Trauma 1991; 31: 247–50.

30. Blaivas M. Triage in the trauma bay with the focused abdominal sonography for trauma (FAST) examination. J Emerg Med 2001; 21: 41–4.

31. Harmon JW, Haluszka M. Care of blast-injured casualties with gastrointestinal injuries. Mil Med 1983; 148: 586–8.

32. Mallonee S. Physical injuries and fatalities resulting from the Oklahoma City bombing. JAMA 1996; 276: 382–7.

33. Wightman J, Gladish S. Explosions and blast injuries. Ann Emerg Med 2001; 37: 664–78.

34. Patterson J, Hamernik R. Blast overspressure induced structural and functional changes the auditory system. Toxicology 1997; 121: 29–40.

35. Garth RJN. Blast injury of the ear. In: Cooper GJ, Dudley HAF, Gann DS, et al., eds. Scientific foundations of trauma. Oxford, UK: Butterworth-Heinemann; 1997: 225–35.

36. Ziv M, Philipsohn NC, Leventon G, Man A. Blast injury of the ear: Treatment and evaluation. Mil Med 1973; 138: 811–13.

37. Kronenberg J, Ben-Shoshan J, Modan M, Leventon G. Blast injury and cholesteatoma. Am J Otol 1988; 9: 127–30.

38. Cohen JT, Ziv G, Bloom J, et al. Blast injury of the ear in a confined space explosion: Auditory and vestibular evaluation. Isr Med Assoc J 2002; 4: 559–62.

39. DePalma RG, Burris DG, Champion HR, Hodgson MJ. Current concepts: Blast injuries. N Engl J Med 2005; 352: 1335–42.

40. Leibovici D, Gofrit ON, Shapira SC. Eardrum perforation in explosion survivors: Is it a marker of pulmonary blast injury? Ann Emerg Med 1999; 34: 168–72.

41. Mines M, Thach A, Mallonee S, Hildebrand L, Shariat S. Ocular injuries sustained by survivors of the Oklahoma City bombing. Ophthalmology 2000; 107: 837–43.

42. Mimran S, Rotem R. Ocular trauma under the shadow of terror. Insight 2005; 30: 10–2.

43. Brunette D. Ophthalmology: Ocular trauma. In: Marx J, Hockberger R, Walls R, eds. Rosen's Emergency Medicine: Concepts and Clinical Practice. 5th ed. Philadelphia, PA: Mosby; 2002: 802–13.

44. Wolf YG, Rivkind A. Vascular trauma in high-velocity gunshot wounds and shrapnel-blast injuries in Israel. Surg Clin North Am 2002; 82: 237–44.

17
Orthopedic Injury in Urban Terrorism

MEIR LIEBERGALL and RAMI MOSHEIFF

Mechanism of Injury and Epidemiology

Mass-casualty events in civilian settings have recently become more frequent due to various geopolitical reasons. Terrorism that involves the use of conventional weapons is still the most common form of urban terrorism, resulting in a high-casualty event. The easy accessibility to high-quality explosives has made it the most popular mode of terror worldwide. The unique pattern of the ensuing injuries, both in their magnitude and severity is completely different from the more familiar blunt trauma scenario. Events like the massive terror attack in London in 2005, the attack on the train in Madrid in 2004, and the continuous terrorist attacks in Israel in 2000–2005,[1,2] and the Gulf War in Iraq have exposed new patterns of injury not recognized before.[3-5]

Most of the research describing penetrating limb injuries relates to military conflicts rather than terrorism. However, even in modern warfare most of the penetrating limb injuries are connected to the detonation of explosives such as bombs, mortars, grenades, or land mines rather to other mechanisms such as gunshot injury.[6-9] According to the studies, the proportion of limb injuries ranges from 40% to 70% of all injuries in civilian and military conflicts and are often described as the major reason for surgical treatment.[8,10-12]

Blast is caused by detonation of an explosive. The harm it causes in human tissues has been traditionally classified as primary (direct effect of pressure), secondary (effects of projectiles), tertiary (effects due to wind and motion of air), or quaternary (burns, asphyxia, and exposure to toxic inhalants),[13] (see Chap. 11 and Table 19.1).

Studies on the suicide bombings in civilian Israeli settings show that special attention should be given to the location and setting of the explosion causing the blast injuries.[1,14] It is evident that morbidity and mortality from terror-related injuries was far worse when the attack took place in a confined area such as a bus and not in open space.[1]

As for the orthopedic manifestations of blast injuries, primary blast usually affects air–fluid interfaces and rarely has a direct effect on the limbs. Hull and Cooper studied primary blast effects on the extremities, resulting in traumatic amputations in Northern Ireland.[15] Only 9 out of 52 victims with traumatic amputation

S.C. Shapira et al. (eds.), *Essentials of Terror Medicine*,
DOI: 10.1007/978-0-387-09412-0_17, Springer Science+Business Media, LLC 2009

survived, demonstrating the high level of energy involved. In all 52 patients, the lower extremity amputation was at the level of the tibial tuberosity, and the limb was avulsed through the fracture site rather than through the joint. The coaxial forces produced the fracture, and dynamic forces (i.e., blast wind) caused the avulsion of the fractured limb.

Secondary blast effects comprise the core of the orthopedic injuries encountered in the Middle Eastern practice.[16–19] Secondary blast effects are related to penetrating injuries caused by fragments erupted from the explosives or the foreign bodies impregnated inside the bomb. The secondary effect of fragments and penetrating foreign bodies depends on the victim's distance from the detonation center, the shape and size of the fragments, and the number of foreign bodies implanted in the bomb or created by the explosion. In contrast to most warfare injuries, the improvised explosives used by terrorists have multiple additional fragments, such as screws, bolts, nails, and other objects, which increase the damage caused by penetrating injuries.[20] Open fractures, severe soft tissue injuries, and multiorgan penetrating injuries are the more common patterns found in the severely injured victim.[20]

Tertiary blast injury is actually the blunt trauma component of the explosion. Flying objects or the fall can cause additional traumatic elements. Along with structural collapse, a high-casualty and -mortality event occurs.[13] Our experience in Israel did not demonstrate a significant proportion of additional blunt trauma. However, reports from other parts of the world, such as the collapse of the Twin Towers in New York and the Oklahoma City explosion report, state this as the primary mechanism of the injury.

The quaternary blast effect includes the thermal and chemical damage caused by fire and noxious substances occurring in the vicinity of the explosion. Confined-space explosions significantly increase these types of injury.[1]

Finally, the fact that more and more suicide bombers are involved in modern terrorism can increase the risk of biological contamination of the victims with tissues, such as bone fragments, originating from the terrorists themselves.[21] The concern for blood-borne infections such as Hepatitis B/C and HIV should be kept in mind when dealing with suicide bombers.[21]

Evaluation

Patient Evaluation

It should be borne in mind that no prospective randomized trial regarding the preferred diagnosis or treatment of these injuries is known. The experience is being studied retrospectively in primarily uncontrolled descriptive trials. In addition, most of the descriptions come from military settings where tertiary facilities with modern surgical equipment and experienced personnel are often far away from the scene of action.

As for other high-energy trauma patients, a systematic approach relying on Advanced Trauma Life Support should be applied as early as possible.[6,20] In military settings, the average time interval from evacuation to surgery may be about 5 h.[9] This is not the case in urban terrorism. On the contrary, in case of mass-casualty incident this scenario delay can be caused by disorganization in the trauma center. It should be remembered that a patient suffering from a major penetrating limb injury such as an open fracture has a high chance of having an additional life-threatening-associated injury.[20] Therefore, maximal effort to detect these additional injuries in the primary medical instance should be carried out.

Limb Evaluation

The physical examination of the open wound should consider several important points.[22] Fragments do not travel in straight lines, therefore for those injuries where tumbling of the fragment occurs, the entry and possible exit wound can be far apart or in unexpected areas. Also, the exit wound is generally larger than the entrance wound, as in gunshot injuries. Finally, special attention should be addressed to certain anatomical areas of injuries: near joints or in proximity to major vessels (e.g., in the groin or axilla) or nerves (e.g., the sciatic nerve in the buttock or posterior thigh), and mandate further diagnostic studies.[23]

Soft tissue evaluation of penetrating blast limb injury should be carefully performed. To date, no unique classification exists for this type of injury. The Red Cross E.X.C.V.F.M. Wound Scores, originally designed for gunshot injuries, may be applied with some modifications. (Each letter designates a category of injury for which points are assigned: entry wound, exit wound, presence of a cavity, vital structure injury, fracture, metallic foreign body.) Bowyer et al.[24] used it for the treatment of 63 injured patients during the Gulf War and suggested that it should include an assessment of neurological injuries as well. The Gustillo and Anderson classification can be used for the evaluation of open fractures. However, as for gunshot wounds, it seems that all of these injury types should be considered as type 3 open fractures.[6]

In recent years, radiology has played an important role in the medical evaluation of terrorist attack victims. Imaging examinations, including plain radiographs, computed tomography (CT), ultrasound, and angiography, are used to asses the site and extent of the injury. These examinations also play an important role in determining each patient's need for immediate versus late surgery.[25] These types of procedures are unique to urban setups since they are not available in the military scenario.

Plain radiographs, which are routinely obtained in cases of skeletal trauma, are in most cases sufficient for determining the presence and location of shrapnel as well as the diagnosis of bone fractures. Generally, no additional studies are necessary.

Computed tomography is useful for identifying the precise anatomic location of most metal shrapnel and may add information about the missile's tract. However, since it is a static study it does not contribute to the understanding of the dynamic relationship of the shrapnel to other structures. Ultrasound, on the contrary, is useful for diagnosing shrapnel in soft tissues; it demonstrates the dynamic relationship with other structures like proximity to tendons or movement within a joint.

Ultrasound equipment is portable and available for intraoperative localization and is also used to detect nonmetal shrapnel. Anecdotally, ultrasound has been reported as a useful tool in the detection of depleted Uranium.[26]

Fluoroscopy is useful for diagnosis, placement, and intraoperative use in cases of shrapnel injury. The multiple projections of the image intensifier enable three-dimensional localization of the shrapnel, based on two-dimensional projections. In mass-casualty events, there is an overwhelming exhaustion of imaging resources.[27] The availability of fluoroscopy both reduces the need for other imaging resources and facilitates case handling. In most of the cases, MRI is contraindicated due to the unknown magnetic properties of the shrapnel.

The constant trade-off between tissue damage as a complication of surgery and the benefits of nonacute shrapnel removal lead to the search for minimally invasive removal approaches. Recently, other high-tech modalities have been added to the arsenal of the intraoperative imaging and detecting scenario, like the employment of computerized surgical navigation based on real-time acquisition of fluoroscopic data. An accurate spatial location of the foreign object can be seen on images displayed on the computer screen. An infrared camera tracks down the position of a surgical probe on the patient's anatomy and continuously updates its three-dimensional position, simultaneously on all displayed images until the shrapnel is located.[28]

Treatment

Soft Tissue Management

The cornerstone of the treatment of war and terror limb injury lies in aggressive and meticulous debridement, and prevention of contamination. On the basis of treating 12,000 open fractures, Coupland, in his expert opinion review paper for the International Committee of the Red Cross,[29] stated that complete removal of all necrotic tissue, fat, foreign material, and contamination was much more imperative than fixation of fractures. By adequate wound excision, closure of most fracture sites can be achieved in most cases 5 days later. In more modern conflicts remote from first-level trauma care hospitals as in Afghanistan, wound closure in tertiary centers with comparatively good results was achieved within an average period of 10 days.[10] Beyond the evidence known from bacteriological studies on colonization in necrotic tissue, the importance of early wound debridement and excision cannot be overstated.[30] Jacob et al.,[11] in their study of open fractures during Operation Just Cause, reported a threefold increase in the infection rate (66% vs 22%) in patients who did not undergo debridement before their arrival at a tertiary medical facility as compared with those who underwent early debridement. Lin et al. [10] report an almost threefold lower incidence of repeated orthopedic procedures in patients undergoing adequate initial wound treatment before arriving at a tertiary military facility. The authors concluded that the recent relocation of experienced general and orthopedic surgical teams to the front, and the improvement of airborne evacuations are equally responsible for the decrease in infections detected in war injuries. Recently, an important device, the VAC system, has been introduced; this system may add to the armamentarium of soft tissue debridement and coverage, it may serve as a draining system and delay definitive closure.[31]

These issues are less significant when dealing with civilian populations suffering from similar injuries in level I trauma centers, since evacuation is faster in most cases. It should be noted that the minimal debridement that may be adequate for low-energy gunshot wound most probably is not enough under these circumstances. Free vascularized flaps may be used later for wound coverage.[32]

Fracture Fixation

Regarding fracture fixation, there is a discrepancy between modern trauma care standards and fixation methods traditionally described in war injury literature.

In almost all the studies dealing with fracture care either external fixation or casting was used for treating fractures.[6,8,10,11,22,29,33] Coupland[29] stated that fixation with an external fixator has advantages in soft tissue care since it provides union by callus formation and thus internal fixation is entirely unnecessary. He suggests, splinting with casts and/or traction as an alternative. The Swedish Army reported on their positive experience with a simplified external fixator in a primary military hospital in Somalia. They recommend the use of this procedure due to its simplicity.[34] In treating patients injured in recent US campaigns, there are no reports on internal fixation with intramedullary nailing or plating.[10,33] Intramedullary nailing has proved to be very effective in treating long bone fractures caused by gunshot wounds in civilian settings.[35–37] We applied this technique as well as external fixation, when treating terror-related penetrating long bone extremity fractures, and achieved a similar degree of success in our treatment of gunshot injuries.[20] This discrepancy may be related to the unavailability of advanced orthopedic equipment, including the necessary setup such as fluoroscopy, and experienced personnel in primary military medical facilities. Thus, terror-related blast injuries differ not only in mechanism but also in the availability of different treatment modalities.

It should be noted that in both situations late reconstruction of bone and soft tissue may be staged and prolonged due to soft tissue and bone loss, deformation, nonunion, and deep infection. A recent Turkish study describes a series of 225 patients requiring 108 bone grafts, 14 distraction osteogenesis, and 208 free flaps as late reconstructive efforts to treat war limb injuries. In our series, 15% of the patients treated for long bone fractures caused by terror, required secondary procedures including exchange nails, conversion of external fixators to internal fixators, bone grafting, and application of Ilizarov apparatus for segmental bone transport.

Fragment Management/Removal

Fragment management/removal is chronologically divided into acute, subacute, and late phases.

Acute Phase

The acute phase deals with fragment removal at the time of injury. The fundamental principles guiding fragment wound management are proper evaluation and excision of necrotic or contaminated tissue. Although war surgery literature stresses the need for complete wound debridement, it is a mistake to assume that it is an easy task. We are often aware of how frequently it is performed inadequately.[38]

Most physicians believe that high-velocity projectiles cause more tissue damage than low-velocity projectiles. Unfortunately this is not exactly true on our case, since many bullets do not efficiently impart all of their velocity into the victim.[39-41] In fact, high-velocity military bullets are less damaging to soft tissue, particularly when bursting from body. Bowyer et al.[42] indicated that most casualties who reach surgical facilities alive were struck by fragments with initial velocities of <600 m/s. The aerodynamic drag of these irregularly shaped projectiles results in an outward deceleration from the point of detonation.[43-45] Thus, depending on the distance from the blast, when fragments strike the body, they can range from high to low velocity. Upon striking tissues, even at low velocities, these fragments may exhibit the tumbling or so-called shimmy effect which can increase the amount of tissue damage. Moreover, these fragments usually carry environmental debris into the wound, frequently causing more severe tissue injury than low-velocity bullets. These are the reasons why modern authorities have abandoned the concept of mandatory, wide debridement of high-velocity wounds. However, this information has not yet trickled down the mainstream of surgical literature.[46,47]

Fragment and projectile wounds should be treated on a case by case basis using the fundamental principle guiding the management of these wounds: evaluation and excision of the necrotic or contaminated tissues. The four Cs of muscle viability (color, consistency, capacity to bleed, and contractility) are used to assess what should be excised, although this is subjective and greatly depends on the surgeon's former experience.[48] Serial debridement is often necessary in high-risk injuries, that is, excision of muscle which is merely questionable at the initial assessment but can become necrotic at a later stage. Fragments in the wound tract is usually removed during the acute stage. Other shrapnel is left for delayed removal or be retained in the tissue for life.

It is sometime difficult to predict whether a penetrating fragment injury has a high potential for infection and therefore debridement is inevitable. This decision requires experienced clinical judgment. However, certain guidelines can assist in making the right clinical decision. There are certain factors which help the surgeon decide whether the wound is of a high or low risk; time to treatment, path of the projectile, bone involvement, and the number of projectiles are all taken into account.[48]

It should be emphasized that in the acute phase, damage control principles are applied, and only life-saving procedures are performed to stabilize the patient hemodynamically.[1] After the patient is stabilized, shrapnel, even if initially planned to be removed, should be left untouched in the tissue, up to a later stage, after the emergency condition has subsided.

Subacute Phase

In certain cases, retained shrapnel removal is indicated following the acute phase such as when infection is suspected; in the presence of periarticular involvement, in weight bearing areas, superficial placement or proximity to neurovascular structures. Significant large fragments which can interfere with normal functioning should also be removed.

Periarticular involvement: High-energy projectiles are likely to carry foreign material into the joint. The surgeon should not hesitate to explore the wound surgically. Apart from posing an infection hazard, any foreign material in the joint can cause mechanical abrasion and joint destruction, whereas fragments passing through the joint can cause ligament or meniscus injury.[48–50] Fragments in the periarticular area, as in bursae, should also be removed. Other indications for removal are cases of superficial shrapnel under the skin or cases of weight-bearing surfaces which become painful when touched or when exposed.

Nerve involvement: Nerve palsy is a common finding following shrapnel injury and is usually temporary, thus neouropraxy in itself is not an indication for exploration. However, if shrapnel is located near nerve structures and there is irritation of the nerve with progressive neurological signs or symptoms appear, nerve exploration accompanied by shrapnel removal is indicated. Omer[51] reported a recovery rate of up to 70% usually within 6–9 months following injury for gunshot wounds with nervous symptoms. A transected nerve should be repaired after the inflammatory phase has subsided and when all signs of infection have disappeared. Shrapnel removal is indicated whenever exposure of the nerve is performed. Twenty-five percent recovery rage after nerve repair is reported.

Late Phase

Retained fragments are usually benign and the surgeon should not try to remove them.[50] Metal shards do not usually call for surgical excision, since the metal pieces remain inert inside the tissue and do not cause any long-term damage. After recovery from the preliminary injury, most people are asymptomatic. The fragment gradually become encased in fibrous tissue and are considered inert.[49,52] However, in rare cases, fragments can cause harm after a long time, either systemic damage as a result of a degrading of the shrapnel or due to a local foreign body reaction. Large lead fragments retained in soft tissue can result in plumbism.[53] Chronic plumbism should be considered in patients with retained lead material.

The first widespread use of depleted Uranium occurred in the early 1990s during the Gulf War. The kidney Uranium concentration in some individuals reached its peak 6 years after the war.[54] It was found that depleted Uranium degrading caused multiorgan toxicities. Malignant processes have been reported in conjunction with the prolonged presence of shrapnel.[40,55] Cases of delayed aneurisms and abscesses in the site of a retained foreign body have been described[56,57] as well as foreign body granulomas and reactions. Nevertheless, considering the morbidity involved in surgical removal, these rare incidents do not justify the surgical removal of fragment in all cases.[50] A relatively new indication for fragment removal is the clinical indication for an MRI study. This examination cannot be safely performed on patients with retained metallic fragments, since patients with retained metal who undergo MRI examination may suffer from magnetic effects on the fragments (pain, bruises, and even injury to nerve or blood vessels located in the vicinity of the shrapnel). Removal of such material is thus indicated before performing the MRI study.

After Care

Casualty treatment does not terminate upon discharge following initial hospitalization. Continuing treatment may take place either in a primary health care setting or in rehospitalization. Treatment may include additional surgery, physician follow-up, physical therapy, and so on. Nearly 50% of terror victims who were hospitalized immediately after injury and survived were rehospitalized. The total number of recurrent hospitalization days amounts to 80% of the first hospitalization period for all casualties. The probability rate of recurrent referral during the first 3 months varied between different population groups.

Patients who were severely injured (injury severity score, ISS, of 16 or more) or were hospitalized in the ICU during their initial hospitalization had a greater than 40% chance for returning within 3 months. Recurrent hospital referrals are a heavy burden on health systems, on the patients themselves, and on their families. The severity of the injury of a terror victim is greater than that of other casualties, thereby necessitating longer hospitalization periods, particularly in the ICU. Their in-hospital mortality rate is also greater.[58]

Conclusion

Despite the lack of randomized control trials in the treatment of war- and terror-related penetrating injuries, there are some consistent findings in the literature on the topic. Most terror- and war-related injuries involve limbs and are primarily due to blast injuries rather than gunshot. These can include additional life-threatening-associated injuries which may involve heavy contamination, soft tissue and bone loss; and should therefore be diagnosed early. Prompt, thorough, and meticulous wound debridement is the key to the treatment of these devastating injuries, followed by achievement of skeletal stability. Late reconstructions and attainment of functional results are a great challenge for the surgical team.

References

1. Almogy G, Beltzberg A, Mintz Y, Pikarski A, Zamir G, Rivkind A: Suicide bombing attacks update and modifications to the protocol. *Ann Surg.* 2004;239(3):295–303.
2. Kluger Y, Peleg K, Daniel-Aharonson L, Mayo A: The special injury pattern in terrorist bombings. *J Am Coll Surg.* 2004;199(6):875–879.

3. Nelson TJ, Clark T, Stedje-Larsen ET, et al.: Close proximity blast injury patterns from improvised explosive devices in Iraq: a report of 18 cases. *J Trauma.* 2007;11; [Epub ahead of print].

4. Ramalingam T, Pathak G, Barker P: A method for determining the rate of major limb amputations in battle casualties: experiences of a British Field Hospital in Iraq, 2003. *Ann R Coll Surg Engl.* 2005;87(2):113–116.

5. Gawande A: Casualties of war–military care for the wounded from Iraq and Afghanistan. *N Engl J Med.* 2004 9;351(24):2471–2475.

6. Covey D: Blast and fragment injuries of the musculoskeletal system. *J Bone Joint Surg (A).* 2002;84(7):1221–1234.

7. Spalding TJ, Stewart MP, Tulloch DN, Stephens KM: Penetrating missile injuries in the Gulf war 1991. *Br J Surg.* 1991;78(9):1102–1104.

8. Hodalic Z, Svagelj M, Sebalj I, Sebalj D: Surgical treatment of 1,211 patients at the Vinkovci General Hospital, Vinkovci, Croatia, during the 1991–1992 Serbian offensive in east Slavonia. *Mil Med.* 1999;164(11):803–808.

9. Marshall TJ Jr: Combat casualty care: the Alpha Surgical Company experience during Operation Iraqi Freedom. *Mil Med.* 2005;170(6):469–472.

10. Lin DL, Kirk KL, Murphy KP, McHale KA, Doukas WC: Evaluation of orthopaedic injuries in Operation Enduring Freedom. *J Orthop Trauma.* 2004;18(5):300–305.

11. Jacob E, Erpelding JM, Murphy KP: A retrospective analysis of open fractures sustained by U.S. military personnel during Operation Just Cause. *Mil Med.* 1992;157(10):552–556.

12. Ramalingam T: Extremity injuries remain a high surgical workload in a conflict zone: experiences of a British field hospital in Iraq, 2003. *J R Army Med Corps.* 2004;150(3):187–190.

13. DePalma RG, Burris DG, Champion HR, Hodgson MJ: Blast injuries. *N Engl J Med.* 2005;352(13):1335–1342.

14. Leibovici D, Gofrit ON, Stein M, et al.: Blast injuries: bus versus open-air bombings—a comparative study of injuries in survivors of open-air versus confined-space explosions. *J Trauma.* 1996;41(6):1030–1035.

15. Hull JB, Cooper GJ: Pattern and mechanism of traumatic amputation by explosive blast. *J Trauma.* 1996;40(Suppl 3):S198–S205.

16. Peleg K, Aharonson-Daniel L: Letter: blast injuries. *N Engl J Med.* 2005;352:2651–2653.

17. Barham M: Letter: blast injuries. *N Engl J Med.* 2005;352:2651–2653.

18. Ashkenazi I, Olsha O, Alfici R, Peleg K, Aharonson-Daniel L, Barham M, DePalma RG, Burris DG, Champion HR: Blast injuries. *N Engl J Med.* 2005;352(25):2651–2653(correspondence).

19. Langworthy MJ, Sabra J, Gould M: Terrorism and blast phenomena: lessons learned from the attack on the USS Cole (DDG67). *Clin Orthop.* 2004;422:82–87.

20. Weil Y, Petrov K, Liebergall M, Mintz Y, Mosheiff R: Long bone fractures caused by penetrating injuries in terrorists attacks. *J Trauma.* 2007;62(4):909–912.

21. Leibner E, Weil Y, Gross E, Liebergall M, Mosheiff R: A broken bone without a fracture: traumatic foreign bone implantation resulting from a mass casualty bombing. *J Trauma.* 2005;58(2):388–390.

22. Covey DC, Lurate RB, Hatton CT: Field hospital treatment of blast wounds of the musculoskeletal system during the Yugoslav civil war. *J Orthop Trauma.* 2000;14(4):278–286.

23. Gray R: War wounds: basic surgical management. Geneva: International Committee of the Red Cross; 1994.

24. Bowyer GW, Stewart MP, Ryan JM: Gulf War wounds: application of the Red Cross wound classification. *Injury* 1993;24(9):597–600.

25. Shaham D, Sella T, Makori A, Appelbum, L, Rivkind AI, Bar-Ziv J: The role of radiology in terror injuries. *Isr Med Assoc J*. 2002;4:564–567.
26. Kalinich JF, Ramakrishnan N, Mc-Clain DE: A procedure for the rapid detection of depleted uranium in metal shrapnel fragments. *Mil Med*. 2000;165:626–629.
27. Avitzour M, Liebergall M, Assaf J, et al.: A multicasualty event: out-of hospital and in-hospital organizational aspects. *Acad Emerg Med*. 2004;11:1102–1104.
28. Mosheiff R, Weil Y, Khoury A, Liebergall M: The use of computerized navigation in the treatment of gunshot and shrapnel injury. *Comput Aided Surg*. 2004;9:39–43.
29. Coupland RM: War wounds of bones and external fixation. *Injury*. 1994;25(4):211–217.
30. Tian H, Deng G, Huang M, Tian FG, Suang GY, Liu YG: Quantitative bacteriological study of the wound track. *J Traum*. 1988;28(S):S215–S216.
31. Ullmann Y, Fodor L, Ramon Y, Soudry M, Lerner A: The revised "reconstructive ladder" and its applications for high-energy injuries to the extremities. *Ann Plast Surg*. 2006;56(4):401–405.
32. Chattar-Cora D, Perez-Nieves R, McKinlay A, Kunasz M, Delaney R, Lyons R: Operation Iraqi freedom: a report on a series of soldiers treated with free tissue transfer by a plastic surgery service. *Ann Plast Surg*. 2007;58(2):200–206.
33. Johnson BA, Carmack D, Neary M, Tenuta J, Chen J: Operation Iraqi Freedom: the Landstuhl Regional Medical Center experience. *J Foot Ankle Surg*. 2005;44(3):177–183.
34. Hammer RR, Rooser B, Lidman D, Smeds S: Simplified external fixation for primary management of severe musculoskeletal injuries under war and peace time conditions. *J Orthop Trauma*. 1996;10(8):545–554.
35. Nowotarski P, Brumback RJ: Immediate interlocking nailing of fractures of the femur caused by low to mid-velocity gunshots. *J Orthop Trauma*. 1994;8(2):134–141.
36. Tornetta P, Tiburzi D: Anterograde interlocked nailing of distal femoral fractures after gunshot wounds. *J Orthop Trauma*. 1994;8(3):220–227.
37. Nicholas RM, McCoy GF: Immediate intramedullary nailing of femoral shaft fractures due to gunshots. *Injury*. 1995;26(4):257–259.
38. Lindeman G, McKay MJ, Taubman KL, Bilous AM: Malignant fibrous histiocytoma developing in bone 44 years after shrapnel trauma. *Cancer*. 1990;66:2229–2232.
39. Marcus NA, Blair WF, Shuck JM, Omer GE Jr: Low-velocity gunshot wounds to extremities. *J Trauma*. 1980;20:1061–1064.
40. Coupland RM: Technical aspects of war wound excision. *Br J Surg*. 1989;76:663–667.
41. Santucci RA, Chang YJ: Ballistics for physicians: myths about wound ballistics and gunshot injuries. *J Urol*. 2004;171:1408–1414.
42. Bowyer GW, Cooper GJ, Rice P: Small fragment wounds: biophysics and pathophysiology. *J Trauma*. 1996;40(3 suppl):S159–S164.
43. Ryan JM, Cooper GJ, Haywood IR, Milner SM: Field surgery on a future conventional battlefield: strategy and wound management. *Ann R Coll Surg Engl*. 1991;73:13–20.
44. Bowyer GW, Cooper GJ, Rice P: Management of small fragment wounds in war: current research. *Ann R Coll Surg Engl*. 1995;77:131–134.
45. Wightman JM, Gladish SL: Explosions and blast injuries. *Ann Emerg Med*. 2001;37:664–678.
46. Fackler ML: Gunshot wound review. *Ann Emerg Med*. 1996;28:194–203.
47. ChartersACIII, Charters AC: Wounding mechanism of very high velocity projectiles. *J Trauma*. 1976;16:464–470.
48. Volgas DA, Stannard JP, Alonso JE: Current orthopaedic treatment of ballistic injuries. *Injury*. 2005;36:380–386.

49. Sclafani SJ, Vuletin JC, Twersky J: Lead arthropathy: arthritis caused by retained intra-articular bullets. *Radiology*. 1985;156:299–302.
50. Rhee JM, Martin R: The management of retained bullets in the limbs. *Injury*. 1997; 28(suppl 3):SC23–SC28.
51. Omer GE Jr: Injuries to nerves of the upper extremity. *J Bone Joint Surg Am*. 1974; 56:1615–1624.
52. Eylon S, Mosheiff R, Liebergall M, Wolf E, Brocke L, Peyser A: Delayed reaction to shrapnel retained in soft tissue. *Injury*. 2005;36:275–281.
53. Stromberg BV: Symptomatic lead toxicity secondary to retained shotgun pellets: case report. *J Trauma*. 1990;30:356–357.
54. Squibb KS, Leggett RW, McDiarmid MA: Prediction of renal concentrations of depleted uranium and radiation dose in Gulf War veterans with embedded shrapnel. *Health Phys*. 2005;89:267–273.
55. Kalinich JF, Emond CA, Dalton TK, et al.: Embedded weapons-grade tungsten alloy shrapnel rapidly induces metastatic high-grade rhabdomyosarcomas in F344 rats. *Environ Health Perspect*. 2005;113:729–734.
56. Lee JH, Kim DG: Brain abscess related to metal fragments 47 years after head injury: case report. *J Neurosurg*. 2000;93:477–479.
57. Chedid MK, Vender JR, Harrison SJ, McDonnell DE: Delayed appearance of a traumatic intracranial aneurysm: case report and review of the literature. *J Neurosurg*. 2001;94:637–641.
58. Peleg K, Aharonson-Daniel L, Stein M, Michaelson M, et al.: Gunshot and explosion injuries: characteristics, outcomes, and implications for care of terror-related injuries in Israel. *Ann Surg*. 2004;239(3):311–318.

18
Terror-Inflicted Burn Injury

Tomer Tzur and Arieh Eldad

Burn injuries are common among victims of terrorism. Since bombs are the most common weapon used by terrorists all over the world, the inevitable results are a combination of blast injuries, penetrating injuries, and burns. This type of injury is very similar to injuries seen in wars. The main difference between war and terrorist attacks is in the targeted population – soldiers in the former, civilians in the latter. Civilians are less protected compared to soldiers and therefore are more suscepti- ble. The fact that acts of terrorism harm the very old and the very young confronts the medical system with a case-mix that is utterly different from the one expected in war. The extreme age groups are special populations in terms of morbidity and mortality from burns, and this adds a new dimension to the treatment of burns caused by terrorist attacks, compared to war injuries.

The development of weapons has had a colossal impact on the frequency and severity of burns in war. Similarly, the creation of new explosives with the addition of common items such as fuel, cooking gas cylinders, and other volatile materials in terrorists' bombs has further increased the severity of burns caused by terrorist attacks in the last few decades.

Terrorist attacks are usually perpetrated in highly populated areas and therefore in close proximity to medical centers. Both in war and in a terrorist attack, there are usually multiple casualties within a very short time. This puts a much heavier load than usual on the medical system, which is used to coping with only a few cases of accidental burns at any given time in peacetime.

During the past decade, Israel has experienced two waves of terrorism (1994– 1996 and "The Al-Aqsa intifada" that began in October 2000 and gradually dimin- ished after 2003) and the difference in the prevalence of burns in these two periods is significant. This change is due to the different components used in the bombs carried by suicide bombers during these two periods. The 1994–1996 terrorist wave included 12 suicide bombings, most of which occurred in closed environments, 9 on buses. Most of the injuries were characterized by a combination of blast injuries and severe burns, accompanied by inhalation injuries. Of the 144 people killed in these attacks, 52 (42%) had severe burns (mean 32% total body surface area, TBSA); and of the 760 people injured, 97 (12.7%) had burns with a mean of 15% TBSA. During the second wave of mass murders by suicide bombers that started in October 2000, more than 650 people were killed and more than 4,500 injured. Many of the attacks

S.C. Shapira et al. (eds.), *Essentials of Terror Medicine*,
DOI: 10.1007/978-0-387-09412-0_18, Springer Science+Business Media, LLC 2009

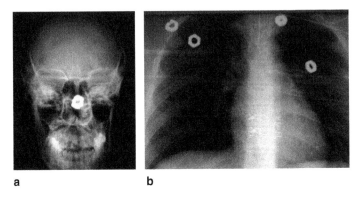

a   b

FIG. 18.1. Fifteen-year-old female with shrapnel injury. **a** Skull X-ray showing a bolt penetration in the root of the nose. **b** Chest X-ray indicating bolt penetration in each lung.

took place in malls, outdoor restaurants, or other open areas. Only 6.2% of the survivors sustained burns. Most of the bodies examined in this period had some burns, but the major cause of death was multiple penetrating injuries from nails, bolts, screws, and other metal objects added to the bombs to intensify the injuries (Fig. 18.1a and b). Since this added to the killing effect of these bombs, there were fewer surviving burn casualties admitted to the hospitals. In most cases, the burns were superficial, and involved a small percentage of the TBSA. The casualties who were closer to the bomber and sustained deeper and more extensive burns died of the penetrating injuries caused by the metal particles.

The explosives used during 1994–1996 were mainly homemade (usually made with agricultural fertilizers and other chemicals purchased legally), while in the second "intifada" standard military explosives (like, trinitrotoluene, TNT) were used.

Analysis of data published by the Israel National Trauma Registry on hospitalized victims of terrorism between October 1, 2000 and December 31, 2005 includes 2,446 casualties. 2002 was the year with maximum number of casualties. Since 2003, there has been a continued and significant decline in the number of casualties. About half of them occurred as a result of an explosion. Again, many of the attacks took place in malls, outdoor restaurants, or other open areas. The percentage of severely injured among the casualties of terrorism is significantly higher than other casualties recorded in the Trauma Registry (29% compared with 10%, respectively). The in-patient mortality caused by terrorist acts was three times as high as that of other trauma casualties (6% compared to 2%, respectively).[1]

Until recently, Hadassah University Hospital in the Ein-Kerem Campus had been the only level I trauma center in Jerusalem, and the only one with a burn unit. Data obtained from the Trauma Registry regarding hospitalized casualties with burns sustained from terrorist acts were analyzed. The data were classified as belonging to two periods: January 1, 1997 to September 30, 2000 (the 3 years of the first terrorism wave) and October 1, 2000, the beginning of the second wave, to December 31, 2005.

% TBSA

■ <20
■ 20-29
□ 30-39
▨ >40

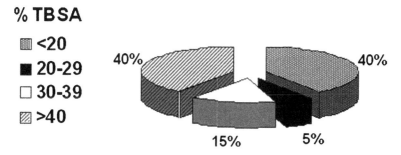

FIG. 18.2. Burn case distribution of total body surface area in the First Terror Wave 1997–August 31, 2000.

%TBSA
▨ <20
■ 20-29
□ 30-39
■ >40

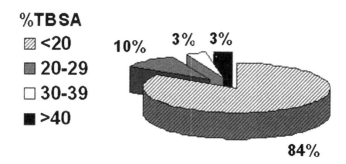

FIG. 18.3. Burn case distribution of total body surface area in % "Al- Aqsa" Intifada September 1, 2000 – December 31, 2005.

During the first period, 63 terrorism casualties were hospitalized, most of them injured in explosions, of whom 20 patients (32%) had sustained burns. Most casualties (60%) had major burns involving more than 20% TBSA and 40% sustained burns involving more than 40% TBSA (Fig. 18.2).

In the second period analyzed, 649 casualties were hospitalized, of whom 61 (9%) suffered from burns. The majority (84%) had burns involving less than 20% TBSA (Fig. 18.3). Only 10 casualties (16% of the burn patients) had burns as their only injury. Most were injured in more than one body region. Data published by the Israel National Trauma Registry from October 2000 to December 2004 showed that a total of 16.6% of casualties had sustained burns, of whom 70.5% had an additional penetrating or blunt injury (Fig. 18.4).[2].

In both periods, the majority of the casualties suffered multiple trauma of varying severity, with an Injury Severity Score (ISS) of 16 or more (Fig. 18.5).

Children under the age of 15 account for half of the nonterrorism-related burns. In contrast, people in their most productive decades (15–60 years) comprised the main group of terrorism-related victims, 75% and 86% in both periods, respectively, as a result of the public nature of these attacks (Fig. 18.6).

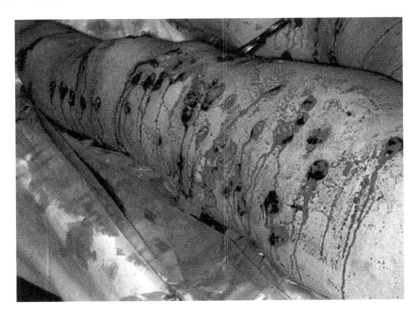

FIG. 18.4. Lower left limb of a 14-year-old female who sustained multiple penetrating shrapnel injuries with extensive soft tissue damage.

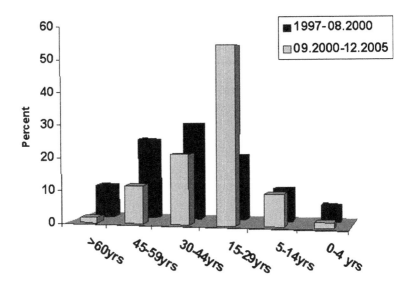

FIG. 18.5. Age distribution of casualties.

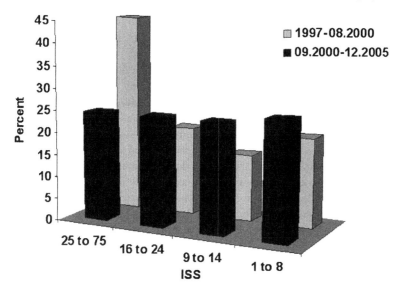

FIG. 18.6.   Injury Severity Score (*ISS*) distribution of casualties.

Management of Casualties

The essentials of the management of patients with burn injuries from terrorism-related incidents are the same as those for any burn patients. Nevertheless, the complexity of the injuries and the related trauma require some special considerations. Before addressing these considerations, a typical terrorism-related burn casualty case is presented.

Case Report

One August morning, on a number 26 bus in Jerusalem, LY, a 31-year-old computer worker in the Ministry of Justice, was on her way to work when a suicide bomber standing 3 yards away exploded with a 4 kg TNT bomb worn under his shirt.

This was a summer morning in Jerusalem. The bus windows were open, reducing the severity of blast injuries. Only five people were immediately killed. (Later that year, in the fall, Jerusalem experienced more suicide bombers on busses and many more died as a result of severe blast injuries.) Thirty-five casualties were evacuated from the scene; 14 of them, the most severe cases, were brought to Hadassah Ein-Kerem, the regional level I trauma center, located some 15–20 minutes away. Eight of them suffered burns as part of their multiple injuries.

Most of the casualties had blast injuries to their lungs, abdominal viscera and ears, penetrating shrapnel injuries, fractures, and burns, including airway thermal injuries and smoke inhalation.

The mass-casualty situation should be described, as it may have had some impact on the clinical decisions taken that morning. It was early and the regular operation rooms (OR) list had not begun as it had been put on hold as soon as the bomb notification was delivered. When LY was brought to the emergency department, there were already six or seven casualties in the trauma unit and hers did not seem to be the most severe case. She was already intubated and sedated and only a month later did she show signs of hemodynamic shock: a tender abdomen, with penetrating injuries, bilateral pneumohemothorax, comminuted open fracture of her right knee and traumatic amputation of a few toes in her left foot. She sustained burns involving 50% TBSA, covering her face, neck, chest, back, and right upper and lower extremities.

She had chest drains put in and was rushed to the OR. Laparotomy revealed severe lacerations in her spleen. LY had a splenectomy. Lacerations of the mesenterium were sutured. A feeding jejunostomy was deferred in light of her hemodynamic instability. The orthopedic surgeons tried to put her right knee together and a muscle flap was rotated to cover it. She was not stable, and hypothermic, so no attempts at early excision and grafting of her third degree burns were made during this first operation. Instead, wet gauze was used for mechanical debridement of all the burns that appeared to be of partial thickness: over her face, chest, and back. Cryopreserved cadaver homograft from the national skin bank was stapled to cover her burns.

The next day, when she was more stable, she was returned to the OR, to excise all the burns that were definitely of full thickness: over her right arm, right leg, and left foot. No autologous skin was harvested, so as not to add trauma to this complicated case, and the excised areas were covered with cryopreserved homograft.

Over the next few days, gradual peeling of the homograft that covered partial-thickness burns was observed, with new epidermis growing beneath it. The narrow gaps between the homograft sheets that were not protected by the grafts took longer to heal and eventually became hypertrophic, as they desiccated and turned to full thickness. Most of her face healed spontaneously under the homograft cover. During the next months, the homograft over the excised areas was exchanged with autologous skin.

The patient had several septic episodes including Candida sepsis. At that point, Candida was isolated from her right knee, as well as from her blood. A decision was made not to amputate the leg and to try to save it. The knee joint seemed to be destroyed: open, infected with exposed patella and tendons, and with no skin cover. An irrigation system was put into the joint and it was irrigated alternately with Betadine solution and Amphotericin B. Eventually the infection subsided.

Despite the severe infection, the leg was not amputated, based on the assumption that long-term ambulation would be better compared to prosthesis. The cartilage was totally destroyed in this joint, but now the patient is completely ambulatory, walking without any aid except a walking stick, and surprisingly, has no pain in her leg.

Pre-hospital Treatment

In urban areas, medical teams arrive quickly at the scene of a terrorism-related mass-casualty incident. Time spent at the scene is brief; only emergency, life-saving procedures are conducted on-site and a "scoop and run" policy is usually implemented, leaving a short warning time for hospital medical staff. The first casualty would be expected to arrive at the emergency department about 15–20 minutes after the attack, depending on the distance of the scene from the hospital.[3]

While all hospitals should be able to treat severely injured patients, pre-hospital personnel should be familiar with triage criteria to determine which patient should be taken to a level I trauma center. Not all patients will go to a trauma or burn center, however. In rural areas, such a center may not exist. Many patients will be self-transported to the nearest facility. In large burn catastrophes, effective patient distribution to a regional network requires active planning efforts. Survivors arriving at a less than optimal medical facility often require secondary transfers. Fortunately, experience with the US military's Critical Care Air Transport Team (CCATT) shows that even severely burned patients "travel well" and can be transported long distances[4].

Acute Lung Injuries

More than half of the victims of these suicide bombings had some type of acute lung injury. Burns were found to be one of the specific external signs of trauma in these terrorist attacks, associated with a high rate of blast lung injuries.[5] As described in the literature, injuries following closed-space explosions were worse compared with open-space explosions.

A decrease in pulmonary function can occur in patients with severe burns without evidence of inhalation injury from the bronchoconstriction caused by humoral factors such as histamine, serotonin, and thromboxane A2. A decrease in lung and tissue compliance is a manifestation of a reduction in pulmonary function.

The respiratory management of patients with severe blast lung injury who present with burns is challenging because these entities may require somewhat contradictory therapies.[3,6]

Hemodynamic Support

In the case of patients whose burns exceed 30% of TBSA, cytokines and other mediators are released into the circulation system, to play a major role in the systemic inflammatory response. Because vessels in burned tissue exhibit increased vascular permeability, an extravasation of fluids into the burned tissues occurs. Hypovolemia is the immediate consequence of this fluid loss and accounts for decreased perfusion and oxygen delivery. In patients with serious burns, release of catecholamines, vasopressin, and angiotensin causes peripheral and splanchnic bed vasoconstriction which can compromise in-organ perfusion. Myocardial contractility also may be reduced by the release of inflammatory cytokine tumor necrosis factor-alpha.

Among the survivors of terrorism attacks, hypovolemic shock, resulting from blast and penetrating injuries, is frequent in the acute stage. Massive burns contribute to this condition because of fluid lost through the affected body surface area and into the interstitium. Fluid resuscitation is the primary therapy. The problem is that such large volumes of fluid resuscitation might result in respiratory deterioration in the presence of acute lung injuries.[2,3]

Patients suffering severe blast injuries, especially blast lung, as well as penetrating injuries from shrapnel, in combination with burns, benefit from invasive monitoring. Invasive monitoring optimizes fluid management. A central venous pressure (CVP) catheter is routinely placed. Pulmonary artery catheters are placed only in those patients showing significant hemodynamic instability. Another method used to optimize fluid management is the use of transthoracic or transesophageal echocardiogram, usually in conjugation with a CVP catheter.[6]

Infections

The human population is not germ free. The skin is man's most significant defense, and any alternations of the integument disturb the balance with the microbial flora. The open burn wound is a favorable target for bacterial colonization either from the environment or from the patient himself. This colonization or "contamination" of the burn wound does not imply a local or systemic infection. If the microorganisms actively reach viable tissue, they will produce a local infection or a systemic one by hematological or lymphatic dissemination of the microorganisms themselves or their toxic products.

Repeated showers with running water and cleansing agents and topical antibiotics decrease microbial growth and reduce invasive infection. Prophylactic systemic antibiotics, however, are not recommended because they do not prevent wound or systemic sepsis. The use of prophylactic antibiotics increases the risk of opportunistic infection. Burn eschar has no microcirculation, hence there is no mechanism for the local delivery of systemically administered antibiotics.

As mentioned already, most terrorism-related burn casualties also suffered from penetrating or blunt injury. These complex injuries necessitated broad-spectrum antibiotic treatment in cases of penetrating abdominal trauma and penetrating brain injury. The unavoidable use of catheterization, sometimes through the burned tissue, was another potential cause of infection. The use of broad-spectrum antibiotics and catheterization increased the incidence of burn wound infections and systemic infections with resistant microorganisms (mainly MRSA, MRSE, pseudomonas aeruginosa, and acinetobacter species).

The incidence of mycotic invasion has doubled since the use of topical antimicrobial agents to control bacterial colonization. Candida species is the most common. Early diagnosis is difficult as clinical symptoms resemble low-grade bacterial infections. The burn wound is the most commonly infected site. Candida infections occur most commonly in patients who are hospitalized for long periods of time with large burns and receive multiple courses of antibiotics.

In a study done by the department of clinical microbiology in Hadassah University Hospital, a cluster of candidemia among patients who had sustained injuries in a bomb blast at a marketplace was investigated. Candidemia occurred in 30% of the patients between 4 and 16 days after the injury and was the single most frequent cause of bloodstream infections. Inhalation injury was the strongest predictor for candidemia in multivariate analysis. These findings suggest a role for an exogenous, environmental source in the development of candidemia in some trauma patients.[7]

One of the major goals of the burn surgeon is to prevent microbial invasion, and when contamination occurs, to reduce the microbial levels so that wound healing will not be impaired. The burn wound should be inspected at least once daily for any signs of local infection, such as black or dark brown focal areas of discoloration, conversion of partial-thickness injury to full thickness, edema of skin around the margins of the wound, and enhanced sloughing of burn tissue or eschar. Quantitative burn wound cultures may differentiate infection from colonization, and can identify sensitivities, but does not correlate well with the histopathological examination and does not predict outcome of skin grafting.[8]

Burn wound sepsis is suspected when the wound is the site of proliferating microorganisms and when there is invasion of subjacent unburned tissue. The clinical diagnosis is made when clinical symptoms appear and a septic source can be identified. When the patient exhibits signs of sepsis, immediate institution of antibiotics is obligatory, even in the absence of confirmatory cultures.

Maintaining the wound at low contamination levels reduces the frequency and duration of septic episodes. This is accomplished by cleansing the wounds twice daily by showering the patient. The showers wash the exudate that has accumulated between dressing changes.

Debridement of the burn wound is one of the important methods of lowering the bacterial load and reducing the incidence of septic episodes. Definitive wound closure may take time in cases with extensive injury. For these patients, topical antibiotics are the single most important factor in minimizing septic complications. Mechanical wound care is a very important adjunct to the application of topical antibiotics, allowing maximal penetration to the wound surface.

Burn Wound Management

Early burn excision and skin grafting are standard care for full-thickness burn wounds. The concept of early excision was popularized in the early 1970s by Janezovic.[9] The benefits of early excision are clear and well documented. Early excision and grafting result in increased survival, decreased infection rates, and decreased length of hospital stay. It appears that early excision may also decrease the incidence of hypertrophic scars.[10]

Early-stage excision of full-thickness burns should start as early as possible (usually at post burn day 3). As mentioned, most terrorism-related burn casualties have additional injuries, mainly blast injury and penetrating injury, and are severely injured (ISS > 16). The complexity of injuries makes these casualties unstable, and emergency operations are usually abbreviated laparoscopy and/or thoracotomy and damage control.[11] Patients' instability usually delays early excision, and in a few cases, when we managed to enter the operating theater for excision of burns which were clearly full thickness, grafting was postponed to decrease the trauma to the patients.

Early treatment of partial-thickness burn wound was mechanical debridement by rubbing it thoroughly with chlorhexidine wet gauzes without surgical excision. Burns involving small BSA were treated conservatively with silver sulfadiazine or mafenide. Large areas of partial-thickness burns were treated with homografts stapled to the wounds. Homografts adhered to the wound for 10–14 days and peeled off when the burn was healed (Fig. 18.7a–c). This protected the wound from desiccation and infection. Less deepening of the burns was observed in the homograft-treated wounds as compared to burns treated with silver sulfadiazine. No vascular bridges are formed and the homografts serve as a biological dressing. In some cases, we could observe the narrow gaps between the homografts deepening and eventually becoming hypertrophic bands, while the areas that were properly covered with homografts healed

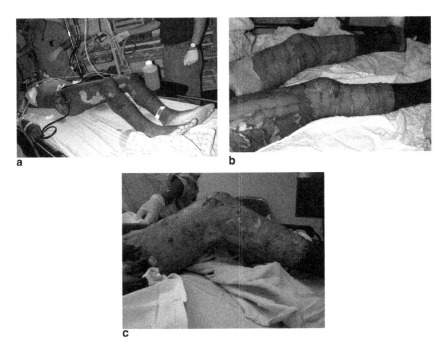

Fig. 18.7 Lower limbs of a 21-year-old soldier who sustained injuries by a suicide bomber. a Deep partial burns as seen upon arrival at trauma center. b Homografts application after mechanical debridement of wounds. c Reepithelization of burns underneath as seen after removal of homografts.

uneventfully. Similar results were reported when glycerolized (nonviable) homografts were used for partial-thickness injuries.[12]

Open wounds left after deep burns eschar excision was also covered with homografts until the patients became stable enough for skin harvesting and autografting.

Early excision and grafting of special areas should be performed if possible. In patients suffering blast lung injury or smoke inhalation, who are expected to be ventilated for a long time, the anterior neck should be considered for early grafting to lower the chance of infections, should a tracheostomy be required.[13]

The Israeli National Skin Bank at Hadassah University Hospital has sufficient supplies to provide skin to all the burn units in Israel for everyday use. The amount of cadaver skin stored (for wartime or mass-casualty situation) has made it unnecessary to use any occlusive dressing or skin substitute for temporary coverage of burn wounds. Such products were used after the 2002 Bali bomb blast due to the lack of cadaver skin.[14]

However, with a skin bank for long-term storage, the question arose: How long can skin be stored and remain a viable skin substitute? A literature search did not provide any answers, most probably because most skin banks store only for short periods as the demand is always greater than the supply.

In a series of experiments, we established an in vivo immunocompetent mice model to assess the efficacy of human cryopreserved skin grafts after short-term transplantation. We compared the performance of nonviable glycerolized skin stored in 90% glycerol at room temperature to cryopreserved skin and to fresh skin.[15] Various modalities of cryopreservation were also compared.[16] Storage in $-180°C$ liquid nitrogen was compared to storage in $-80°C$ in an electric freezer, and gradual cooling by $-1°C/min$ was compared to stepwise cooling to $-20°C$, $-40°C$, $-80°C$, and $-180°C$, respectively. We found that fresh homografts are the best skin substitutes and should be considered the "gold standard."

Cryopreserved homografts perform better than nonviable glycerolized skin. Gradual cooling by $1°C/min$ is preferable to stepwise freezing for long-term storage, and liquid nitrogen storage is superior to $-80°C$ in an electric freezer. However, if only a short-term storage is desired (up to 1 month), an electric freezer is as effective as liquid nitrogen, without the complicated logistics of liquid nitrogen storage. We compared batches of skin cryopreserved for several months to samples that were cryopreserved for several years, the longest being 7 years. This long-term experiment demonstrated that skin can still act as a viable tissue after being stored for 5 years, after which time the deterioration makes it similar to nonviable biological dressing.[17]

Reports of the successful engraftment of cultured keratinocytes in burn casualties suggested a new horizon for the treatment of extensive burns.[18] Our clinical experience with autologous or homologous cultured keratinocytes to treat burns was not very satisfying.[19] Better engraftment was demonstrated in partial-thickness burns when the keratinocytes were engrafted over viable dermis. Storing large amounts of banked skin may provide us with vast quantities of expired skin that can be a source for dermis. In a series of experiments with nude mice and domestic pig models, we tried to evaluate the performance of fresh and old human dermis as the dermal substrate for cultured keratinocytes to reconstitute a whole skin.[20] These still ongoing experiments will hopefully produce some chimera of autologous and homologous definitive skin substitute.

Conclusion

Burns are a common form of injury among terrorist-attack victims. In the past decade, a gradual shift in the nature of terrorist attacks has occurred, and a larger proportion of attacks are performed by suicide bombing rather than random shooting. There is also a change in the nature of bombs. A new type of bomb is being used by the suicide bomber: standard military explosives in a belt or a back pack, with nails, bolts, small metal balls, and other fragments. These explosions result in a combination of penetrating, blast, blunt, and burn injuries.

The thermal component in terrorism-related trauma is more common compared to nonterrorism-related trauma.[21] This should serve as a guideline in the planning of future medical services wherever terrorist attacks might be expected. The number of patients with multidimensional burns, complicated by other injuries, is likely to increase. Burn care facilities and personnel should be prioritized accordingly.

References

1. Trauma Injuries in Israel 1998–2005, data from 10 trauma centers in Israel. The Israel National Center for Trauma and Emergency Medicine Research—Gertner Institute. Israel Center for Disease Control (ICDC)—Trauma Section, Ministry of Health; Apr 2007: 42–50.
2. Aharonson-Daniel L, Klein Y, Peleg K. Suicide bombers form a new injury profile. Ann Surg. 2006 Dec; 244(6): 1018–23.
3. Shamir MY, Rivkind A, Weissman C, Sprung CL, Weiss YG. Conventional terrorist bomb incidents and the intensive care unit. Curr Opin Crit Care. 2005 Dec; 11(6): 580–4.
4. Renz EM, Cancio LP, Barillo DJ, et al. Long range transport of war-related burn casualties. J Trauma. 2008 Feb; 64: 5136–145.
5. Almogy G, Luria T, richter T, et al. Can external signs of trauma guide management?: Lessons learned from suicide bombing attacks in Israel. Arch Surg. 2005 Apr; 140(4): 390–3.
6. Aschkenasy-Steuer G, Shamir M, Rivkind A, et al. Clinical review: the Israeli experience: conventional terrorism and critical care. Crit Care. 2005 Oct 5; 9(5): 490–9. Epub 2005 Jun 29.
7. Wolf DG, Polacheck I, Block C, et al. High rate of candidemia in patients sustaining injuries in a bomb blast at a marketplace: a possible environmental source. Clin Infect Dis. 2000 Sep; 31(3): 712–6. Epub 2000 Oct 4.
8. D'Avignon LC, Saffle JR, Chung KK, et al. Prevention and management of infections associated with burns in the combat casualty. J Trauma. 2008 Mar; 64: 5277–286.
9. Janzekovic Z. A new concept in the early excision and immediate grafting of burns. J Trauma. 1970 Dec; 10(12): 1103–8.
10. Heimbach D. Early burn excision and grafting. Surg Clin North Am. 1987 Feb; 67(1): 93–107.

11. Almogy G, Belzberg H, Mintz Y, Pikarsky AK, Zamir G, Rivkind AI. Suicide bombing attacks: update and modifications to the protocol. Ann Surg. 2004 Mar; 239(3): 295–303.

12. Eldad A, Ad-El D, Chaouat M, Ben Bassat H. Cryopreserved cadaveric allografts for treatment of unexcised partial thickness flame burns. Clinical experience with 12 patients. J Burn Care Rehabil. 1997; 18: S94.

13. Ad-El DD, Eldad A, Mintz Y, et al. Suicide bombing injuries: the Jerusalem experience of exceptional tissue damage posing a new challenge for the reconstructive surgeon. Plast Reconstr Surg. 2006 Aug; 118(2): 383–7; discussion 388–9.

14. Chim H, Yew WS, Song C. Managing burn victims of suicide bombing attacks: outcomes, lessons learnt, and changes made from three attacks in Indonesia. Crit Care. 2007; 11(1): R15.

15. Cinnamon U, Eldad A, Chaouat M, Wexler MR, Zagher U, Ben Bassat H. A simplified testing system to evaluate performance after transplantation of human skin preserved in glycerol or in liquid nitrogen. J Burn Care Rehabil. 1993; 14: 435–9.

16. Ben Bassat H, Strauss N, Ron M, et al. Transplantation performance of human skin cryopreserved by programmed or stepwise freezing and stored at −80 or −180. J Burn Care Rehabil. 1996; 17: 421–8.

17. Ben Bassat H, Chaouat M, Segal N, Zumai E, Wexler MR, Eldad A. How long can cryopreserved skin be stored to maintain adequate graft performance? Burns 2001; 27: 425–31.

18. Gallico GG, O'Connor NE, Compton CC, et al. Permanent coverage of large burn wounds with autologous cultured human epithelium. N Engl J Med. 1984; 311: 448.

19. Eldad A, Burt A, Clarke J. Cultured epithelium as a skin substitute. Burns 1987; 13: 173–80.

20. Ben Bassat H, Eldad A, Chaouat M, et al. Structural and functional evaluation of modifications in the composite skin graft: cryopreserved dermis and cultured keratinocytes. Plast Reconstr Surg. 1992; 89: 510–20.

21. Haik J, Tessona A, Givon A, et al. Terror-inflicted thermal injury: a retrospective analysis of burns in the Israeli-Palestinian conflict between the years 1997 and 2003. J Trauma. 2006 Dec; 61(6): 1501–5.

19
Neurosurgical Injury Related to Terror

Jeffrey V. Rosenfeld

The signature weapons of the terrorist are the improvized explosive device (IED) and suicide bomb blast which cause complex combinations of blast injury, multiple penetrating injuries, and burns to multiple casualties.[1,2] Mines, mortars, rocket propelled grenades, and bullets have also all been used in terrorist attacks.

The treatment of missile and blast injury to the head and spine has evolved during the wars of the twentieth century by military surgeons working in austere conditions and is currently being further refined by military neurosurgeons operating in the combat surgical hospitals of Iraq in Operation Iraqi Freedom and in Afghanistan.[3] The recommended treatment of these injuries is now directly applicable to the civilian setting where terrorist events are increasingly frequent but disparate events. Most civilian neurosurgeons have little knowledge or exposure to these horrific injuries. In this chapter, we aim to familiarize our civilian colleagues with these injuries and how to manage them. The pathology and management of gunshot injuries to the head and spine are well covered in the literature[4] and will not be reviewed in this chapter.

We should remember the pioneering work of Dr. Harvey Cushing in the First World War when the mortality of penetrating brain injury fell from 54.4% to 28.8% which astonishingly was in the pre-antibiotic and pre-diathermy era. Cushing brought neurosurgery close to the battle front, classified head injury and developed surgical techniques of craniectomy, debridement, and dural closure.[5] Osteoplastic craniotomy became standard practice in the Second World War and Sir Hugh Cairns developed mobile neurosurgical units ("Head Units") which were formed and trained in Oxford and provided small well-trained and well-equipped units which could deploy and supplement regular medical formations.[4]

Less-extensive surgical procedures were recommended for penetrating head wounds in the Israel Lebanon conflicts of 1982–1985. Brandvold et al. described early neurosurgery, less-aggressive debridement, leaving bone fragments in situ, intracranial pressure (ICP) monitoring, and the use of CT for military surgery.[6] Taha et al. described simple debridement for missile injuries.[7] Amirjamshidi et al. described minimal or no surgery in wartime head-injured patients with low- to moderate-velocity missile or shell fragment injury in Iran with good results.[8] This minimalist approach would not be suitable for the severe blast injuries being encountered in Iraq and after civilian bomb blast where more extensive procedures

S.C. Shapira et al. (eds.), *Essentials of Terror Medicine*,
DOI: 10.1007/978-0-387-09412-0_19, Springer Science+Business Media, LLC 2009

including craniectomy, extensive debridement, duroplasty, and skull base dural repair and ventriculostomy are frequently required.

Epidemiology

The head and neck are vulnerable in a bomb blast. In a postmortem study Gofrit et al. found 19.6% of shrapnel injuries were to the face, 6.6% were to the head, and 3.4% were to the neck.[9] In terror-related injuries secondary fragments injured the face in 49.5% cases, the head in 33.7% cases, and the neck in 13% cases.[10] Following the terrorist bombing in Madrid in 2004, 52% of victims sustained head trauma.[11] Suicide bombings in Israel resulted in the head being the most common site of penetrating injury in survivors.[12] Wearing a Kevlar helmet, body armor with neck extension, and industrial eye goggles offers some protection. However, in US military hospitals in Iraq, 65/127 (51%) blast, gunshot wounds (GSW), and fragmentation injuries involved the head and neck, and 64% of projectile deaths involve head or neck, with exposed parts of the head and neck of some soldiers being a target of snipers.

Pathology of Blast Injury to the Head, Neck, and Spine

The effects of bomb blast injury to the head vary widely in severity and may result in burns, concussion, brain contusions, petechial hemorrhages, subdural hematoma, intracerebral hematoma, intraventricular hemorrhage, subarachnoid hemorrhage (SAH), brain swelling, raised ICP, and penetration of metal and bone fragments into the brain.

Reducing the neurological, cognitive, behavioural, and psychological sequelae of blast brain injury is a high priority in military health care, and it is therefore important to understand the pathophysiology of blast injury to the brain. The exact mechanism of structural brain injury due to blast is unknown. It is tempting to assume that it is due to the effects of the overpressure wave, but other components of the blast such as acoustic energy and electromagnetic radiation may also be contributors and this is the subject of intense study at present. There are the direct effects of the blast on the brain, and there also is experimental evidence that a thoracic or extremity blast injury causes secondary oscillating high-frequency shock waves to the brain and spinal cord which may cause chromatolysis of neurons, an increase in microglia, shrinkage of axoplasm, SAH, and multiple petechial hemorrhages.[13] Whole-body and local chest blast exposure of rats results in ultrastructural and biochemical changes in the hippocampus, and causes cognitive deficit,[14] and at a cellular level blast causes free-radical–mediated oxidative stress which contributes to blast injury.[15] There may be a short period of apnea accompanied by bradycardia and hypotension immediately following the blast which is postulated to be due to a blast wave effect on the brain stem,[16] or to a vago-sympathetic reflex activated from the chest.[17,18]

Pulmonary blast injury may also result in alveolar-venous fistulae and air embolism which contributes to the brain injury. This has been rarely observed in humans probably because of its transient course.[13] The true incidence of air embolism following blast and its contribution to blast brain injury is unknown.[19]

The size and velocity of debris and fragments vary considerably following a bomb explosion. The bomb may contain metal fragments of varying size including ball bearings, nails, bolts, and other metal objects which can cause devastating penetrating injuries. Secondary fragments of dirt, gravel, glass, wood, fragments of clothing, skin and hair, and tissue from other victims may also enter the wounds so that all wounds following bomb blast must be regarded as contaminated. Penetrating metallic fragment injury varies widely in severity but cannot be assumed to be low velocity and benign. The distance of the victim from the blast as well as the magnitude of the blast and whether it occurs in a confined space are all critical factors. The typical fragment injuries following bomb blast have a small entry wound with gross internal damage due to pressure wave vacuum cavitation effect, devitalized tissue, and gross contamination.

Blast injury to the head is often accompanied by cervical, facial, skull base, and intracranial vascular injuries with trajectories of bomb fragments passing anteriorly up through the face, orbits, and sinuses and laterally and posteriorly through the neck to pierce the skull base and the brain. The skull base fractures and penetrations will cause cerebrospinal fluid (CSF) leak which will increase the risk of infection. The pharynx, larynx, and esophagus may be injured by penetration through the neck. The mandible, tongue, palate, orbits and eyes, maxilla, teeth, nasopharynx, and paranasal sinuses may be injured in facial penetrations.

The brain swelling which follows bomb blast and diffuse axonal injury is due to combinations of cerebral edema and vascular engorgement and often occurs in the first few hours following the blast but may also be delayed 24 hours or even several days after the injury justifying an early craniectomy at the first point of neurosurgery particularly if there are long evacuation distances to more definitive care (Fig. 19.1).

The extracranial and intracranial vascular injury includes carotid and vertebral artery dissection, rupture, and thrombosis to late pseudoaneurysm formation. Intracranial vasospasm is an under-recognized problem in patients with bomb blast injury to the head. Armonda et al. described 47.4% of patients had traumatic vasospasm of 57 patients with traumatic brain injury most of whom had bomb blast injury.[20] The onset was at 24–48 hours postinjury by transcranial Doppler (TCD) and the duration was an average of 14.3 days with a range up to 30 days. The commonest vessel to be affected was the supraclinoid internal carotid artery followed in descending order by the middle cerebral artery, anterior cerebral artery, basilar artery, and the vertebral artery. The presence of SAH, Glasgow Coma Scale score (GCS) < 8, pseudoaneurysm, and the number of lobes injured were associated with vasospasm. The early outcome was worse in those with traumatic cerebral vasospasm (TCV).[20]

The blast commonly injures the eyes and ruptures the tympanic membranes.[1] The ear is extremely vulnerable to blast injury and almost all victims of blast have some degree of ear injury.[19] Rupture of the ear drum is common and results in deafness,

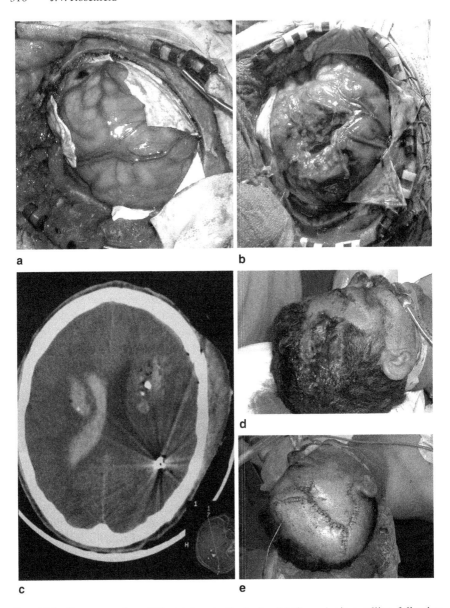

FIG. 19.1. Four examples of blast injury to the brain: (a) Gross brain swelling following blast injury. Note the engorgement of the cerebral vessels. (b) Penetrating injury to the fronto-parietal region with gross surrounding brain swelling and vascular engorgement. (c) Axial CT scan showing a typical blast injury with multiple metal fragments and a scattered intracerebral and intraventricular hemorrhage, brain swelling, and mild ventricular dilatation. (d) Tangential blast wound. (e) Following primary repair of tangential blast wound with craniectomy, extensive debridement of lacerated cortex, primary scalp closure, and insertion of ventriculostomy drain. (b) From Rosenfeld, JV,[3] Reprinted with permission from Elsevier.

tinnitus, and vertigo. Dislocation of the ossicles and damage to the cochlea may also occur and cause permanent hearing loss.[21] The eyes are vulnerable in a blast if not protected. Conjunctival hemorrhage is the most common sign of eye injury.[19] More severe eye injuries occur in up to 28% of blast injury survivors including ruptured globe and hyphema.[1] Air emboli can sometimes be seen in retinal vessels.[19]

Bomb blast injury to the spine results in penetrating wounds which may traverse the spine and cause spinal fractures and injury to nerve roots and the spinal cord ranging from spinal cord concussion and neuropraxia to spinal cord transection and complete division of nerve roots (axonotmesis). CSF leak and secondary CNS infection may result. The fractures are classified the same way as blunt injuries and the surgeon will need to decide if the fracture is stable or unstable. The trajectory of the fragments may also pass through the neck, chest, abdomen, pelvis, or perineum to reach or traverse the spine adding further complexity to these injuries. For instance, a fragment passing through the perineum may perforate the rectum and pass into the sacral spinal canal injuring sacral nerve roots and causing a recto-spinal fistula with fecal contamination of the spine. Metallic or other foreign bodies and bone fragments from comminuted fractures may be lodged in the spinal canal or nerve root foramina causing compressive injury to the spinal cord and nerve roots. Blunt injury to the spine including fracture/dislocations may also occur when the victim is thrown against a fixed object by the force of the blast, where they are struck by falling objects or where there is a deceleration injury with torsion, hyper-flexion, or hyperextension injury.

Bomb blast injury has been divided into four components[1] which can be applied specifically to the head, neck, and spine to delineate the clinical patterns of blast injury (Table 19.1).

Principles of Management of Blast Injury to the Head and Neck

Pre-Hospital Management

The resuscitation and early management of the bomb blast victim follows the principles of Advanced Trauma Life Support (ATLS) and is covered elsewhere in this text. The acute management of head trauma has been covered in more detail in evidence-based guidelines published by the Brain Trauma Foundation.[22] Although these are specifically written for conventional domestic head trauma, they also pertain to the treatment of casualties received following a terrorist bomb blast event in civilian settings.

In-hospital Management

Coordination of the flow of casualties is a critical element of successful mass casualty management. Following a mass casualty event the duties of the Incident Commander, Operations chief, and Disaster Control Officer include having knowledge of the current resources available in the hospital, triage of the casualties, and coordination of the cases for the operating rooms. A senior trauma surgeon is

TABLE 19.1. Clinical Patterns of Blast Injury to the Head, Neck, and Spine

Primary blast injury

Concussion – diffuse axonal injury (DAI) ranging from mild to severe
Intracranial hemorrhage – petechial, intracerebral, intraventricular, subdural, epidural
Early brain swelling with hyperemia and or edema → intracranial hypertension
Delayed brain swelling > 24–48 hours
Subarachnoid hemorrhage (SAH) and secondary vasospasm
Air embolism following pulmonary blast injury
Ear injury – eardrum, ossicles, cochlea

Secondary blast injury

Penetrating trauma – compound skull fractures
Depressed fractures with brain injury
Fragmentation injuries: multiple metal and bone fragments in the brain, face, neck with dirt, gravel,
    hair contamination.
Variable velocity of fragments
Skull base fractures with CSF leak
Intracranial vascular injury: rupture, dissection, thrombosis, pseudo-aneurysm
Severe hemorrhage from cervical and facial vascular injury
Pharyngo-laryngeal injury
Esophageal injury
Orbit and ocular injury
Facial/mandibular fractures
Penetrating spine injury with spinal fractures and nerve root and spinal cord injury

Tertiary blast effect

Victims thrown against fixed objects causing traumatic brain and spine injury
Structural collapse of buildings and vehicles causing crush and entrapment injuries
Penetrating injuries due to exploding objects and buildings with glass, metallic, wood, and cement
    foreign bodies
Coup and contrecoup TBI
Spine fracture/dislocation

Quarternary blast effect

Burns – chemical and thermal to skin and respiratory tract
Toxic inhalation
Asphyxiation (carbon monoxide, cyanide)
Radiation
Napalm in incendiary bombs

involved in making decisions on the priority of cases for surgery. It may be appropriate to undertake simultaneous surgery to different regions of the same patient, for example, craniotomy and laparotomy or limb exploration and control of vascular injury. The timing and extent of the neurosurgery must be balanced against the relative priorities of the other injuries and the state of physiological stabilization of a patient. The neurosurgeon needs to give timely and clear advice to the chief trauma surgeon about the relative urgency and likely prognosis of brain and craniofacial injuries so that the patients can receive urgent treatment or perhaps be triaged to nonoperative supportive or palliative care.

Damage Control Neurosurgery

The neurosurgical strategies should embrace the principles of damage control surgery which is now standard practice for the initial care of severely injured patients with polytrauma. The priority is vigorous replacement of blood loss and correction of hypothermia and acidosis which cause coagulopathy and a higher mortality if not corrected. Correction of coagulopathy is of vital importance in being able to undertake effective neurosurgery. Coagulopathy is defined as elevated International Normalized Ratio (INR > 1.3) or partial thromboplastin time (PTT) greater than 34 seconds. Clinical or laboratory evidence of coagulopathy should be treated urgently with clotting factors including fresh frozen plasma, platelets, and blood transfusion. The administration of Recombinant Factor VIIa (rFVIIa) is currently under investigation in patients with severe trauma including severe brain injury and coagulopathy. The optimal indications, timing, and dosage are yet to be defined. We should await further published data before rFVIIa can be recommended as a routine treatment. Damage control neurosurgery includes rapidly executed neurosurgery to stop major bleeding, evacuate hematomas, decompress the brain with craniectomy flaps, obtain a watertight dural closure, and insert an ICP monitor.[23] Prolonged micro-neurosurgical procedures including plastic reconstructive flaps should not be undertaken in the initial surgery. Returns to theatre for secondary and tertiary procedures including reconstructions are preferable. The neurosurgeon should work closely with ENT, faciomaxillary surgeons, and ophthalmologists where there is craniofacial and cervical trauma and decide on the priority and timing of management of these injuries. The conjoint team approach to managing these complex injuries rather than disjointed sequential management by different specialists cannot be overemphasized.

Go to CT or OR?

One of the early and important decision nodes is whether the patient should go to CT scan or straight to the operating room. Unless the patient is bleeding uncontrollably, has urgent torso injury, or needs urgent tracheostomy, a CT scan should be obtained prior to surgery especially if there is penetrating head and neck trauma. The CT scan of blast injury may show brain swelling similar to a diffuse axonal injury with loss of gray white differentiation, petechial hemorrhages, effacement of the subarachnoid space and basal cisterns and small ventricles often with midline shift if there is focal pathology. Orbital and faciomaxillary blast injuries are also assessed on CT. The location of metal and bone fragments will also be seen on CT. The neurosurgeon and other members of the head and neck team will depend on the CT to plan the type and extent of surgery required. CT angiography is indicated when cervical vascular injury is suspected and is much quicker than taking the patient to an angiography suite for digital subtraction angiography (Fig. 19.2).

Operative or Nonoperative Care?

Patients are often sedated and intubated and no relatives are available to obtain consent, and perhaps the patient cannot be assessed neurologically. There is often pessimism about the prognosis in patients with GSW to the brain and a low GCS,[4] but we have found the prognosis for brain injury following blast is better than comparable penetrating GSW and the degree of damage to the brain caused by penetrating fragments is not as predictable as it is for bullets and may be less in many cases because

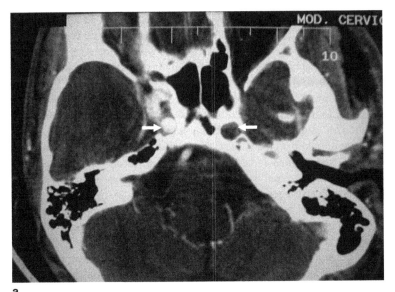

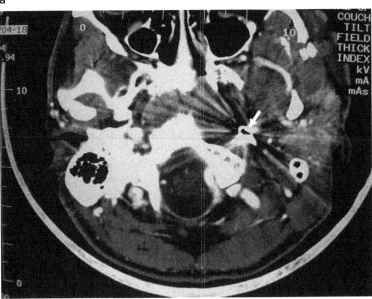

Fig. 19.2. CT angiography to investigate carotid artery injury. (a) Axial CT of the cranio-cervical junction showing a metal fragment in the vicinity of the left internal carotid artery. (b) Axial CT with contrast, that is, CT angiogram showing lack of filling of the left internal carotid in the carotid cannel and normal enhancement of the right internal carotid artery in the carotid cannel and the cavernous sinus.

of lower energies imparted to the brain than bullets. We therefore recommend exploration of penetrating brain injury caused by blast except where the prognosis is clearly hopeless to the neurosurgeon. We generally have found that families desire operative intervention to be performed if there is a chance of a recovery. Fixed dilated pupils may not necessarily indicate a hopeless prognosis in patients with blast injury to the head and who are in shock. These patients should be resuscitated and assessed in relation to all their injuries and the CT appearance of their brain injury. Orbital and ocular trauma may cause mydriasis. Profound shock due to severe chest injury may be associated with low GCS and dilated pupils and be reversible.[24] Information on the pre-intubation GCS can be helpful in making this decision. If the patient has had a GCS of 3 since the injury, has developed fixed and dilated pupils, and has a CT scan showing severe brain injury then there is no chance of survival and the treatment should be expectant (Table 19.2).

The Surgery

Complex airway problems are common with craniofacial and cervical blast injury and early securing of the airway is essential. Orofacial swelling is often rapid and is compounded by facial and airway burns. There should be a low index for early tracheostomy. This is often done as the first procedure for those with craniofacial trauma. Early nasal packing can be used to control epistaxis (Fig. 19.3).

TABLE 19.2. Principles of Management of Craniofacial Blast Injury

Low index for early tracheostomy
Vigorous replacement of blood loss and correction of coagulopathy
Nasal packing
Neck exploration and management of carotid artery injury
Broad spectrum antibiotics
Close an open eye injury within 24 hours
Enucleate a destroyed globe within 14 days to avoid sympathetic ophthalmia
General principles of surgical management of severe blast TBI
CT is essential for planning the extent of the neurosurgery
CT angiography is useful when cervical vascular injury is suspected
The timing and extent of the neurosurgery must be balanced against the relative priorities of the other injuries and the state of physiological stabilization.
Early wide decompressive craniectomy for GCS < 9, brain swelling on CT, deep or multiple penetrations, multiple lobe involvement, diffuse hemorrhage
Evacuate intracranial hematomas
Washout and debride brain wound
Remove accessible in-driven bone and metal fragments
Consider lobectomy (us. temporal and frontal) esp. if brain stem compression
Watertight dural closure ± Duroplasty
Dural repair of the skull base
± Scalp advancement in burns
Ventriculostomy and CSF drainage
Place bone in subcutaneous abdominal pocket
Monitor for vasospasm and treat with angioplasty or topical intra-arterial nicardipine, papaverine

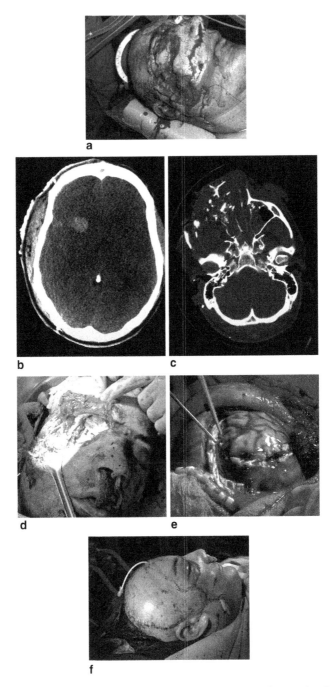

Fig. 19.3. Severe blast injury to the face and cranial cavity. (a) Penetrating injury to the right maxilla, orbit, anterior cranial fossa, and brain. (b) Axial CT image with brain windows showing cerebral swelling with effacement of subarachnoid space, general hypodensity within the cerebral hemispheres, a small intracerebral hemorrhage, and a small metal

A generous decompressive craniectomy is performed for those with GCS < 9, brain swelling on CT, deep or multiple penetrations, multiple lobe involvement, or intracranial hematomas. This is usually a large unilateral fronto-temporo-parietal flap to the side with the predominant pathology. If there is diffuse frontal lobe pathology a bifronto-temporal flap can be raised. A bilateral craniectomy is required with two separate flaps is required for bilateral hematomas. Small craniectomies are ineffective for reducing ICP when extensive brain swelling is present.

The dura is opened widely, epidural and subdural hematomas are evacuated, and active hemorrhage stopped by coagulation of bleeding vessels and tamponade using Surgicel and Gelfoam. Large intracerebral hematomas are evacuated and if associated with penetrating fragments, these are also removed. Bleeding from the venous sinuses or cavernous sinus is technically challenging to control and may require tamponade with a segment of crushed muscle and direct pressure in some circumstances but further details are beyond the scope of this chapter. If the brain is congested, swollen, and tight and there is evidence of upper brain stem compression with a dilated pupil, the surgeon should consider temporal lobectomy and resection of the uncus. Lobectomy may also be indicated if there is extensive damage with devitalized cerebral tissue, fragment penetration, and hemorrhage in that lobe. Intravenous mannitol (0.5–1 g/kg) can be helpful intra-operatively in order to reduce cerebral swelling provided the patient has been adequately resuscitated.

The degree of debridement is controversial but we favor a more aggressive approach in bomb blast injury.[2,3] These penetrating wounds often damage the brain extensively and are heavily contaminated and minimal superficial debridement would not be adequate to treat the injury or decompress the brain. Accessible in-driven bone fragments and metallic and other foreign bodies are removed, devitalized cerebral tissue debrided, and the resultant cavity irrigated with Ringer's or equivalent solution. Deeper fragments are not pursued because the chance of cerebral injury and neurological deficit outweighs the advantage of foreign body removal at the initial surgery. The decision as to what extent to pursue fragments depends on the judgement and experience of the neurosurgeon, and the duration of the procedure must also be considered to conform to damage control principles. There is no correlation between the presence of retained fragments and the subsequent development of epilepsy and infection.[6,25] Bone fragments have a greater chance of causing late infection than metallic fragments and scalp wound dehiscence greatly increases the chance of intracranial infection.[26]

---

fragment near the midline posteriorly. (c) Axial CT image with bone windows showing gross destruction of facial skeleton. (d) Orbital exenteration and packing of the orbit with Vaseline gauze. Debridement of the maxillary wound. (e) Swollen engorged right frontal lobe with a frontal lobectomy proceeding. (f) Postcraniectomy and repair of the anterior cranial fossa floor using pericranium, the facial lacerations, right orbital exenteration and packing, insertion of ventriculostomy drain, and nasal packing. Note the Penrose drain from the maxillary wound.

More targeted local surgery may be sufficient for a focal injury such as a depressed fracture or isolated epidural hematoma. A ventriculostomy is placed if there is a severe brain injury (GCS < 9) and/or the patient will remain sedated and intubated postoperatively. The ventriculostomy will allow for CSF drainage and help control the ICP in the intensive care unit. Intraparenchymal ICP monitors such as Camino[R] or Codman[R] can be inserted as an alternative to ventriculostomy but the therapeutic advantage of CSF drainage is lost. The intraparenchymal ICP monitor can also be inserted in addition to the ventriculostomy. Intradural suction drains are not usually necessary or desirable. Subgaleal drains may be used if the dura is closed.

The dura is closed watertight to avoid CSF leak and secondary infection. Duroplasty using pericranium or temporalis fascia may be used to close dural defects and also serves the purpose of accommodating a swollen brain beneath. Commercial dural substitutes are avoided if there is heavy contamination. Tissue glues are helpful to secure a watertight closure. Skull base defects should be identified and repaired if technically feasible at the first procedure to prevent postoperative CSF leaks. This can be achieved with a pericranial flap for the anterior cranial fossa and temporalis fascia for the temporal bone in the middle cranial fossa and the use of tissue glue. A compound fracture of the frontal sinus may require exenteration of the sinus. The risks to the patient of minimal debridement and nonwatertight dural closure are much greater compared with a watertight dural closure.[27] The bone flaps are not replaced because of the possibility of worsening brain swelling or inability to close the scalp. The bone flaps may be placed in a subcutaneous abdominal pocket or stored in a $-70\,^{\circ}$C freezer for later cranioplasty. Contaminated pieces of skull are discarded (Fig. 19.4).

Initial scalp closure over the injured area should be the goal of the initial surgery. Dura and bone should not remain exposed in the injured area. Extensive scalp loss due to blast injury or scalp burns is not uncommon and may render it difficult or impossible to close the scalp primarily. Scalp advancement or rotation flaps may be required to cover the primary wound area in the first operation. The secondary defects created in the uninjured areas of scalp can be grafted at later procedures. The exposed skull covered with pericranium in these secondary defects can be initially covered with moist dressings.

As distinct from stab wounds to the neck, penetrating neck injuries require exploration for adequate debridement and assessment of the internal injuries. Certain intracranial and cervical vascular injuries such as dissections and carotid-cavernous fistulas may require neuroradiological endovascular therapy.

An intravenous phenytoin loading dose is administered to prevent seizures and this is continued postoperatively for 1 week. There is no evidence that anticonvulsants beyond this period prevent late onset of seizures.[28]

Prophylactic Antibiotics

Guidelines for antibiotic prophylaxis for penetrating brain injury have been published.[29,30] Blast wounds must be regarded as heavily contaminated and should be assumed to contain organic material such as soil and plant matter so that a broad

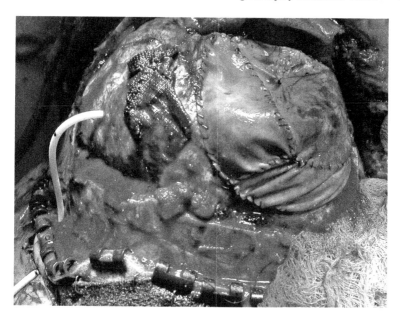

FIG. 19.4. Extensive surgery for blast injury showing extensive bi-fronto-temporal craniectomy, partial right frontal lobectomy, duroplasty, and insertion of left ventriculostomy drain.

cover of antibiotics should be used including Gram positive and negative bacteria and anerobes, for example, cephazolin or flucloxacillin, gentamycin, and metronidazole or timentin alone. These are continued postoperatively for 7 days. In infected cases unusual bacteria such as Acinetobacter may be isolated and are often resistant to standard antibiotics. Fungi may also be a cause of infection.

Treatment for Traumatic Cerebral Vasospasm and Intracranial Vascular Injury

Cerebral vasospasm is detected by regular TCD examinations and cerebral angiography is indicated if TCD is positive for vasospasm. Cerebral angiography is also indicated in blast or penetrating injury patients with intracerebral hemorrhage, or a traversing fragment or where there is new unexplained neurological deficit (Table 19.3). Balloon angioplasty may be indicated for vessels in spasm. Intra-arterial nicardipine or papaverine may also be used but tend to be shorter in duration of effect than balloon angioplasty.[20] The outcome of this therapy following blast injury is uncertain and still under investigation but aggressive surgical and endovascular treatment strategies may improve outcome.[20] Angioplasty with microballoon significantly lowers middle cerebral artery and basilar flow velocities. However, clinical outcomes are worse for those with traumatic vasospasm.[20] There is not sufficient

TABLE 19.3. Indications for Diagnostic Angiography in Blast and Penetrating Injury to the Head

Penetrating injury (pterional, transorbital, posterior fossa)
Known cerebral vessel injury (e.g., seen at operation)
CT evidence of traumatic subarachnoid hemorrhage
TCD evidence of vasospasm
Blast injury with presenting GCS < 8
Known surgically treated traumatic aneurysm
Spontaneous decrease in partial pressure brain tissue O_2 or CBF
Lack of improvement in GCS without explanation

CT computed tomography, GCS Glasgow Coma Scale score, TCD transcranial Doppler, O_2 oxygen, CBF cerebral blood flow.

evidence that "HHH" (hypertension, hypervolemia, hemodilution) therapy, or intravenous or oral nimodipine improve outcome in posttraumatic vasospasm and therefore they are not recommended.[31] The operative clipping or interventional coiling of psedoaneurysms may be indicated.

Ocular Trauma

Of all patients (including military personnel and civilians) treated in the 332nd Expeditionary Group US Airforce Field Hospital in Balad, Iraq in 2004, 16% had ocular trauma and 40.6% of these had an open globe injury. The emergency care of eye injuries includes the application of a clean dressing without pressure. Patients with blast injury occurring in a remote location should reach an eye surgeon <18 hours after the injury and an open globe should be closed within 24 hours. Lateral canthotomy is a simple bedside procedure to relieve tension on the globe when there is gross swelling of the lids and orbit. Deep anesthesia is required for the repair so that the intraocular pressure remains controlled. An enucleation should be performed within 14 days to avoid sympathetic ophthalmia. The details of the repair of penetrating eye injuries are beyond the scope of this chapter.

Postoperative Intensive Care

Intensive care management should follow the Brain Trauma Foundation Guidelines which have recently been revised.[28] Brain PO_2 monitoring and cerebral blood flow (CBF) monitoring are available in more advanced settings and may be helpful for the ongoing management of the patient with severe brain injury.

Air Transportation of the Blast Injury Victim

The details of aero-medical evacuation have been outlined.[32] The patient is intubated if GCS < 12. An intraventricular catheter is inserted if the GCS < 8T. The management of raised ICP in an aircraft is difficult, and it is preferable to have the pressure controlled before the journey, that is, the neurosurgical management should be optimized before the journey. Hematomas of significance should be evacuated and a decompressive craniectomy helps to lower the ICP and maintain it for the journey. The medical management of ICP in flight is limited to the use of head of bed elevation, increased sedation, thiopental, ventricular drainage, and temporary mild hyperventilation. Loading the patient head-of-bed first limits the effects of takeoff on ICP. If there is intracranial air or the air in the eye, the aircraft would need to fly at low altitude to avoid expansion of the air with tension.

Late Reconstruction

Bone flaps removed from bomb blast victims with penetrating injury to that part of the skull placed in the abdominal wall have a high risk of subsequent infection when replaced in the cranial defect. The option used for the injured soldiers from Iraq is to construct an acrylic replica of the defect based on the CT reconstructions. The neurosurgeon should place multiple holes the cranial flap for drainage. Complex reconstruction with free vascularized skin flaps may be required for larger areas of scalp loss. Ocular prostheses will need to be fitted following eye removal and further nasal, plastics, faciomaxillary, orthodontic, and prosthodontic procedures are required following penetrating facial injury.

Large scalp defects and damaged scalp from burns are not uncommon problems requiring late reconstruction. Balloon expansion of the scalp similar to what is done in the pediatric population can be used successfully to gain more length in the scalp when it is advanced into the defect.[33]

Minor Traumatic Brain Injury and Concussion Following Bomb Blast

Cognitive, behavioural, neurological, and psychiatric disorders are common after moderate and severe blast and penetrating brain injury, and there have been many US troops evacuated from Iraq with these problems who will require long-term rehabilitation and therapy following these injuries.[34] The symptoms of mild traumatic brain injury (TBI) may also occur when the main impact of the blast is distant from the head. A study of patients with blast injury to the lower extremities found that 51% (665/1303) had neurological symptoms consistent with TBI. Of these, 36% had electroencephalographic (EEG) abnormalities during the acute stage and both the EEG and neurological abnormalities became chronic in 30% of this group.[35]

The neuropsychiatric impairment after bomb blast seems to be similar to that reported after other trauma such as accidents and assaults.[36] Postconcussion symptoms increase in frequency after multiple exposures to blast and include headache, vertigo and balance problems, poor memory, inability to concentrate, irritability, excessive fatigue, sleep disturbance, tinnitus, and blurred vision. These patients require a full neuropsychological assessment. The Defense and Veterans Brain Injury Center (DVBIC) in the USA is working collaboratively to provide and improve TBI care for defense members and veterans.[37] This Center has developed a Military Acute Concussion Evaluation (MACE) which would also be applicable in a civilian setting. It consists of a structured history, examination, and diagnosis and a score is obtained. The evaluation can be repeated to assess clinical progress. This Evaluation is not yet fully validated but is proving useful in the military setting. It was derived from the standard assessment of concussion (SAC), a widely used tool in sports medicine.[38] MR imaging has an increasing role in the assessment and prognostication of TBI patients. The MR is usually performed 1 week postinjury when the patient is stable and the numbers of casualties permit access.

The postconcussion syndrome is well recognized.[39] Mild postconcussional symptoms will usually resolve over a few months. Rest, gradual return to normal activities, avoidance of alcohol and drugs, avoidance of contact sport and recreational sport that may lead to a further concussion, relaxation techniques for irritability, are all sensible strategies to improve the rate and completeness of recovery. Guidelines for the pharmacological treatment of neurobehavioral sequelae of TBI have been recently published.[40] There may be overlap of postconcussional symptoms with posttraumatic stress disorder (PTSD) and psychological and psychiatric evaluation will be required to distinguish the relative contribution of each. Hoge et al. recently surveyed 2,525 US Army infantry soldiers 3–4 months after their return from a year-long deployment in Iraq and reported that mild TBI (i.e., loss of consciousness and concussion) was strongly associated with PTSD and physical health and that PTSD and depression are important mediators of the relationship between mild TBI and physical health problems.[41] This may also apply to civilians with mild TBI following terrorist bombings. Psychological factors account for many postconcussive symptoms.[42]

The Outcome of Blast Injury to the Brain

The detailed outcome data of severe blast injury to the brain have not yet been reported in the civilians injured in terrorist bomb blasts or in injured military personnel from Iraq or Afghanistan. Some idea of outcome can be obtained from reviewing the outcome of military and civilian GSW. Of the penetrating head injuries in Vietnam, 20% of soldiers had very severe wounds and died without surgery soon after admission. The other 80% had surgery with a mortality of 10% and most returned to productive lives. The incidence of epilepsy was 51% at 15 years postinjury.[43] The survival of civilians with GSW is GCS 3–5: 8.1%, GCS 6–8: 35.6%, GCS 9–15: 90.5%. The incidence of epilepsy is 1.3–24%.[4]

A preliminary report of 433 injured military personnel from Iraq and Afghanistan treated at Walter Reed Army Medical Center between January 03 and April 05 gives an indication of the overall impact of neurotrauma from this hostile environment. Sixty-eight percent of injuries were due to blast and 88.5% of these patients had closed TBI. Seventy-nine percent had loss of consciousness <1 hours and 79% had posttraumatic amnesia of <24 h. Twenty-five percent had a skull fracture, 18.7% had a subdural hematoma, and 1.5% had an epidural hematoma. The mortality after reaching Walter Reed Medical Center was 0.29%. Six percent had seizures. Ninety-one percent reported postconcussive symptoms with headache (47%), memory deficits (46%), irritability/aggression (45%), and attention/concentration difficulties (41%) and of 43% with a psychiatric disorder noted, depression was the most common (27%).[44]

Decompressive craniectomy has potential serious morbidity with which the neurosurgeon should be familiar. Aarabi et al. reported hydrocephalus (10%), ipsilateral, hemorrhagic swelling (16%), and subdural hygroma (50%).[45] The incidence of infection ranges from 2% to 20% requiring removal of bone flap (3–15%), 3% to 15% with meningitis/encephalitis, and 9–29% hydrocephalus requiring ventriculo-peritoneal shunt.[46] Metal fragments in the brain may rarely migrate over the long term.

The mortality of injured US soldiers reaching hospital has progressively improved from 30% in Second World War, to 24% in Vietnam and the Persian Gulf War 1990–1991, to 10% in Iraq and Afghanistan.[47] This is due to a combination of factors including improved resuscitation and stabilization in the pre-hospital phase, head and neck teams performing early surgery using damage control techniques including neurosurgery, advances in intensive care, aggressive control of ICP, and rapid evacuation to specialist facilities. All these factors are directly transferable to the civilian health sector and are important to include in disaster plans.

Penetrating Spine Injury

The intraspinal neural structures may be injured by missile penetration or cavitational/concussional effects of penetration close to the spine, and indirectly as a result of fractures and dislocations. Bony fragments from the spine may also lodge in the spinal canal or neural foramina and cause neural injury. The two types of clinical presentation are immediate and complete sensori-motor loss or incomplete or nonprogressive neurological deficit. The first group has a poor prognosis for neurological recovery and a much better prognosis for the second group.[48] CT and MR have an important role in the diagnosis of penetrating spinal injury.

Damage control techniques can be used for penetrating spine injury.[49] Maintaining an adequate mean arterial blood pressure and oxygenation are vital for any patient with spinal cord injury. The strategies for the surgery include initial vigorous debridement of the associated missile wounds. More urgent attention may need to be applied to the contiguous injuries to the adjacent body cavities and viscera. Hammoud et al. has reported a series of 64 patients injured by bullets and shell fragments, and there was no significant advantage in performing laminectomy for patients with complete and partial (fixed and stable) deficit groups.[48] This remains controversial and will depend on the nature of the wound and how this is managed. Decompressive laminectomy is definitely indicated for the small group with progressive neurological deficit and laminectomy is required for CSF fistula. Removal of metallic fragments from the spine is not necessary unless this is part of a decompression procedure. It should be noted that retained metal fragments may rarely migrate in the spinal canal.

The usual approach to the decompression of the spine is dorsal via laminectomy but alternative approaches such as costotransversectomy or trans-thoracic and retroperitoneal approaches may be required depending on the wounding pattern. Neural structures are decompressed by removal of in-driven bone fragments and metallic and other foreign bodies. The spinal cord is manipulated as little as possible to avoid compounding the injury. Dural closure should be attempted and use of fascial graft and tissue glue are helpful. Internal fixation may be used for unstable fracture dislocations but there needs to be vigorous debridement of all contaminated and devitalized tissue. Shattered vertebrae may require vertebrectomy and reconstruction with a cage, plate, and screws in addition to a posterior fixation. The timing of this more extensive surgery will depend on the other clinical priorities. A vacuum dressing may be used if there is no CSF leak. The wounds are packed with regular changes of dressing as an alternative. These penetrating wounds should not be closed primarily. Broad spectrum antibiotics are administered as for the penetrating brain injury (Fig. 19.5).

Application of skull callipers and skeletal traction may be indicated for unstable cervical fractures until internal fixation is available and the wounds are clean. The administration of methyl prednisolone to patients with penetrating spinal missile injuries does not significantly improve functional outcome.[50,51] This probably applies to blast injury to the spine as well as GSW but there is no published evidence available.

Rehabilitation

Prolonged periods of intensive rehabilitation are required for the victims of bomb blast. The rehabilitation program is often disrupted because these patients are also often returning to the operating room multiple times for revisional surgery especially if they have burns. Severe TBI due to bomb blast frequently results in cognitive deficits affecting memory, concentration, attention, speed of processing, and other domains. Chronic epilepsy, personality change, neurological deficits, and wound healing and plastic reconstruction issues are also frequently encountered. Chronic infection may add further challenge. Psychiatric disorders including depression and PTSD are common and psychosocial issues including family breakdown requiring intervention from social workers, psychologists, and psychiatrists. The aftermath of mild to moderate blast TBI may also have profound effects on cognitive function, mood, and personality and require ongoing support from psychologists, psychiatrists, and social workers.

Bomb blast victims also often have multiple other injuries including amputations with other specific rehabilitation needs. Difficult decisions will have to be made about

---

→

Skin marking in the midline for the laminectomy site. (b) A–P X-ray showing a large metallic foreign body at the level of T12/L1. (c) Lateral X-ray showing the fragment to be within the spinal canal. (d) Laminectomy performed revealing metal fragment impacted in the spinal canal with transsection of the cauda equina and adjacent roots of the cauda equina. (e) The foreign body removed. (f) Postremoval of the metal fragment showing transsected lower conus and severed roots of the cauda equina. The patient remained paraplegic following this injury.

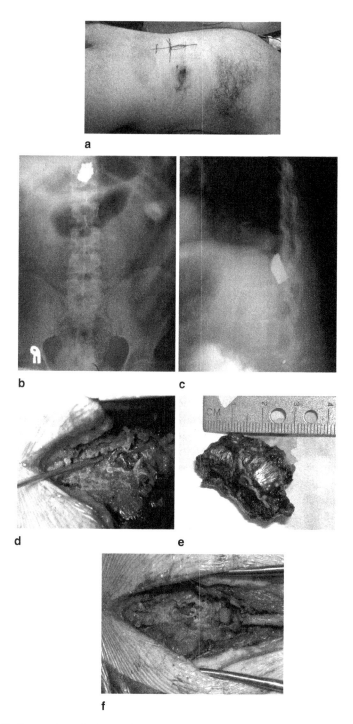

Fig. 19.5. Penetrating spinal wound. (a) Patient lying prone on the operating table. Ragged entry wound in the right flank. Note the surrounding skin contusions. (*continued on the opposite page*)

the future employability of the victim. Patients with retained metal fragments in the brain or spine may require long-term monitoring of serum lead levels.

Future Research

There is a strong need for ongoing research to better understand the pathophysiology and optimal treatment of blast injuries to the head and spine. Some of the specific areas that need further investigation include: the elucidation of the mechanisms of brain injury and correlation with the imaging, pathology, and outcome; a detailed audit of the early treatment of blast injuries to the head and spine and correlation with outcome; better definition of the indications for craniectomy, quality of life, and outcome analysis including neuropsychology and psychosocial adjustment; the incidence and outcome of brain abscess/meningitis, the prevention of infection by Acinetobacter and other resistant organisms; the incidence and outcome of early and late epilepsy and how it can be better prevented; a controlled clinical trial of treatment for TCV and to further develop simple screening tools for mild blast TBI; and evaluation of the management and outcomes.

Conclusion

War has always provided an impetus to advance the practice of medicine. This is no less so than the treatment of bomb blast and penetrating trauma which has been dramatically improved over the last 4 years by the exceptional care provided in Iraq and Afghanistan and then on to Germany and the United States by the many teams of dedicated medics, nurses, physicians including trauma surgeons, rehabilitation specialists, and allied health personnel all working seamlessly to save the lives of injured soldiers and civilians and achieving the best outcome possible. Bomb blast injury creates the most horrific injuries of all and requires supreme efforts on the part of health systems, hospitals, and individual health professionals to get the best outcomes.

The signature weapons of the terrorist are the IED blast and suicide bomber resulting in mass casualties. The explosions cause combinations of blast injury, multiple penetrating injuries, and burns. The injury pattern to the head and neck includes intracranial hemorrhage, brain swelling with multiple intracranial metal and bone fragments, cervical and facial vascular injury, pharyngo-laryngeal injury, acute airway compromise, facial and scalp burns, large scalp defects, extensive skull base fractures, profound shock, and multiple other systemic injuries. Head and neck teams consisting of neurosurgeon, head and neck (ENT) surgeon, ophthalmologist, and facio-maxillary surgeon are an integral part of the US Combat Surgical Hospitals in Iraq treating these often horrific injuries and serve as an excellent model of care for the civilian system.

Lessons pertaining to the management of these injuries include

- Rapid treatment of blast injury to the head and spine in proximity to the event by specialist head and neck teams including neurosurgeons who are able to aggressively control ICP will help to ensure the best results.
- The timing and extent of the neurosurgery must be balanced against the relative priorities of the other injuries and the state of physiological stabilization.
- The neurosurgery follows the principles of damage control surgery and is generally more extensive and aggressive than that which has been described for penetrating brain injury in the literature from previous wars.
- Acute neurosurgery includes early generous craniectomy, intracranial hematoma evacuation, removal of accessible fragments and debridement of devitalized cerebral tissue, ventriculostomy, duroplasty, and use of broad spectrum antibiotics.
- CT is essential for planning the extent of the neurosurgery and CT angiography is useful when cervical vascular injury is suspected.
- There is a low index for early tracheostomy
- Vigorous replacement of blood loss and correction of coagulopathy
- Early neck exploration and management of carotid injury
- Repair of ocular injury or eye removal is often deferred.
- Cerebral vasospasm is common and is detected with regular TCD examinations and cerebral angiography if TCD is positive. Balloon angioplasty may be indicated.
- Maintaining an adequate mean arterial blood pressure and oxygenation are vital for any patient with spinal cord injury.
- The strategies for penetrating spine surgery include initial vigorous debridement of the associated missile wounds.
- Decompressive laminectomy is indicated for progressive neurological deficit and laminectomy is required for CSF fistula repair.

Bomb blast injuries are uncommon in the advanced countries but these are the typical injuries that we would encounter following a terrorist attack so it is important that health professionals who treat trauma patients including those who manage head and neck, spine injury, and neurotrauma become familiar with their management.

References

1. DePalma RG, Burris DG, Champion HR, Hodgson MJ. Current concepts: blast injuries. New Eng J Med 2005; 352(13): 1335–1342.
2. Neuhaus SJ, Sharwood PF, Rosenfeld JV. Terrorism and blast explosions: lessons for the Australian surgical community. Aust N Z J Surg 2006; 76: 637–644.
3. Rosenfeld JV. A neurosurgeon in Iraq: A personal perspective. J Clin Neurosci 2006; 13(10): 986–990.
4. Rosenfeld JV. Gunshot injury to the head and spine. Review. J Clin Neurosci 2002; 9(1): 9–16.
5. Cushing H. A study of wounds involving the brain and its enveloping structures. Br J Surg 1918; 5: 558–684.

6. Brandvold B, Levi L, Feinsod M, George ED. Penetrating craniocerebral injuries in the Israeli involvement in the Lebanese conflict 1982–1985. Analysis of a less aggressive surgical approach. J Neurosurg 1990; 72: 15–21.

7. Taha JM, Saba MI, Brown JA. Missile injuries to the brain treated with simple simple wound closure: results of a protocol during the Lebanese conflict. J Neurosurg 1991; 29: 380–383.

8. Amirjamshidi A, Abbassioun K, Rahmat H. Minimal debridement or simple wound closure as the only surgical treatment in war victims with low-velocity penetrating head injuries. Indications and management protocol based upon more than 8 years follow-up of 99 cases from Iran–Iraq conflict. Surg Neurol 2003; 60: 105–111.

9. Gofrit ON, Kovalski N, Leibovici D, Shemer J, O'Hana A, Shapira SC. Accurate anatomical location of war injuries: analysis of the Lebanon war fatal casualties and the proposition of new principles for the design of military personal armour system. Injury 1996; 27: 577–581.

10. Sheffy N, Mintz Y, Rivkind AI, Shapira SC. Terror-related injuries: a comparison of gunshot wounds versus secondary-fragments-induced injuries from explosives. J Am Coll Surg 2006; 203: 297–303.

11. Gutierrez de Ceballos JP, Turegano-Fuentes F, Perz-Dias D, Sanz-Sanchez M, Martin-Llorente C, Guerrero-Sanz JE. 11 March 2004: The terrorist bomb explosions in Madrid, Spain-an analysis of logistics, injuries sustained and clinical management of casualties treated at the closest hospital. Crit Care 2005; 9: 104–111.

12. Almogy G, Luria T, Richter E et al. Can external signs of trauma guide management? Lessons learned from suicide bombing attacks in Israel. Arch Surg 2005; 140: 390–393.

13. Guy RJ, Glover MA, Cripps NPJ. Primary blast injury: pathophysiology and implications for treatment Part III: injury to the central nervous system and limbs. J R Nav Med Serv 2000; 86: 27–31.

14. Cernak I, Wang Z, Jiang J, Bian X, Savic J. Ultrastructural and functional characteristics of blast-induced neurotrauma. J Trauma 2001; 50: 695–706.

15. Elsayed NM. Toxicology of blast overpressure. Toxicology 1997; 121: 1–15.

16. Axelsson H, Hjelmqvist H, Medin A, Perrson JKE, Suneson A. Physiological changes in Pigs exposed to a blast wave from a detonating high-explosive charge. Mil Med 2000; 165: 119–126.

17. Guy RJ, Kirkman E, Watkins PE, Cooper GJ. Physiological responses to primary blast. J Trauma 1998; 45: 983–987.

18. Sapsford W. Penetrating brain injury in military conflict: does it merit more research? J R Army Med Corps 2003; 149: 5–14.

19. Mayorga MA. The pathology of primary blast overpressure injury. Toxicology 1997; 121: 17–28.

20. Armonda RA, Bell RS, Vo AH, Ling G, DeGraba TJ, Crandall B, Ecklund J, Campbell WW. Wartime traumatic cerebral vasospasm: recent review of combat casualties. Neurosurgery 2006; 59, 1215–1225.

21. Leibovici D, Gotfrid ON, Shapira sc. Eardrum perforation in explosion survivors: is it a marker for pulmonary blast injury? Ann Emerg Med. 1999; 34: 168–72.

22. Knuth T, Letarte PB, Ling G, et al. Guidelines for the field management of combat-related head trauma. New York, New York: Brain Trauma Foundation. 2005.

23. Rosenfeld JV. Damage control neurosurgery. Injury 2004; 35: 655–660.

24. Bushby N, Fitzgerald M, Cameron P, Marasco S, Bystrzycki A, Rosenfeld JV, Bailey M. Prehospital intubation and chest decompression is associated with unexpected survival in major thoracic blunt trauma. Emerg Med Australas 2005; 17: 443–449.

25. Levi L, Linn S, Feinsod M. Penetrating craniocerebral injuries in civilians. Br J Neurosurg 1991;5: 241–247.
26. Taha JM, Haddad FS, Brown JA. Intracranial infection after missile injuries of the brain: report of 30 cases from the Lebanese conflict. Neurosurgery 1991; 29: 864–868.
27. Carey ME. The treatment of wartime brain wounds: traditional versus minimal debridement. Surg Neurol 2003; 60: 112–119.
28. Brain Trauma Foundation. Guidelines for the management of severe traumatic brain injury. 3rd edition. J Neurotrauma 2007; 24(1 Supplement): S1–S106.
29. Anon. Antibiotic prophylaxis for penetrating brain injury. J Trauma 2001; 51:S34–S40.
30. Bayston R, de Louvois J, Brown EM, Johnstone RA, Lees P, Pople IK. Use of antibiotics in penetrating craniocerebral injuries. Review. Lancet 2000; 355: 1813–17.
31. Langham J, Goldfrad C, Teasdale G, Shaw D, Rowan K. Calcium channel blockers for acute traumatic brain injury. Cochrane Database Syst Rev 2000; (2): CD000565.
32. Burris DG, Dougherty PJ, Elliot DC et al. (Editors). Emergency War Surgery. 3rd Edition. Borden Institute. Department of Defence, United States of America. Chapter 15.15–16, 2004.
33. Miyazawa T, Azuma R, Nakamura S, Kiyosawa T, Shima K. Usefulness of scalp expansion for cranioplasty in a case with postinfection large calvarial defect: a case report. Surg Neurol 2007; 67: 291–295.
34. Okie S. Traumatic brain injury in the War Zone. New Eng J Med 2005; 352: 2043–47.
35. Cernak I, Savic J, Ignjatovic D, et al. Blast injury from explosive munitions. J Trauma 1999; 47: 96–103.
36. Taber KH, Warden DL, Hurley RA. Blast-related traumatic brain injury: what is known? J Neuropsychiatry Clin Neurosci 2006; 18(2): 141–145.
37. Defense and Veterans Brain Injury Center Web site. Availabe at: http:/www.DVBIC.org. Accessed September 30, 2008.
38. McCrea M, Kelly J, Randolph C. Standardized assessment of concussion (SAC): Manual for administration, scoring and interpretation. 2nd Edition. Waukesa, WI. 2000.
39. Ryan LM, Warden DL. Post concussion syndrome. Int Rev Psychiatry 2003; 15(4): 310–316.
40. Neurobehavioral Guidelines Working Group, Warden DL, Gordon B, McAllister TW, et al. Guidelines for the pharmacological treatment of neurobehavioral sequelae of traumatic brain injury. J Neurotrauma 2006; 23: 1468–1450.
41. Hoge CW, McGurk, Thomas JL, Cox AL, Engel CC, Castro. Mild traumatic brain injury in US Soldiers returning from Iraq. New Eng J Med 2008; 358: 453–63.
42. Bryant RA. Disentangling mild traumatic brain injury and stress reactions. Editorial. New Eng J Med 2008; 358: 525–27.
43. Salazar AM, Schwab K, Grafman JH. Penetrating injuries in the Vietnam War. Traumatic unconsciousness, epilepsy and psychosocial outcome. Neurosurg Clin N Am 1995; 6: 715–726.
44. Warden DL, Ryan LM, Helmick KM et al. War neurotrauma: the Defense and Veterans Brain Injury Center (DVIBC) experience at Walter Reed Army Medical Center (WRAMC). (Abstract). J Neurotrauma 2005; 22:1178.
45. Aarabi B, Hersdorffer DC, Ahn ES, Aresco C, Scalea TM, Eisenberg HM. Outcome following decompressive craniectomy for malignant swelling due to severe head injury. J Neurosurg 2006; 104: 469–79.
46. Cooper DJ, Rosenfeld JV, Murray L et al. Early decompressive craniectomy for patients with severe traumatic brain injury and refractory intracranial hypertension: a pilot randomised trial. J Crit Care. 2008 Sep; 23(3): 387–93. Epub 2007 Dec 11.

47. Gawande A. Casualties of war-military care for the wounded from Iraq and Afghanistan. New Eng J Med 2004; 351: 2471–2479.
48. Hammoud MA, Haddad FS, Moufarrij NA. Spinal cord missile injuries during the Lebanese civil war. Surg Neurol 1995; 43(5): 432–437.
49. Kossmann T, Trease L, Freedman I, Malham, G. Damage control surgery for the spine. Injury 2004; 35(7): 661–670.
50. Levy ML, Gans W, Wijesinghe HS et al. Use of methyl prednisolone as an adjunct in the managenment of patients with penetrating spinal cord injury: outcome analysis. Neurosurgery 1996; 39: 1141–1149.
51. Heary RF, Vaccaro AR, Mesa JJ et al. Steroids and gunshot injuries to the spine. Neurosurgery 1997; 41: 576–584.

20
Crush Injury, Crush Syndrome

Moshe Michaelson

Crush injury (CI) is defined as a direct and local injury to the limbs that is caused by continuous prolonged pressure, basically causing damage to the muscle cells. Crush syndrome (CS), or reperfusion syndrome, is the systemic manifestation of CI (systemic pathopysiological and biochemical clinical picture, e.g. renal failure). As the definition indicates, a victim must be either buried or pinned down for a substantial period of time for CI to develop. The minimal time for this process, as delineated by Bywaters, is 2 hours.[1,2] While one report mentions less than 1 hour,[3] the usual time is much longer. This limits the cases of developing CI to patients whose extrication is delayed, and the obvious scenarios are mine accidents, tunnel accidents, earthquakes, and bombed buildings.[3–6] It is also highly relevant to terrorist attacks. In each of these scenarios, extrication may take a long time because of technical problems.

History

The first to describe CI and CS in the literature in English was Bywaters, in 1941.[1,2] He was not only the first to describe the symptoms but also the first to collect cases (about 100), to try to define the pathology and the treatment. He also set up a laboratory model for CI to better understand the pathophysiology of the process. He understood that these patients, specifically survivors of the London blitz who were buried under the rubble, appeared to have minor or no physical injuries at the outset, but later developed shock, with no blood loss and with severe hemo concentration. Armed with the knowledge that this was a different and unknown injury and syndrome, he researched the literature and found it described as far back as 1910 by von Colmers in the literature in German,[1] describing civilians buried in Messina during an earthquake. Muscle necrosis was also described by von Colmers[1] in 1916 during the First World War in soldiers buried after mine explosions, while anatomic changes in the kidney were described by Hackradt in 1917.[1] Although crush injuries were described sporadically between the First and Second World Wars, it was Bywaters, with his colleagues, who gathered the information and named it CI.

From the 1940s to the 1980s, there were only sporadic papers dealing with this injury, mostly anecdotal. In 1968, Bentley and Jeffreys[7] described CS in three

S.C. Shapira et al. (eds.), *Essentials of Terror Medicine*,
DOI: 10.1007/978-0-387-09412-0_20, Springer Science+Business Media, LLC 2009

miners who were buried for 7 hours in a coal mine. Brown and Nicholls[5] described two victims trapped for 7.5 and 13 hours during an accident in the Moorgate tube in London.

In the 1980s, new interest arose in the subject, with papers by a group from Rambam Medical Center in Haifa, Israel, which had the opportunity to treat two groups each of eight CI patients, and to describe in detail their experience and understanding of the syndrome.[3,8–11] The treatment of the first group led to writing a protocol for the treatment of the local injuries (CI) and a protocol to prevent the devastating results of the systemic manifestations of CI (CS). The second group was treated according to the suggested protocols and had a much better outcome. Since then, there have been other publications about larger groups of patients. Nineteen patients with CS caused by an earthquake in northern Italy were described by Santangelo,[4] and many articles have been written summarizing the knowledge and treatment of CI and CS.[11]

In the 1990s and early twenty-first century, more reports appeared on the subject. Two papers from China and Japan describe the injury in earthquake casualties.[12–15] Since the beginning of this century, there have been a number of reports from Turkey, written by Sever and colleagues, describing in detail CI patients treated at several hospitals during the Marmara earthquake in 1999.[16–19]

Crush Injury

CI is an injury caused by continuous and prolonged pressure. The main damage is to the muscles, although no damage is visible macroscopically. While many injuries come under the name of CI in the literature in English—usually dealing with mangled extremities after agricultural or industrial accidents and characterized by extensive physical injury of the limbs, including the skin, muscle, and bone—it is important to stress that CI is a very specific injury. CI occurs in patients who are pinned down for an extended period. The minimal time which can cause this injury remains in dispute, and 1–2 hours is considered by some to be the shortest time.

CI is also described in drug addicts who lie motionless on their hands.[18] From this, we can conclude that the factor of weight is less important than the length of time that the limb is immobilized. Patients suffering from CI report that they found themselves pinned down by a weight and that they experienced pain in the trapped limb; after some time, the limb became numb and the pain dissipated.[20]

Theoretically, we should see CI of the trunk as well; however, this has not been described, perhaps because prolonged pressure on the chest or abdomen results in death from respiratory failure.

The victims suffering from CI will commonly present a distinctive clinical picture. While exhibiting no other evident injuries, they will be agitated and frightened because of the extended period of entrapment during which they were unsure that they would survive. After rescue they usually do not complain of pain because the injured limbs are numb. Ironically, the limbs show no sign of traumatic injury and the skin is intact although there may be a dimple on the surface at the site of maximum pressure. The pulses distal to the injuries are palpated (in correlation with the blood pressure). It is vital to remember that lack of a pulse is not a necessary part of CI. If the pulses are not palpated, shock or vascular injury must be ruled out.

The affected limb is paralyzed and may present with patches of anesthesia and hypoesthesia. Strangely, patients often fail to mention the paralysis, perhaps due to the relief of the mental stress that was intense prior to the extrication. The patients will have a high pulse rate and low blood pressure. They are in hemodynamic shock. The urine is dark in color, ranging from pink to dark brown, depending on its pH.

The clinical picture changes dramatically during the first hours after extrication. The affected limb swells greatly and the skin becomes taut and shiny. The muscular compartment becomes severely tense. The pulses may not be palpated because of severe edema. Alternatively, they should be detected by Doppler measurements, because the pressure in the limb is not high enough to occlude the arteries.

Pre-Hospital Treatment

After the patient is extricated, priority should be given to the assessment and treatment of life-threatening conditions according to the Advanced Trauma Life Support (ATLS) protocols of the American College of Surgeons (http://www.facs.org/trauma/atls/index.html). This generally does not include CI. Active treatments for CI should be considered only after more severe injuries have been addressed, usually during a secondary survey. At the same time, it is essential to realize that the patient may be suffering from CI. So, to try to avoid the CS phase, an IV infusion of crystalloids should be started at the scene even before extrication.

The important point is to suspect the presence of CI. Medical personnel at the scene of an incident, whether in the aftermath of a terrorist attack or some other devastating event, are best suited to know how many hours the victim has been pinned down. This information should be entered on the patient's medical chart. By the time the victim is transferred to a hospital, that facility may already have received large numbers of victims with more obvious injuries. It then becomes all the more important and challenging not to overlook the more subtle characteristics of CI and to make a proper diagnosis. In this regard, it is also helpful for receiving hospitals to be notified by incident-site personnel that a patient with a possible diagnosis of CI is on the way. By doing so, the chances that victims will be given proper attention for CI immediately upon arrival, including placement in the intensive care unit, are improved.

Table 20.1 shows the only active treatment that should be administered at the scene.

TABLE 20.1. Active Treatment for crush injury (CI) at the Scene

a. Exclude life-threatening injuries (Advanced Trauma Life Support – ATLS)
b. Suspect CI according to the history of the injury
c. Note the suspicion in the patient's notes and notify the hospital if possible
d. Start IV fluids
e. Organize rapid evacuation to an appropriate hospital

Hospital Issues

By the time patients reach the hospital, they may have received a large volume of IV fluid, in which case their presenting symptoms may have changed. They might have a massive edematous limb with stretched and shiny skin. The muscular compartments may be tense, as in compartment syndrome. The limb will be paralyzed with anesthetic or hypoesthetic areas. The pulses should be palpable or traced by Doppler. The main treatment for CI is to try to avoid CS, as will be discussed later.

The appearance of a limb afflicted by CI and one by compartment syndrome can be so similar that a physician could wrongly conclude that both injuries are essentially the same. But they are significantly dissimilar and warrant distinctive treatments. Compartment syndrome occurs from pressure in a confined space, usually caused by inflammation after an injury. The space is bounded by thick connective tissue (fascia) and the blood supply is impaired. If not treated quickly by cutting open the facia (fasciotomy) the result will be death of nerve and muscle tissue.

In the case of crush, however, the mechanism of injury is different. In CI, the muscle cells die and then the swelling of the dead muscle cells causes edema, raising the pressure in the compartment. The edema is a result of the cells being dead, and not the other way round. This fact is crucial to understanding the rationalization of the treatment (Fig. 20.1). Thus, performing a fasciotomy on a limb that has suffered a CI would be akin to closing the gate after the horse has fled.

In their series, Michaelson and Reis[10,21] showed that avoiding fasciotomy yields much better results in terms of mortality and morbidity. Similar results have also been reported in other later works.[14,15]

Fasciotomy of a CI limb is often unnecessary and could actually be harmful. Dead muscle tissue, exposed to the open air, may foster infection that can lead to amputation. (Antibiotics cannot reach the dead muscle.) Additionally, the procedure could become a source of continuous oozing of blood. The vascular bed, although intact, bleeds because the venules and arterioles are dilated because of the acidotic environment, and it is very difficult to stop the oozing. Patients who undergo fasciotomy need repeated debridement until all the dead muscle is removed, which can lead to massive blood transfusions.[10]

During fasciotomy or debridement, physicians face the problem of identifying dead muscle. Dead muscle tissue is usually identified as tissue that does not bleed when cut, but this is not the case in CI. Here the muscle bleeds profusely, and there is no injury to the blood supply. In CI, the muscle loses its shiny color and tone.

- Compartment syndrome: injury → high pressure in the compartment → death of muscle cells

- Crush injury: injury → death of muscle cells → high compartment pressure

---

FIG. 20.1. Mechanisms of injury.

It does not react to physical or electrical stimuli by retracting. It is frail and can be torn easily.

This brings us to the mechanisms that cause such vast damage to the muscles in CI. There are three mechanisms to consider: vascular injury, neural injury, and direct pressure.

Vascular Injury

The injury caused to a limb when a major artery is occluded is well documented. The first sign is a skin lesion with demarcation of the ischemic zone and death of all tissue in that zone. In CI, there is no damage to the skin, so major vessel occlusion is not the cause of the damage, especially since the distal pulses can be palpated.

Neural Injury

The injury caused to a limb by severing a main nerve is well known. Although it may cause paralysis and areas of skin anesthesia, the severing of a nerve does not cause immediate damage to the muscle with swelling and disintegration of the cells. On the other hand, survivors describe feeling that the limb "fell asleep" and the recovery period is characterized by pain and hypersensitivity, showing that neural injury plays a part in this injury.

Direct Pressure

Although it is not entirely understood how direct pressure damages the muscle cells and causes their death, experimental models have shown that CI can result from continuous pressure on the muscle.[22]

In sum, the damage to a limb in CI is caused by direct pressure on the muscle and nerves. Pressure on the small vessels in the muscle may also play a role, but not pressure on the large arteries.

Crush Syndrome

CS is the systemic manifestation caused by CI or, more precisely, by the contents of the dead muscle cells that pour into the blood system. It is also a reperfusion syndrome, which means that the symptoms of the syndrome start only after the victim is extricated from the pressure. Therefore, the time of entrapment has no direct correlation to the severity of the symptoms. Most of the symptoms are a direct result of the mass of muscular dead cells. The larger the mass, the more severe are the symptoms. This syndrome is very well known as traumatic rhabdomyolysis.[21] Rhabdomyolysis from nontraumatic etiology is well documented in nephrologic literature and is caused by the nontraumatic death of muscle cells.[23-25]

Etiology

When the limbs are entrapped for a few hours, the pressure on the muscle cells, especially on the membranes, causes a change in the cation pump that eventually leads to cell death. Once the cell is dead, the cell membrane becomes permeable, unable to maintain the osmolar gap and the anion/cation differences in concentration between the intracell and the extracell environment. This causes a large shift of fluids into the cell with the swelling of the cell and, on the other hand, a large shift of anions/cations out of the cell. As a result, the swelling cells cause an elevation in the muscle compartment pressure (resembling classical compartment syndrome) and depletion of fluids in the vascular system. If not treated, this will lead to hypovolemic shock. This is documented by the high hematocrit concentration found in the results of the first blood test taken from CI patients.

For reasons still unknown, this sequence starts only after the patient is extricated from pressure. As noted earlier, the process starts at extrication and continues for some hours until a state of equilibrium is achieved. At the same time, the contents of the dead muscle cells pour into the vascular system as the pumps that kept them in place no longer work, and they move freely according to the anion/cation concentration gap, until they reach equilibrium.

Among them are mainly potassium (K), calcium (Ca), magnesium (Mg), phosphorus (P), and cell breakdown products such as myoglobin and creatinine phosphorus kinase (CPK). The first and most dangerous one is potassium. In blood, its normal range is 3.3–4.5 mequiv./L but during the first few hours it can reach as high as 8–9 mequiv./L, which endangers the life of the victim by causing malignant arrhythmias. The second major problem arises from the combination of three components (listed in Table 20.2).[3,26]

The combination of these three elements has been known for many years to be toxic to the tubular cells of the kidney and the cause of acute renal failure.[2] The signs in a CI patient who may develop CS are shown in Table 20.3.

Once CI has occurred, the muscle is dead and one must try to avoid the devastating results of CS. In the past, mortality was high and a high percentage of survivors had their limbs amputated.[4,8]

There are two ways to approach this problem. The first is to treat the symptoms of CS and the second is to prevent these symptoms from occurring. There is no doubt that acute renal failure can be treated successfully by hemo or peritoneal dialysis. Although dialysis is universally appreciated as standard treatment, the procedure is still associated with some risk of morbidity and mortality.[14] Furthermore,

TABLE 20.2. Three Components that, When Combined, are Toxic to Tubular Cells of the Kidney, and Can Cause Acute Renal Failure

1. Hypovolemia – influx of fluids into the dead muscle cells, causing depletion in the vascular bed
2. Acidemia – caused mainly by phosphorus anions pouring into the blood
3. Myoglobulinemia – myoglobin is the main pigment in the muscle cell; when the cell dies, it reaches the blood stream in large amounts and is toxic to the kidney

TABLE 20.3. Signs that a CI Patient May Develop Crush Syndrome (CS)

1. Hypovolemic shock
2. Oliguria/anuria – the color of the first urine may range from dark brown to pink and will show traces of myoglobin
3. Blood test will reveal:
   a. high hemoglobin and hematocrit levels (if there is no bleeding and the patient has not yet received a large amount of fluids)
   b. high concentration of potassium (K) in the blood
   c. high blood level of creatinine phosphorus kinase (CPK) (usually a quantitative marker for cell damage)
   d. high levels of phosphorus (P)

suitable facilities to treat large numbers of patients are absent in many locations, and even when the necessary equipment and facilities are available, the high cost of dialysis treatment is yet another consideration. As in any other illness, the best and cheapest strategy is prevention.

In the 1980s, a group from Rambam Medical Center in Haifa, Israel, summarized its experience in treating two groups of patients with CS.[21,26] In the first group, patients were given dialysis for acute renal failure and fasciotomies for CI. Because of the poor results, it was decided to develop a prevention strategy. This strategy was tried on a second group a few years later with very promising results. The prevention strategy has one problem: It needs to be initiated as early as possible, preferably at the catastrophe site. The prevention plan has three elements:

1. Hydration – fill the intervascular space and keep it full
2. Forced diuresis
3. Alkalinization of urine

The rationale behind these elements is the following:

1. Hydration – as the leak of fluids into the dead cells continues for a few hours until equilibrium is achieved, hypovolemic shock develops. This by itself can cause acute renal failure. It was found that some patients were in a positive fluid balance of more than 12 kg in the first 24 hours, most of which accumulated in the injured limbs.[3]
2. Forced diuresis – it was hypothesized that diuresis would flush out and dilute the myoglobins, thereby preventing acute renal failure
3. Alkalinization of urine – pH above 6.5 was found to protect the kidney cells from the toxic effects of myoglobins[11]

The suggested protocol for preventing acute renal failure (ARF) in CI patients is shown as an algorithm in Fig. 20.2.

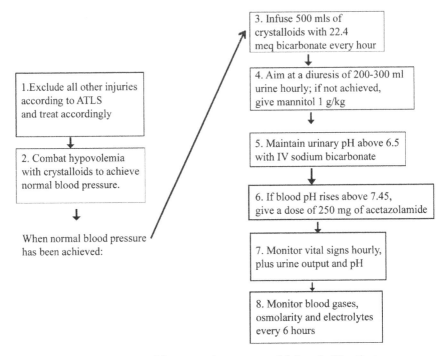

FIG. 20.2.   Suggested protocol for preventing acute renal failure in CI patients.

As can be seen, the patient needs to be hospitalized in an intensive care unit for this regime. The Rambam group experience showed that this regime not only prevented the development of acute renal failure but also affected the hyperkalemia so that the potassium level declined to almost normal in the second measurement and that no other treatment was necessary. This regime is generally well accepted but can only work if started early. The problem is that CS develops in victims during catastrophes such as earthquakes or possibly in the event of a mass casualty terrorist attack, during which the medical system could be overly taxed. In such cases, treatment is given first to victims with immediate life-threatening injuries. By the time the medical staff is free to treat CI patients, the window of opportunity for prevention may have closed and acute renal failure established.

Conclusion

CI and CS are the result of body entrapment for several hours. Damage to the muscle cells is mainly a result of direct pressure, and the severity of the syndrome is correlated to the amount of muscle damage. The lack of professional literature on the subject is probably because these injuries occur during catastrophes when the medical system is overwhelmed by patients with immediate life-threatening injuries. By the time CI patients reach the hospital, their injured muscles are dead and there is no benefit in performing fasciotomies. On the contrary, fasciotomy may result in bleeding and uncontrolled infection, which can in turn lead to amputation.

The best way of dealing with CS is to prevent acute renal failure. This can be done if the patient reaches hospital early, before acute renal failure has set in. Those who arrive after the onset of this syndrome should be treated as quickly as possible by performing dialysis, as their acute renal failure is usually transitory.

References

1. Bywaters EG. Ischemic muscle necrosis. JAMA. 1944;124:1103–1109.
2. Bywaters EG, Beall D. Crush injuries with impairment of renal function. 1941. J Am Soc Nephrol. 1998;9:322–332.
3. Ron D, Taitelman U, Michaelson MM, Bar-Joseph G, Bursztein S, Better OS. Prevention of acute renal failure in traumatic rhabdomyolysis. Arch Intern Med. 1984;144:277–280.
4. Santangelo ML, Usberti M, Di Salvo E, et al. A study of the pathology of crush syndrome. Surg Gynecol Obstet. 1982;154:372–374.
5. Brown AA, Nicholls RJ. Crush syndrome: a report of 2 cases and a review of the literature. Br J Surg. 1977;64:397–402.
6. Jones RN. Crush syndrome in a Cornish tin miner. Injury. 1984;15:282–283.
7. Bentley G, Jeffreys TE. The crush syndrome in coal miners. J Bone Joint Surg Br. 1968;50:588–594.
8. Michaelson M, Taitelman U, Bshouty Z, Bar-Joseph G, Bursztein S. Crush syndrome: experience from the Lebanon War, 1982. Isr J Med Sci. 1984;20:305–307.
9. Michaelson M, Taitelman U, Bursztein S. Management of crush syndrome. Resuscitation. 1984;12:141–146.
10. Reis ND, Michaelson M. Crush injury to the lower limbs. Treatment of the local injury. J Bone Joint Surg Am. 1986;68:414–418.
11. Better OS, Michaelson M, Taitelman U, Zinman C, Reis DN. Rescue and salvage operations for casualties with the crush syndrome. Postgrad Gen Surg. 1990;2:189–196.
12. Shimazu T, Yoshioka T, Nakata Y, et al. Fluid resuscitation and systemic complications in crush syndrome: 14 Hanshin-Awaji earthquake patients. J Trauma. 1997;42:641–646.
13. Zui-Yong Z. Medical support in the Tangshan earthquake: a review of the management of mass casualties and certain major injuries. J Trauma. 1987;27:1130–1137.
14. Matsuoka T, Yoshioka T, Tanaka H, et al. Long-term physical outcome of patients who suffered crush syndrome after the 1995 Hanshin-Awaji earthquake: prognostic indicators in retrospect. J Trauma. 2002;52:33–39.
15. Shimazu T, Yoshioka T, Nakata Y, et al. Fluid resuscitation and systemic complications in crush syndrome: 14 Hanshin-Awaji earthquake patients. J Trauma. 1997;42:641–646.
16. Sever MS, Erek E, Vanholder R, et al. Renal replacement therapies in the aftermath of the catastrophic Marmara earthquake. Kidney Int. 2002;62:2264–2271.
17. Sever MS, Erek E, Vanholder R, et al. Lessons learned from the Marmara disaster: time period under the rubble. Crit Care Med. 2002;30:2443–2449.
18. Sever MS, Erek E, Vanholder R, et al. Treatment modalities and outcome of the renal victims of the Marmara earthquake. Nephron. 2002;92:64–71.
19. Sarisozen B, Durak K. Extremity injuries in children resulting from the 1999 Marmara earthquake: an epidemiologic study. J Pediatr Orthop B. 2003;12:288–291.

20. Kikta MJ, Meyer JP, Bishara RA, et al. Crush syndrome due to limb compression. Arch Surg. 1987;122:1078–1081.
21. Michaelson M, Reis ND. Crush injury – crush syndrome. Unfallchirurg. 1988;91:330–332.
22. Reis ND, Better OS. Mechanical muscle-crush injury and acute muscle-crush compartment syndrome. J Bone Joint Surg. 2005;87-B:450–453.
23. Better OS. Traumatic rhabdomyolysis ("crush syndrome") – updated 1989. Isr J Med Sci. 1989;25:69–72.
24. Better OS, Stein JH. Early management of shock and prophylaxis of acute renal failure in traumatic rhabdomyolysis. N Engl J Med. 1990;322:825–829.
25. Gabow PA, Kaehny WD, Kelleher SP. The spectrum of rhabdomyolysis. Medicine (Baltimore). 1982;61:141–152.
26. Michaelson M. Crush injury and crush syndrome. World J Surg. 1992 ;16:899–903.

21
Maxillofacial Injury Related to Terror

Eran Regev and Rephael Zeltser

September 11, 2001, prompted a marked increase in concern about terrorism in most parts of the western world. But even before then, several countries, Israel among them, had become sensitive to the issue because of their experiences with terrorist attacks. The frequency of terrorist assaults had already heightened concerns about security and medical responses.

Terrorism-related injuries have some unique attributes that are not encountered in other trauma. Most of these incidents, caused by bombs or other explosives, are multi-casualty or mass-casualty events. The injuries cause "multi-trauma," affecting several organs and systems, and the treatment is usually multidisciplinary. An important facet is that they involve the special characteristics of blast injuries, which require particular attention.

Dobson and his colleagues studied the trends in maxillofacial injuries in war between 1914 and 1986 and found that 16% of all war injuries involved the maxillofacial area. However, when considering only terrorism-related injuries, the involvement rose to 21%.[1] Frykberg reviewed the medical management of disasters caused by terrorist bombings and concluded that head and neck injuries occur more frequently than would be expected on the basis of the 12% body area exposed to the environment.[2]

Injuries of the oral and maxillofacial region are seldom life-threatening, though they can be highly debilitating. They may cause both severe functional disability and esthetic disfigurement. Therefore, this relatively small, though highly visible, area requires special attention.

Four types of terrorism-related maxillofacial injuries are recognized: stab wounds, gunshot wounds (GSW), stone-related injuries, and blast injuries. The first two have been thoroughly described, with voluminous literature available on civilian-related injuries. Although stones are used mainly in civilian uprisings and riots, they have become a popular terrorist weapon, causing potentially severe injuries. This was patently the case during the first Palestinian intifada (1987–1993).

During the more recent intifada (beginning in 2000), blast injuries, which had been traditionally part of military medicine, became a growing concern for civilian victims. In particular, suicide bombings in confined places such as buses and restaurants, as well as foreign objects added to the explosives, brought new and unique aspects to these injuries.

S.C. Shapira et al. (eds.), *Essentials of Terror Medicine*,
DOI: 10.1007/978-0-387-09412-0_21, Springer Science+Business Media, LLC 2009

Epidemiology

The literature on maxillofacial injuries caused by terrorist attacks is sparse and limited to reports on isolated events. Data from multiple events were available mainly from Northern Ireland and Israel. In recent years, although terror attacks with explosives have increased sharply in Iraq and Afghanistan, little relevant data from these events have so far been published. Consequently, most of the epidemiological data presented here is based on the Israeli experience.

Reviews of the literature by Dobson[1] and Frykberg[2] suggest that maxillofacial injuries from a terrorist incident are more numerous than in non-terror trauma incidents. Adler and his colleagues[3] reported 19.3% head and neck injuries in 500 casualties in a series of bomb blasts in Jerusalem in the 1970s. It is important to note that during that period, bombs typically were smaller and placed on the ground or under bus seats and not carried on the bodies of suicide bombers.

But a review of data from the National Israeli Trauma Registry from 2000 to 2003 reveals a different picture. In a period of 33 months, during which 1,811 terrorism-related casualties were reported, 493 (27.2%) involved facial injuries.[4]

From October 2000 through February 2004, terrorist attacks in the Jerusalem area were especially intense. Scores of assaults by stabbing, firearms, and suicide bombs occurred in markets, buses, restaurants, and other public locations. The most severely wounded generally were sent to the Hadassah University Hospital, the only level I trauma center in Jerusalem. Of the 577 patients admitted to that hospital due to terrorism-related injuries, 172 (29.8%) had maxillofacial injuries (excluding isolated eye and ear injuries). Seventy-five of these patients had maxillofacial fractures. During that same period, 6,298 patients were admitted due to non-terrorism-related trauma, but only 1,108 (17.6%) had maxillofacial injuries.

Upon examining the epidemiology of terrorism-related maxillofacial injuries compared with non-terrorism maxillofacial trauma, differences could be noted on several scales. Terrorism-inflicted maxillofacial injuries affected both genders almost evenly (M:F 60:40 in terrorist attacks vs. 70:30 in non-terrorist cases); there were more patients with maxillofacial injuries who were above 18 years in terrorist incidents (>80%) than in non-terrorist incidents (59%); injuries in terrorist incidents were also more severe according to the injury severity score (ISS); length of hospital stay (LOS) was longer; and the death rate was higher. These parameters are similar to those for terrorism-related general trauma.[5,6]

The death rate was 4% among terrorism victims with injuries to the maxillofacial area, which was three times the rate among those suffering from non-terrorism maxillofacial trauma (1.3%), though the maxillofacial injuries were not the cause of death.

Since almost 50% of the patients suffered from multi-trauma, the higher ISS and death rate could be attributed to the other injuries.

Of the 172 patients admitted with maxillofacial injuries, 87 (50.1%) were injured from explosions, mainly suicide bombs; 50 (29.1%) sustained gunshot wounds; 23 (13.4%) were hit by stones; and 5 (2.9%) were stabbed in the head and neck area.

Seven patients were terrorists or participants in riots and sustained maxillofacial injuries from rubber bullets shot by the army or the police.

The distribution of the different facial fractures (zygoma, maxilla, mandible, and orbit) was not significantly different from that of non-terrorism fractures. Twenty-three percent of the patients required maxillofacial surgical intervention, very similar in proportion to our non-terrorism trauma patients.

Only 37% of the zygomatic complex fractures underwent surgery, compared with 47% of those with a similar fracture among non-terrorism patients. In contrast, almost all the mandibular fractures (88%) required closed or open reduction, while only 50% of the non-terrorism mandibular fractures were fixed surgically. These findings may be explained by the fact that many non-terrorism mandibular fractures are non-displaced, involve the temporo-mandibular joint (TMJ), and affect young children, all of which are treated conservatively.

Unlike mandibular fractures, many zygomatic complex fractures caused by explosions were not or only minimally displaced, so that surgery was not indicated.

Pre-hospital Issues

The aim of terrorism is to intimidate and demoralize the civilian population. Accordingly, most attacks occur in buses and other crowded places, often in the center of a city. Thus, evacuation to a major hospital is commonly accomplished in a matter of minutes.[7,8] If an attack results in only a few victims, the emergency medical services (EMS) can easily perform a "scoop and run" evacuation to the nearest hospital. But if a suicide bomber detonates himself in a crowded bus or restaurant, resulting in many casualties, the scene can be chaotic and management more challenging.

The area will rapidly fill with EMS teams, security and police personnel, and bystanders who wish to help. In this situation, the senior EMS person at the site assumes control as triage commander. He assesses the condition of each victim and decides treatment and evacuation priorities.[8,9] The most seriously injured are sent to a level I trauma center, while the other patients are evenly distributed among hospitals in other areas. These decisions are made very quickly, in accordance with the scoop and run approach, as treatment is best rendered in a hospital and not in a pre-hospital setting. Still, life-threatening conditions such as a blocked airway or heavy bleeding, are aggressively addressed at the site or in transit to the hospital.

There is no need for medical specialists at the site of the attack, though advance reports from the site or from ambulances in transit should be communicated to the receiving hospitals. In this manner, the senior surgeon at the hospital (who will act as triage commander) becomes aware of the estimated number of victims, severity of injuries, and whether an operating room is required immediately.

To avoid transferring patients from one hospital to another, the evacuation of patients with maxillofacial injuries should, when possible, be to the hospital with a maxillofacial surgery service.

Emergency Department

Terrorist attacks are usually unpredictable as to time, location, severity, and the types of injuries that will be inflicted. To minimize the chance of confusion at a receiving hospital, protocols and rehearsed procedures should be in place, and priorities understood for evacuation and distribution.[8] Protocols for triage, evaluation, treatment, and control have been developed at the Hadassah University Hospital[7] and communicated to the oral and maxillofacial surgery service (Fig. 21.1). In fact, the protocol for the command structure at Hadassah is similar to that established

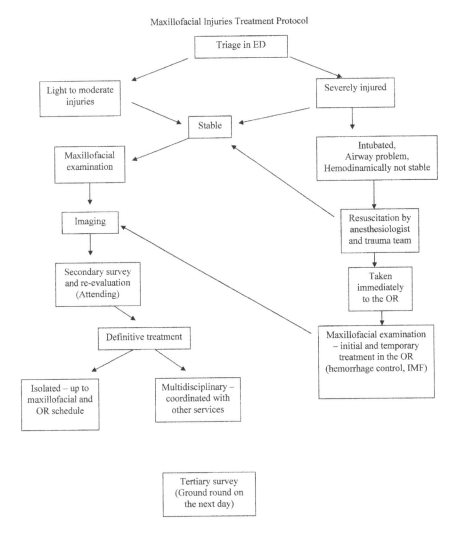

FIG. 21.1. Maxillofacial Injuries Treatment Protocol.

in Northern Ireland and England.[10,11] According to the Hadassah protocol, a senior oral and maxillofacial surgeon is present in the emergency department to assist the resident(s) in diagnosis, complex procedures, and priorities regarding imaging and operating room procedures.

The oral and maxillofacial surgeon should be involved in the initial evaluation and resuscitation of the victims, who may have airway problems due to fractured jaws, foreign bodies, fragments of bones and teeth, and massive oral and nasal bleeding. He may also be needed to assist the anesthesiologist with difficult intubation that requires securing the endotracheal tube to the teeth, as in the case of facial burns.

Most of the emergency endotracheal intubations performed by the EMS or in the emergency department are oral. For a thorough oral and maxillofacial examination and for later surgical procedures, nasal intubation or tracheostomy may be preferable, though not advised in the acute setting. The oral tube can be changed at a later date. Nasal placement of an endotracheal tube is, however, contraindicated in a patient with a closed head injury until a basilar skull fracture is ruled out.

After the initial examination and evaluation, imaging is an essential adjunct for diagnosis and treatment planning. Plain x-rays can be obtained in the trauma room or the emergency department. However, if the head or neck of a patient is seriously injured, the required positioning for optimal x-rays may not be permissible as that would deleteriously affect the quality of the pictures. The gold standard today for multiple facial injuries is a spiral CT scan with thin cuts and three-dimensional (3D) reconstructions, which provide the surgeon with a complete facial picture within a few minutes.[12,13]

We have been very liberal in ordering a full facial CT scan for complicated multiple trauma patients, especially for those undergoing a CT scan of other parts of the body, that is, head, C-spine, lungs, abdomen, and pelvis. But before patients are transferred to the CT scan room, they must have a secured airway and be stable hemodynamically.

Our experience has also demonstrated the value of photographic documentation of the injuries, although this practice has been uneven. We have been involved in the treatment of hundreds of patients but have only limited clinical photographic documentation of the different types of injuries. The reason is that in the tumult of emergency department activity, the focus is on providing care. Also, some might hesitate to take pictures of patients who are unconscious or otherwise unable to grant permission. But the importance of photographs cannot be overstated. They could help confirm the identification of patients who had been reported missing or taken to the OR before family members had the opportunity to see them. In addition, photographs can document pre- and postoperation appearances and can be valuable teaching tools.

Modern technology has made picture-taking quick and easy. Cellular phones now commonly contain digital cameras, which can produce photographs in real time. Assigning a junior resident or student to take photographs in such emergency and hospital settings is therefore warranted.

Keeping records and documentation of all the victims and injuries is crucial in multi-casualty events. Rushed or incomplete examination may lead to wrong or missed diagnosis.[14] Therefore, part of our protocol (Fig. 21.1) is to conduct debriefings at the end of the event. The attending physician responsible, together with the residents, conducts a secondary survey of all the patients with maxillofacial injuries, including reviews of their imaging reports. A tertiary survey is performed the following day, which will include other attending physicians as well. All the admitted patients are seen and evaluated and consideration is then also given to new consultation requests from other services.

Types of Injury

Stones

Stones were one of the first materials used in ancient times as working and hunting tools. Later, they were used as weapons and to carry out executions by pelting ["And David put his hand in his bag, and took thence a stone, and slung it, and smote the Philistine in his forehead; and the stone sank into his forehead, and he fell upon his face to the earth" (Samuel I, 17; 49)]. In modern times also, stones and rocks have been used as weapons, notably by civilians against police or army personnel.[15, 16]

Throwing stones at Israeli soldiers became the Palestinians' most popular form of attack during the uprising that started in 1987 ("First Intifada"). Stones and rocks were also thrown at civilian cars on the roads. This supposedly primitive weapon has turned out to be a dangerous and potentially lethal one. Heering and colleagues[17] described the injuries sustained by Israeli troops in 1987–1989, of which 62% were caused by stones. Although 94% of them were described as light injuries, there was one fatality out of the 673 soldiers injured.

Between 2000 and 2004, the characteristics of terrorism activities changed and the majority of injuries were caused by explosions and gunfire. In that period, only 13% of the injuries were caused by stones.

The mechanism of stone injury is the same as blunt trauma: the impact of the stone on the facial soft tissue and bone causes the injury. The flying stone has a kinetic energy that is directly related to the mass of the stone and the square of its velocity ($E_k = 1/2m \times v^2$). A distinction should be made between two types of victims: those who stood facing the rioters at a "stone throwing distance," and those who were in a car usually moving toward the stone-thrower. The first type was composed almost exclusively of army troops who were facing rioters. Heering[17] described 370 skull, face, and neck injuries among 611 soldiers wounded by stones, 70 of whom sustained jaw injuries. It is not specified whether these were to the soft tissue only or to hard tissue as well. The vast majority of the head and neck injuries in their study were graded as light injuries, despite the authors' comment on the lack of protective equipment that the soldiers should have been wearing.

The second type of victims included drivers and passengers of motor vehicles. When a stone hits a car moving at 60–80 km/h (40–50 miles/h), the velocity at impact is the sum of both the car's and the stone's velocity. The kinetic energy transferred to the body is much higher because it is related to the square of the velocity. Therefore, the severity of injuries sustained even by having a small stone thrown at a moving car can be devastating. The facial fractures are usually open and comminuted as in Fig. 21.2.

In addition, the stone often shatters the car window before hitting the person, adding lacerations from the glass fragments. The head and neck are the areas most frequently affected by stoning injury because these are at window level and unprotected by the door or dashboard.[18] Drivers are almost always injured on the left side of the face and passengers on the right side, because the stone thrower usually is positioned on the side of the road.

Finally, stone throwing increases the risk of secondary injury from a driver's loss of control. Swerving to avoid being hit could result in collision with another vehicle or driving off the road.

Treatment

The patterns of injury caused by stones are similar to those seen by oral and maxillofacial surgeons in blunt trauma and motor vehicle accidents. Nevertheless, in our experience at the Hadassah University Hospital, fractures caused by stones are more complex and comminuted with more soft tissue avulsions and lacerations (Fig. 21.2). Treatment should include cleaning and debridement, preservation of tissue, and bony reconstruction as soon as possible by intermaxillary fixation (IMF) or open reduction internal fixation (ORIF), as described by Nahlieli and colleagues.[18]

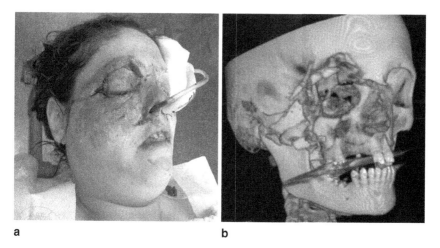

a   b

Fig. 21.2. Car passenger injured by stone (A), the CT scan shows the comminuted fractures of the orbit, zygoma, and coronoid process (B).

Stab Wounds

As with stoning, stabbing of the head and neck is an ancient method of killing. Jael smote a tent peg into Sisera's temple and killed him (Judges 4; 21).

Throughout history, other instruments, especially a variety of knives, have been used for traumatic assault as well. Hanoch et al.[19] mentioned knives as a killing instrument used by the Hashshishins (a secret order of Muslims) in the eleventh century, and by Arabs for murder in the name of family honor. They found a clear distinction between knife attacks as acts of terrorism and other knifings.

The study by Hanoch and his colleagues reviewed 154 patients who were stabbed in acts of terrorism in Israel between 1987 and 1994. Unlike "civilian stabbing," about half of these victims sustained multiple wounds. The most common site was the posterior right thorax, though the head and neck were involved in 49 patients (almost one-third). But in Israel, the use of knives as a terrorist weapon has been relatively infrequent. According to our data, stabbings accounted for only 2.9% of maxillofacial injuries related to terrorism.

In some societies around the globe, civilian stab wounds are much more common. In a hospital in South Africa, for example, 393 cases of head and neck stab wounds were reported in a period of 21 months.[20] A study reported that stab wounds accounted for 26% of the trauma patients admitted to an emergency department in another hospital in South Africa.[21]

The major vessels going to and from the head, and other important anatomical structures, that is, the trachea and the esophagus, are embedded in the neck, which has therefore been a target area for stabbing attacks by terrorists. Stab wounds in the face are much rarer and they, unlike the neck injuries, are not life threatening. Except for a study by Chen et al.,[22] which reported 12 stab injuries out of 78 penetrating face injuries, the majority of the reports are anecdotal.[20,23,24]

Treatment

Our policy for stab injuries is neck exploration for every wound deep to the platysma. Nonetheless, if the patient is hemodynamically stable with no active bleeding, or if the knife or instrument is impacted in the wound, angiography or CT angiography should be performed. The trajectory of the blade and possible damage to blood vessels are thus demonstrated prior to removal of the weapon, which should be performed only in the operating theater. The advantage of formal angiography is the ability to embolize bleeding vessels and perhaps avoid neck exploration and a surgical procedure.

Gunshot Injuries

Firearm injuries are not unique to military or terrorist activity and the vast majority of the available literature is in fact related to civilian incidents.[22,25] The velocity of the bullet used to be the main factor for distinguishing the pattern of injury. Today other more important factors are recognized, such as the bullet's type and shape, the proximity of the victim to the muzzle, the protective equipment that the bullet has penetrated, and the tissue encountered. Powers and Robertson[26] discussed ten common myths relating to ballistics in the area of oral and maxillofacial surgery. They concluded that tissue injury is caused by the design of the bullet and its energy upon striking the tissue, and that the velocity alone cannot be the basis for treatment. For example, a bullet from a low velocity handgun, shot from a short distance and hitting the facial or jaw bones, may cause more damage than a bullet from a high velocity rifle fired from a long distance and penetrating only soft tissue. The Israel National Trauma Registry recorded 36% gunshot wounds out of all the terrorism-related injuries from 2000 to 2004, 25% of them to the head and neck.[27]

Treatment

The immediate treatment protocol is well established. The goal is to preserve life, and the ATLS (Advanced Trauma Life Support) generic approach is applied first. Gunshot wounds to the maxillofacial region may severely damage the upper airway system and require emergency endotracheal intubation. Sometimes this is not feasible because of massive bleeding or anatomical distortion. Alternatively, therefore, a cricothyroidotomy is performed. Once the airway is secured, hemorrhage should be controlled. If one of the major neck vessels is bleeding profusely, local pressure should be applied until the patient is taken to the operating room for exploration.

A dictum common among many authors is "treat the wound, not the weapon." By following this rationale, treatment should be based on the presentation of the wound and not on the type of weapon or projectile that caused it. There are two main treatment protocols for gunshot injuries: immediate and delayed reconstruction.[28,29] Immediate reconstruction is defined as initial treatment of a wound, with the intention to definitively manage all aspects of the injury. The aim is to close the wound in such a way that both hard and soft tissues are restored. This may require the introduction of rigid fixation and then immediate bone grafts and tissue flaps to close soft and hard tissue defects.

In the delayed reconstruction protocol, the initial treatment includes stabilization of bony injuries, maximum tissue preservation, and closure of the wounds with local mucosa and skin. Necrotic tissue and bone fragments that are not attached to the periosteum or soft tissue are excised. Since the maxillofacial region has an excellent blood supply, any part of bone, tooth, or soft tissue that has a chance to remain vital is not removed. Final reconstruction is attempted after edema has resolved and soft tissue covers all the wounds. This may be carried out several weeks or months later, in one or several stages.

Rubber Bullets

In some articles, especially those describing the Northern Ireland conflict, injuries from rubber bullets were included in terrorism-related injuries.[10,30] This kind of weapon is used by the police or by the army against terrorists or rioters and, is, therefore, beyond the scope of this chapter.

Blast Injuries

Among the many and varied weapons that terrorists have used, the most common ones in recent years are those involving explosives. Effects of the detonation of explosive devices in conventional warfare, either on army troops or in urban areas, can be devastating. An aerial bomb may contain as much as one ton of explosive charges encased in metal. The explosive devices used by terrorists are much smaller and in most cases are improvised. The pipe bomb and letter bomb, for example, are uncomplicated and relatively easy to make. Details of construction are freely available in open sources including the Internet, and components can be found in most hardware stores.[31,32] Terrorists have learned to use explosives to maximum effect.

Whitlock[10] reviewed urban guerilla warfare in Northern Ireland after 1969 and described the full spectrum of violent injuries. The terrorists' bombs varied in weight from 1 to 250 kg, but over time they generally became larger and more sophisticated. They were placed in cars, pubs, and hotels and incorporated into various booby-traps such as letter bombs. Charges were packed with nails, bolts, and large nuts and attached to cans of gasoline to maximize the effect. Terrorists in the Middle East have applied all these techniques[33] and in the last 20 years have popularized suicide bombers in particular.

The explosion of a conventional bomb involves the sudden transformation of a solid or liquid material into gas, thus generating a blast wave that spreads out from a point source. The blast wave consists of two parts – a shock wave of high pressure, followed closely by a blast wind. In general, damage produced by the blast wave decreases exponentially with distance.[34] When the explosion occurs in a confined place such as a closed room or a bus, the blast wave is reflected and bounces off the walls, increasing mortality and morbidity.[35,36]

There are four categories of blast injury: primary (direct effect of pressure), secondary (effects of projectiles), tertiary (effect due to wind and motion of air propelling the victim against a stationary object), and quaternary (burns, asphyxia, and exposure to toxic inhalants).[34] (For more information on blast injury types, see Chap. 11 and Table 19.1).

Maxillofacial Blast Injuries

Only a few published studies focus on maxillofacial blast injuries. The wounds caused by a bomb explosion are characterized by their multiplicity and gross contamination. The common basic injuries are a combination of bruises, abrasions, lacerations, and superficial wounds, with few maxillofacial fractures, as described by Whitlock[10] and Hadden[37] in Northern Ireland, Odhiambo in Nairobi,[38] and Holmes in London.[11] This is different from our experience (unpublished data), according to which facial fractures were more common and the severity of injuries was greater. The difference seems attributable to the outdoor versus confined space explosions and to the addition of foreign projectiles to the explosive devices.

Most authors agree that the maxillofacial region is affected by the secondary, tertiary, and quaternary patterns of injuries. The only part of the head and neck region affected by the primary injury is the eardrum. In fact, it is the organ most sensitive to the overpressure wave and thus an indicator of the proximity of the victim to the explosion, though not necessarily correlated to the severity of the injuries.[35,38,39]

An animal model developed by Wang et al.[40] in order to study the effect of the blast wave of a spherical explosive suggests that the wave causes extensive wounds of the soft tissue, skin, and muscle. The bones of the facial skeleton suffer splinter fractures and the fracture sites appear concave. These findings seem in line with those of Shuker[41] based on experiences of the war between Iran and Iraq (1980–1988). He studied three mechanisms of injury by blast wave previously described by Stapczynski[42]: acceleration, spalling, and implosion. Acceleration is the movement of viscera initiated by motion of the body wall in the direction of the blast wave. Spalling is the split or break into flakes that may occur at the interface of two different media when a shock wave moves from a high density to a lower density medium. Implosion is the momentary contraction and burst of the tissue inwards.

Although Shuker's article is not substantially evidence based and he does not provide data on the number of cases that he treated, it is the first and only attempt to describe the typical mechanism of primary blast injuries to the facial skeleton. From the data acquired in our hospital, we have found some cases that conform to the patterns described by Shuker. But the paucity of cases does not allow us to draw definite conclusions.

The middle third of the facial skeleton is composed of strong vertical and horizontal buttresses (naso-maxillary, zygomatico-maxillary, pterygo-maxillary, and palatal) connected by thin cortical bones and containing air spaces or para-nasal sinuses. The thin walls of the maxillary and ethmoid sinuses and the orbits may be subjected to an implosion type of fracture, as described by Shuker.[41] In our patients we have seen comminuted fractures of the walls of the maxillary antrum and the ethmoid sinuses. They exist with and without concomitant zygomatic and Le Fort fractures, which cannot be explained solely by penetrating or external impact trauma. This may also account for the number of radiologically diagnosed zygomatic and maxillary fractures that did not require surgical correction.[34]

The strength of the mandible derives from its U-shaped and thick cortex with little bone marrow in its core. According to Shuker, as opposed to the regular pattern of fracture that is usually vertically oriented, the blast effect on a mandible may cause a horizontal fracture below the mylohyoid line and the apices of the teeth.

In addition to the unique fractures described by Shuker, we have seen some patients, mainly from bus explosions, who had a burst fracture of the mandibular ramus with no penetrating or exit wound and no signs of external impact (Fig. 21.3). Another interesting finding by Shuker is the transection of teeth at the gingival level, which he relates to the blast wave effect. We also found some teeth fractured in a similar fashion, although it is hard to tell whether the cause was the blast wave, a foreign object hitting the teeth, or the impact of the victim against a stationary object.

The consensus is that the secondary mechanism causes the majority of blast injuries to the maxillofacial area. The improvised bombs carried by suicide terrorists in Israel were not usually large: 5–10 kg. To enhance their effect, many metal objects were added, including bolts, nails, screws, and ball bearings. Propelled by the explosive detonation, these projectiles would hit numerous victims in the vicinity.

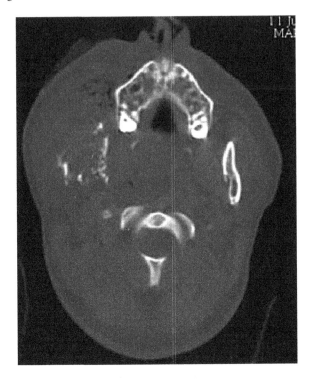

Fig. 21.3. "Burst" fracture of the mandibular ramus in victim of suicide bomb inside bus.

At a velocity of 17 m/s (50 ft/s), skin is easily lacerated and at 133 m/s (400 ft/s), serious wounds are caused by deeper penetration into the body.[42] Depending on the distance from the center of the explosion, the projectiles can penetrate and perforate the hard or soft tissues of the cranio-facial region. These injuries are similar to those caused by pellets from a high-energy shotgun. Like the suicide bomber's projectiles, the gun pellets spread after being shot, with maximum effect close to the muzzle or the center of the explosion. The projectiles can behave as high velocity missiles causing temporary cavitation and indirect damage to adjacent tissues. Koren et al.[14] described indirect VIIth nerve palsy due to a projectile that penetrated the parotid gland, close to the facial nerve.

Figure 21.4 shows foreign bodies located in critical anatomical locations. Figure 21.5 shows the trajectory of a bolt that fractured the mandibular symphysis and penetrated the floor of the mouth. Not all the foreign objects were added to the explosive device; some of them came from other victims or even the terrorist, such as the hand watch in Fig. 21.6 that evidently was torn from someone's wrist by the blast wind (tertiary pattern) and became a projectile.

The blast wind can cause acceleration of the impact of human victims on hard surfaces. Stapczynski[42] concluded that serious injuries should be expected after such an impact from a velocity greater than 5–7 m/s (15–20 ft/s). In addition to

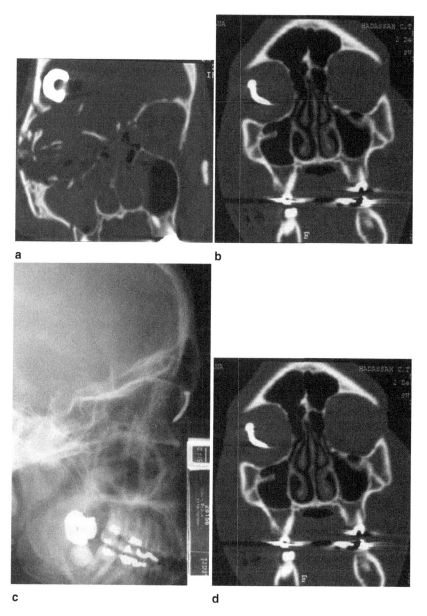

FIG. 21.4. Foreign objects in critical anatomical locations: (A) bolt in the brain after shattering the orbital walls; (B and C) nail in the orbit; (D) metal ball in cervical spine.

the overpressure and wind, the explosion generates a heat wave that is accompanied by fire and gas inhalation. The face, eyes, oral tissues, and upper respiratory system may be seriously affected. Burns of various degrees are encountered, often in combination with other injury patterns. Both the immediate and late effects

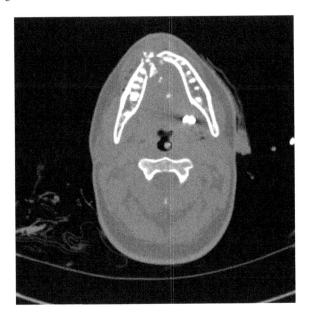

F<small>IG</small>. 21.5. Trajectory of metal bolt that fractured the mandible and penetrated the floor of the mouth.

of the burns call for special attention.[43] One of the difficulties encountered in patients with facial burns is securing the endotracheal tube to the burnt and edematous skin. Our solution for these patients is to secure the tube to the upper teeth (preferably the premolars) with a stainless steel wire.

Treatment

Blast injuries present a full scope of tissue damage and should be treated accordingly. Most patients with maxillofacial injuries suffer from a variety of concomitant injuries such as blast lung, extremity fractures, penetrating wounds, and burns. Therefore, the multidisciplinary treatment should be prioritized, coordinated, and most often staged.

The first priority is life preservation, that is, to secure the airway and gain control of life-threatening hemorrhage. Once the patient is stable from the respiratory and hemodynamic aspects, then the most critical injuries – head, chest, and abdomen – should be attended to.

As mentioned above, maxillofacial injuries are rarely urgent. Nevertheless, early treatment is highly desirable. When feasible, the most definitive treatment should be performed as soon as possible in conjunction with other treatments. If lengthy procedures are contraindicated or the patient is edematous, early maxillofacial intervention should be limited to stabilization of bone segments (e.g., intermaxillary fixation, interosseous or interdental wiring), packing of wounds and sinuses, and closure of soft tissue wounds.

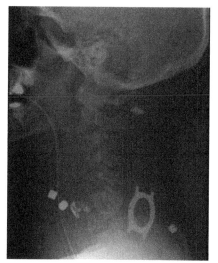
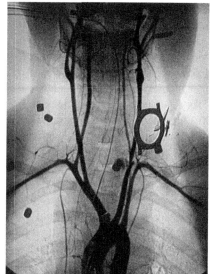
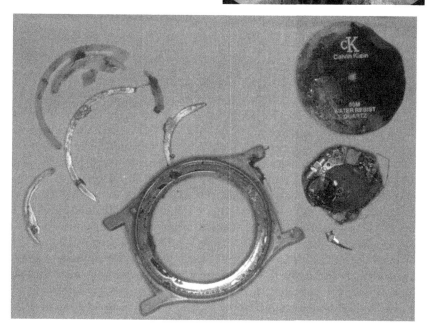

FIG. 21.6. Hand watch and metal balls that penetrated the neck of a victim in a bus explosion; (A) lateral view; (B) angiography with damage to neck vessels; (C) watch fragments after removal. (Part (C) courtesy of Prof. Y. Berlatzky, Hadassah University Hospital).

Since most blast injury victims sustain secondary and tertiary types of injuries, the general principles of oral and maxillofacial surgery treatment should be applied. The treatment of secondary type injuries is similar to the treatment of the three types of gunshot wounds (penetrating, perforating, and avulsive) with the same controversy regarding early and delayed or late reconstruction, although in this case the other injuries may dictate a delayed approach.

As a general rule, for extensive blast injuries, we prefer the more conservative approach. Here the initial treatment includes bone stabilization, usually with intermaxillary fixation, hard and soft tissue preservation, and an attempt to close all the wounds primarily. Because of the excellent vascularity of the head and neck region, supposedly unsalvageable tissue will often be surprisingly viable.

Soft tissue wounds, lacerations, and abrasions may be contaminated with foreign materials, as well as with pieces of human tissue and blood. Thorough and repeated debridement and irrigation with copious amounts of saline should be performed prior to any primary closure attempt. Delayed primary closure may be preferred when the wound margins are too edematous to close. Impacted foreign objects should not be removed unless the risk of leaving them is greater than the risk associated with their removal.

Conclusion

Terrorism-related injuries affect the maxillofacial region to a greater extent than its relative body surface area and more than other causes of trauma. Injuries from blast in particular, often affect several organs and systems and require a multidisciplinary approach. An oral and maxillofacial attending doctor should be on the trauma team and part of the structured protocol in the event of a multi-casualty event. In the pre-hospital and emergency department setting, the immediate concern in maxillofacial injuries is securing the airway and staunching bleeding. After a thorough clinical examination, a complete facial CT scan should be the gold standard adjunct for the diagnosis of maxillofacial injuries.

Of the four types of terrorism injuries recognized here, characteristics of gunshot and stab wounds are similar to those incurred from other civilian injuries. Stones, however, especially those thrown at a moving car, can cause severe facial injuries that may be fatal. Of the four categories of blast injury, mainly the secondary and tertiary types affect the maxillofacial region. But primary blast may also affect the maxillofacial region to some extent. Besides eardrum perforation, fracture of the para-nasal sinuses and splinter fractures of the mandible may result. Because of the nature of multi-casualty events, some maxillofacial injuries may be misdiagnosed or undiagnosed in the primary examination and survey. Therefore, the structured protocol includes secondary survey and debriefing after partial normalization, and tertiary survey the next day.

References

1. Dobson JE, Newell MJ, Shepherd JP. Trends in maxillofacial injuries in war-time (1914–1986). Br J Oral Maxillofac Surg. 1989;27:441–450.
2. Frykberg ER. Medical management of disasters and mass casualties from terrorist bombings: how can we cope? J Trauma. 2002;53:201–212.
3. Adler J, Golan E, Golan J, Yitzhaki M, Ben-Hur N. Terrorist bombing experience during 1975–79. Isr J Med Sci. 1983;19:189–193.
4. Ringler D, Einy S, Giveon A, Goldstein L, Peleg K. Maxillofacial trauma resulting from terror in Israel. J Craniofac Surg. 2007;18(1):62–66.
5. Mintz Y, Shapira SC, Pikarsky AI, Goitein D, Gertcenchtein I, Mor-Yosef S, Rivkind AI. The experience of one institution dealing with terror: the El Aqsa Intifada riots. IMAJ. 2002;4:554–556.
6. Peleg K, Aharonson-Daniel L, Michael M, Shapira SC. Patterns of injury in hospitalized terrorist victims. Am J Emerg Med. 2003;21:258–262.
7. Almogy G, Belzberg H, Mintz Y, Pikarsky AJ, Zamir G, Rivkind AI. Suicide bombing attacks; update and modification to the protocol. Ann Surg. 2004;239:295–303.
8. Einav S, Feigenberg Z, Weissman C, Zaichik D, Caspi G, Kotler D, Freund HR. Evacuation priorities in mass casualty terror-related events; implications for contingency planning. Ann Surg. 2004;239:304–310.
9. Shapira SC, Cole LA. Terror medicine: birth of a discipline. JHSEM. 2006;3:2.
10. Whitlock R. Urban guerilla warfare. In: Rowe NL, Williams JLI, Eds. Maxillofacial Injuries. 1st ed. Churchill Livingstone; 1985:652–682.
11. Holmes S, Coombes A, Rice S, Wilson A. The role of the maxillofacial surgeon in the initial 48 h following a terrorist attack. Br J Oral Maxillofac Surg. 2005;43:375–382.
12. Novelline RA, Rhea JT, Rao PM, Stuk JL. Helical CT in emergency radiology. Radiology. 1999;213:321–339.
13. Shaham D, Sella T, Makori A, Appelbaum L, Rivkind AI, Bar-Ziv J. The role of radiology in terror injuries. IMAJ. 2002;4:564–567.
14. Koren I, Shimonove M, Shvero Y, Feinmesser R. Unusual primary and secondary facial blast injuries. Am J Otolaryngol. 2003;24:75–77.
15. James WV. Riots injuries to policemen: and analysis of 808 policemen injured in rioting between 1969 and 1972 in Northern Ireland. Injury. 1975;7:41–43.
16. Rutherford WH. The injuries of civil disorders. Community Health. 1974;6:14–21.
17. Heering SL, Shohat T, Lerman Y, Danon YL. The epidemiology of injuries sustained by Israeli troops during the unrest in the territories administered by Israel 1987–89. Isr J Med Sci. 1992;28:341–344.
18. Nahlieli O, Baruchin AM, Neder A. Fractures of the mandible caused by stoning – return of and ancient entity. J Trauma. 1993;35(6):939–942.
19. Hanoch J, Feigin E, Pikarsky AJ, Kugel C, Rivkind A. Stab wounds associated with terrorist activities in Israel. JAMA. 1996;276:388–390.
20. Apffelstaedt JP, Müller R. Results of mandatory exploration for penetrating neck trauma. World J Surg. 1994;18:917–920.
21. Hudson DA. Impacted knife injuries of the face. Br J Plast Surg. 1992;45:222–224.
22. Chen AY, Stewart MG, Taup G. Penetrating injuries of the face. Otolaryngol Head Neck Surg. 1996;115:464–470.
23. Scheepers A, Lownie M. The role of angiography in facial trauma: case report. Br J Oral Maxillofac Surg. 1994;32:109–110.

24. Shinohara EH, Heringer L, de Caravalho JP. Impacted knife injuries in the maxillofacial region: report of 2 cases. J Oral Maxillofac Surg. 2001;59:1221–1223.
25. Hollier L, Grantcharova EP, Kattash M. Facial gunshot wounds: a 4 year experience. J Oral Maxillofac Surg. 2001;59:277–282.
26. Powers DB, Robertson OB. Ten common myths of ballistic injuries. Oral Maxillofac Surg Clin N Am. 2005;17:251–259.
27. Peleg K, Aharonson-Daniel L, Stein M, Michaelson M, Kluger Y, Simon D, Noji EK. Gunshot and explosion injuries; characteristics, outcomes, and implications for care of terror-related injuries in Israel. Ann Surg. 2004;239:311–318.
28. Motamedi MHK. Primary treatment of penetrating injuries to the face. J Oral Maxillofac Surg. 2007;65:1215–1218.
29. Ueeck BA. Penetrating injuries to the face: delayed versus primary treatment – considerations for delayed treatment. J Oral Maxillofac Surg. 2007;65:1209–1214.
30. Ellis S. Maxillofacial surgery and the troubles of Northern Ireland. Br Dent J. 1990:411–412.
31. Gibbons AJ, Farrier JN, Key SJ. The pipe bomb: a modern terrorist weapon. J R Army Med Corps. 2003;149:23–26.
32. Rothschild MA, Maxeiner H. Death caused by a letter bomb. Int J Legal Med. 2000;114:103–106.
33. Bamber D. The IRA is teaching Palestinians how to blow up Israelis soldiers in the West Bank. The Daily Telegraph. 2002; April 28.
34. DePalma RG, Burris DG, Champion HR, Hodgson MJ. Blast injuries. N Engl J Med. 2005;352:1335–1342.
35. Kluger Y. Bomb explosions in acts of terrorism – detonation, wound ballistics, triage and medical concerns. IMAJ. 2003;5:235–240.
36. Leibovici D, Gofrit ON, Stein M, Shapira SC, Noga Y, Heruti R, Shemer J. Blast injuries: bus versus open-air bombings – a comparative study of injuries in survivors of open-air versus confined-space explosions. J Trauma. 1996;41:1030–1035.
37. Hadden WA, Rutherford WH, Merrett JD. The injuries of terrorist bombing: a study of 1532 consecutive patients. Br J Surg. 1978;65:525–531.
38. Odhimabo WA, Guthua SW, Macigo FG, Akama MK. Maxillofacial injuries caused by terrorist bomb attack in Nairobi, Kenya. Int J Oral Maxillofac Surg. 2002;31:374–377.
39. Gutierrez de Ceballos JP, Turégano Fuentes F, Perez Diaz D, Sanz Sanchez M, Martin Llorente C, Guerrero Sanz JE. 11 March 2004: The terrorist bomb explosions in Madrid, Spain – an analysis of the logistics, injuries sustained and clinical management of casualties treated at the closest hospital. Crit Care. 2005;9:104–111.
40. Wang Z, Liu Y, Lei D, Bai Z, Zhou S. A new model of blast injury from a spherical explosive and its special wound in the maxillofacial region. Mil Med. 2003;168:330–332.
41. Shuker ST. Maxillofacial blast injuries. J Cranio-Maxillofac Surg. 1995;23:91–98.
42. Stapczynski JS. Blast injuries. Ann Emerg Med. 1982;11:687–694.
43. Bagby SK. Acute management of facial burns. Oral Maxillofac Surg Clin N Am. 2005;17:267–272.

22
Pediatrics and Terrorism

David Markenson

Children have long been known as innocent victims of disasters, public health emergencies, and terrorist attacks. In addition, there is increasing thought being given to the possibility that children could be the primary targets of a group or individual out to undermine morale and destabilize a society. In 2002, for instance, Suleiman Abu Gheith, a senior Al-Qaeda planner, said "We have not reached parity with [the Americans]. We have the right to kill 4 million Americans – 2 million of them children …"* In addition, in 2003 the Singapore government foiled an Al-Qaeda–connected plan to attack the American School (in Singapore) with 3,000 American expatriate children.† And in late 2004 Chechnean terrorists, presumably with Al-Qaeda connections, attacked a strategically unimportant school in Russia.

Terrorism preparedness is a highly specific component of general emergency preparedness. In addition to the unique pediatric issues involved in general emergency preparedness, terrorism preparedness must consider several additional issues, including the unique vulnerabilities of children to various agents, as well as the limited availability of age and weight appropriate antidotes and treatments. While children may respond more rapidly to therapeutic intervention, they are at the same time more susceptible to various agents and conditions and more likely to deteriorate if not carefully monitored. It is imperative to develop, therefore, strategies to protect children from any hazard, including the horrific possibility of an intentional attack on our youngest citizens.

Children have special needs that are not often considered in disaster planning. A determination of the needs of children and planning for their care is essential, including children at home, school, and daycare, in transit, who cannot be reunited with family, or when communication is difficult.

Evaluation of recent natural and man-made disasters has highlighted that there are several categories of potential pediatric victims which can be defined:

---

*Translation of documents seized from Suleiman Abu Gheith and declassified.
†Reported by CNN and Washington Post January 2003 and confirmed by Department of Homeland Security.

S.C. Shapira et al. (eds.), *Essentials of Terror Medicine*,
DOI: 10.1007/978-0-387-09412-0_22, Springer Science+Business Media, LLC 2009

- Primary victims: those children who sustain emergent physical and mental injuries;
- Secondary victims: those children who lost parents, whose access to healthcare and resources such as food, shelter, school, and healthcare was compromised; and
- Tertiary victims: those who saw or heard frequent, graphic, and explicit scenes of the event but were not directly involved in the incident.

It is important to remember that the same public health considerations during disasters which apply to adults are even more important to children due to their increased vulnerability. Examples include the need for maintenance of sanitations and clean water supply. In addition it is important to avoid unnecessary prophylactic antibiotics and vaccines but rather return to normal vaccination schedules and state of the art child care.

Lastly pediatric disaster preparedness includes provision of social services for children. An unfortunate but potential reality is that as a result of a disaster, children may temporarily or permanently loose contact with families. Therefore, during – and following – disasters, it is important to ensure that social service agencies and organizations are available to survivors. Rapid reunification of children with parents, or other appropriate relatives, is an essential goal.

This chapter is designed to provide an overview of key issues with respect to pediatric disaster, terrorism, and public health emergency preparedness. To optimally prepare one needs to become familiar with some key areas of emergency preparedness:

- Unique aspects of children related to terrorism and other disasters
- Emergency, Public Health and Terrorism pediatric preparedness
- Managing family concerns about terrorism and disaster preparedness
- Pediatric hospital preparedness
- Community, government, and public health pediatric preparedness

Unique Aspects of Children Related to Terrorism

Children are uniquely vulnerable to disasters and terrorism events because of anatomic, physiological, and clinical factors, as well as developmental and psychological concerns.[1,2] While children may respond more rapidly to therapeutic intervention, they are at the same time more susceptible to various agents and conditions and more likely to deteriorate if not carefully monitored. The general philosophy of children as victims of disasters, terrorism, and public health emergencies is that

- children are more susceptible to certain injuries or environmental insults than are adults,
- children with acute injuries or illness are more likely to respond to rapid and efficient medical care than do adults, and

- since children are not small adults they require equipment and pharmaceuticals designed for their needs.

Biologic, Chemical, and Radiologic Vulnerabilities

The release of chemical or biological toxins would disproportionately affect children through several mechanisms. For example, because children become dehydrated easily and possess minimal reserve, they are at greater risk than are adults when exposed to agents that may cause diarrhea or vomiting. Agents that might cause only mild symptoms in an adult could lead to hypovolemic shock in an infant.

Another example involves the distinct respiratory physiology of children. Many of the agents used for both chemical and biological attacks are aerosolized (e.g., sarin, chlorine, or anthrax). Because children have faster respiratory rates than do adults, they are exposed to relatively greater dosages and will suffer the effects of these agents much more rapidly than do adults. Children will also potentially absorb more of the substance before it is cleared or diffuses from the respiratory tissues. Many chemical agents, including certain gases such as sarin and chlorine, have a high vapor density and are heavier than air, which means they "settle" close to the ground, in the air space used by children for breathing.

Many biological and chemical agents are absorbed through the skin. Because children have more permeable skin and larger surface area relative to body mass than do adults, they receive proportionally higher doses of agents that either affect the skin or are absorbed through the skin. In addition, because the skin of children is poorly keratinized, vesicants and corrosives result in greater injury to children than to adults. A further concern in children because of their relatively large surface area in relation to body mass is that they lose heat quickly when showered. Consequently, skin decontamination with water may result in hypothermia unless heating lamps and other warming equipment are used.

In addition children may present with different symptoms when exposed to the same agent as adults. An example of such a difference is when children are exposed to nerve agents. While adults usually present with muscarinic symptoms – which are rather typical – children with organophosphate poisoning usually present with rather unspecific central nervous system symptomatology, mainly (hard to control) seizures and coma.

In terms of radiologic exposures, children are also more vulnerable than are adults. First, children have disproportionately higher minute ventilation, leading to greater internal exposure to radioactive gases. Nuclear fallout quickly settles to the ground, resulting in a higher concentration of radioactive material in the space where children live and breathe. Children have a significantly greater risk of developing cancer even when they are exposed to radiation in utero. In addition as radiation has its greatest affects on rapidly growing tissues, children with generally more rapidly developing tissues including bone marrow are particularly vulnerable. Unlike adults, young children's CNS is still developing which makes it susceptible to damage from even low levels of radiation.

Finally, children are particularly vulnerable because of physical developmental limitations. Infants, toddlers, and young children do not have the motor skills to escape from the site of a biological or chemical incident. Even if able to walk, they may not have the cognitive ability to understand the presence of a risk based on a terrorist event and therefore not seek an escape or be able to decide in which direction to flee. Even worse, children may actually migrate toward a disaster event out of curiosity to see the gas, colored agent, or other effects.

Mental Health Vulnerabilities

Disasters and especially terrorist attacks are frightening for adults and can be equally or even more traumatic for children. Feelings of anxiety, sadness, confusion, and fear are all normal reactions. However, if children are anxious, frightened, or confused for long periods of time, it can have devastating long-term emotional effects on their well-being. All children are at risk of psychological injury such as anxiety and post-traumatic stress reactions and disorders from experiencing or living under the threat of chemical or biological terrorism. In addition, their emotional responses are heightened by seeing their parents anxious or overwhelmed. Because children often cannot understand what is happening or the steps being taken to mitigate the event, they will often be even more fearful of the event and also of the potential for future events. In a mass casualty incident, children experience or witness injuries and deaths, possibly of their parents, family, and friends, which would produce both short- and long-term psychological trauma.

How children understand and react to traumatic events such as sudden death, violence, or terrorism is related to age, developmental status, and other factors. A 6-year-old, for example, may react by refusing to separate from parents to attend school. An adolescent, on the other hand, may attempt to hide his or her concern, but become sullen, argumentative, unusually irritable, or show a decline in school performance.

Pre-Hospital and Hospital Pediatric Terrorism Preparedness

Terrorism preparedness presents a unique and specific set of emergency preparedness challenges. In addition to the special pediatric issues involved in general emergency preparedness, terrorism preparedness must consider several additional concerns, including the unique vulnerabilities of children to various agents, as well as the limited availability of age and weight appropriate antidotes and treatments.

Decontamination

Children exposed to biological or chemical agents are likely to require decontamination. Whether or not to use decontamination procedures for asymptomatic individuals after a known or suspected exposure is a decision that must be made before the agent has been identified. Current mass casualty decontamination procedures

TABLE 22.1. Specific Questions One Must Address with Regard to Pediatric Decontamination

Is the water pressure appropriate?
Will it injure a child?
Is the water temperature acceptable?
If water is not warm: may cause hypothermia
Can it handle the nonambulatory child?
Infants, toddlers
Children with special healthcare needs
Does the method and equipment used allow decontamination of a child with a parent or caregiver?
Have mental health concerns been addressed?
Will children follow instructions?
Long-term effects

designed for adults are risky for children. Because children have a higher surface area and a more difficult time with temperature regulation, decontamination with room temperature, or colder water can lead to dangerous hypothermia. Although hypothermia may be a risk, it is less risky than not decontaminating a patient. Young children may be unable to understand the concepts of decontamination and will be unable to comprehend why they must be separated from their family and asked to strip down with strangers. Lastly, ensure that there is clothing for children to be dressed in after decontamination. This includes diapers.

Many shower systems are not suitable for children, who require systems that use warm water and are high-volume but low-pressure. Shower decontamination units designed mostly for young children and infants also must be able to accommodate an adult (parent or caretaker) as well as the child (Table 22.1).

Biological Agent Exposure and the Pediatric Patient

Children may be particularly vulnerable to aerosolized biological weapons because they breathe more times per minute than do adults. As a result, they would get a relatively larger dose of the substance than would an adult in the same period of time. They are also more vulnerable to the biological agents that act through the skin because their skin is thinner, and they will receive a higher exposure because they have a larger surface-to-mass ratio than do adults.

Children are also more vulnerable to the effects of biological agents that produce vomiting and diarrhea because they have less fluid reserves than do adults. This makes them more susceptible to dehydration and shock. They also have less circulating blood volume reserves than do adults, and would be potentially more at risk for hemorrhagic shock than would an adult exposed to viral hemorrhagic fever (VHF).

In addition, children have shorter incubation periods for some of the biological agents. As such, they will become symptomatic earlier, but this also presents a window of opportunity for surveillance systems. They can also present with different symptoms than do an adult.

Anthrax

Signs and Symptoms

Anthrax infection can occur in three forms: cutaneous, inhalational, and gastrointestinal. The symptomology and presentation of these forms is similar in children to adults. The one exception is the less frequent occurrence of inhalational anthrax and a higher incidence of the cutaneous form.

Treatment

In the field, treatment should be supportive. Treatment includes the use of antibiotics. Certain antibiotics are not recommended as first choice drugs in children because of adverse affects; these concerns may be outweighed by the need for early treatment of children exposed to *B. anthracis* after an exposure. Levofloxacin was licensed by the Food and Drug Administration (FDA) for the postexposure treatment/prophylaxis of inhalational anthrax. An oral solution (25 mg/ml) was licensed at that time, along with tablets and an injectable form, although the drug was not specifically given a pediatric indication and no dosing recommendations have been put forth. Nonetheless, in an effort to give clinicians as many options as possible, by extrapolating from available data the recommended dosage is 10–15 mg/kg every 24 hours (Table 22.2).

At this time, anthrax vaccine is not recommended for children younger than 18 years of age but may still be indicated after a bona fide exposure based on assessment of the benefit versus the lack of indication. Consult with the Centers for Disease Control and Prevention (CDC) for current recommended treatments.

Plague

Signs and Symptoms

In the United States, it is usually a rural disease. House cats are also susceptible to plague. Infected cats become sick and may directly transmit plague to persons who handle or care for them. Dogs and cats may also bring plague-infected fleas into the home. Inhaling droplets expelled by the coughing of a plague-infected person or animal (especially house cats) can result in plague of the lungs (plague pneumonia). Presentation of pediatric index cases in an urban setting or outside the normal geographic or seasonal distribution should be reported by medical providers.

Treatment

Treatment options in children include primarily doxycycline or tetracycline (>8 years old).

Tularemia

There are at least nine species of domestic animals including cats that harbor tularemia and could be subjects of vector transmission by ticks, deerflies, and mosquitoes to children.

TABLE 22.2. Recommended Therapy and Prophylaxis of Anthrax

Form of anthrax	Category of treatment (therapy or prophylaxis)	Agent and dosage
Inhalation	Therapy[a]	Ciprofloxacin[b] 10–15 mg/kg IV q 12 h (max 400 mg/dose) *or* Levofloxacin 10–15 mg/kg IV q 24 h *or* Doxycycline 2.2 mg/kg IV (max 100 mg) q 12 h and Clindamycin[c] 10–15 mg/kg IV q 8 h *and* Penicillin G[e] 400–600 k u/kg/d IV divided q 4 h Patients who are clinically stable after 14 days can be switched to a single oral agent (ciprofloxacin *or* doxycycline) to complete a 60-day course[d] of therapy.
Inhalation	Postexposure prophylaxis (60-day course[d])	Ciprofloxacin[f] 10–15 mg/kg PO (max 500 mg/dose) q 12 h *or* Levofloxacin 10–15 mg/kg IV q 24 h *or* Doxcycline 2.2 mg/kg (max 100 mg) PO q 12 h
Cutaneous, endemic	Therapy[g]	Penicillin V 40–80 mg/kg/d PO divided q 6 h *or* Amoxicillin 40–80 mg/kg/d PO divided q 8 h *or* Ciprofloxacin 10–15 mg/kg PO (max 1 g/d) q 12 h *or* Levofloxacin 10–15 mg/kg IV q 24 h *or* Doxycycline 2.2 mg/kg PO (max 100 mg) q 12 h
Cutaneous (in setting of terrorism)	Therapy[a]	Ciprofloxacin 10–15 mg/kg PO (max 1 g/d) q 12 h *or* Levofloxacin 10–15 mg/kg IV q 24 h Doxycycline 2.2 mg/kg PO (max 100 mg) q 12 h
Gastrointestinal	Therapy[a]	Same as for inhalational

From Markenson.[3] This table was created from recommendations developed at the Consensus Conference and in part is based on reviewed reference materials from the American Academy of Pediatrics (AAP), CDC, FDA, and Infectious Disease Society of America.

[a] In a mass casualty setting, in which resources are severely limited, oral therapy may need to be substituted for the preferred parenteral option.

[b] Ofloxacin (and possibly other quinolones) may be acceptable alternatives to ciprofloxacin or levofloxacin.

[c] Rifampin or clarithromycin may be acceptable alternatives to clindamycin as drugs that target bacterial protein synthesis.

[d] Assuming the organism is sensitive, children may be switched to oral amoxicillin (40–80 mg/kg/d divided q 8 h) to complete a 60-day course. We recommend that the first 14 days of therapy or postexposure prophylaxis, however, include ciprofloxacin or levofloxacin and/or doxycycline regardless of age.

[e] Ampicillin, imipenem, meropenem, or chloramphenicol may be acceptable alternatives to penicillin as drugs with good CNS penetration.

[f] According to most experts, ciprofloxacin is the preferred agent for oral prophylaxis.

[g] Ten days of therapy may be adequate for endemic cutaneous disease. We recommend a full 60-day course in the setting of terrorism, however, because of the possibility of concomitant inhalational exposure.

Treatment

In children, the same regimen of antibiotics is used in the treatment of tularemia as is used in the treatment of plague.

TABLE 22.3. Differentiating Smallpox from Chicken Pox

Smallpox	Chicken pox
All lesions in the same stage	Lesions appear in crops in different stages (papules, vesicles, crusted lesions)
Palms and soles involved	Palms and soles rarely involved
Patient appearing moribund or toxic	Patients rarely toxic or moribund
Increased concentration of lesions on face and extremities (centrifugal distribution)	Greatest concentration on face and trunk with relative sparing of the extremities
Lesions develop into pustules that are deeply imbedded in the dermis	Vesicles which are relatively superficial
Significant prodrome	Mild or no prodrome

Smallpox

The greatest difficulty for a medical provider approaching a potential pediatric smallpox victim may be in differentiating smallpox from the common childhood illness of chickenpox. Differences between the rash of smallpox and chickenpox are listed in Table 22.3.

The currently licensed smallpox vaccine makes no mention in its package insert of an approved age range. In practice, until the early 1970s, this vaccine was administered to 1-year-olds. The CDC currently recommends against vaccination of children younger than 1 year. All contraindications to smallpox vaccination are relative. After bona fide exposure or known usage of weaponized smallpox, even the youngest exposed, at-risk infants should be vaccinated. Moreover, future studies of new generation vaccines must include children.

Viral Hemorrhagic Fever

The term VHF describes a syndrome that can occur as a result of a diverse group of diseases including Ebola, Marburg, yellow fever, Rift Valley Fever, and Crimean-Congo hemorrhagic fever. These viruses are contagious, and may be spread through direct contact with body fluids or inhalation of aerosolized droplets. Use of standard body substance isolation precautions have proven to be very effective in protecting healthcare workers from infection.

Signs and Symptoms

The progression and presentation of signs and symptoms will vary depending upon the specific infecting agent. These signs and symptoms may include high fever, chills, headache, weakness, myalgia, nonbloody diarrhea, conjunctival hemorrhage, pharyngitis, epistaxis, hematemesis, hetaturia, bloody stools, petechial hemorrhages, hypotension, bleeding from mucous membranes, and possibly CNS and pulmonary effects. Progression may be similar in children or more rapid.

Treatment

Care is primarily supportive in nature, and may include fluid or vasopressor administration. Avoidance of intramuscular (IM) injections, aspirin, and other medications that could potentially inhibit coagulation is commonly recommended. Patient isolation and strict infection control precautions are needed. Some of the viral hemorrhagic viruses may respond to anti-viral agents such as ribavirin, although data regarding this is limited.

Toxins

Botulism

About 120 children in the United States get botulism each year. Approximately 90 of those victims are infants who obtained *C. botulinum* spores from honey. Symptoms of botulism in adults and children usually begin within 18–36 h of eating the contaminated food. However, symptoms can occur as early as 6 h after eating food or as long as 10 days later.

Treatment

A licensed trivalent (types A, B, E) antitoxin is available through the CDC. This antitoxin is to be used in children of any age known to have been exposed to botulinum toxin of the appropriate serotypes. Licensed pentavalent (types A–E) Botulism Immune Globulin (BabyBIG®) was licensed by the FDA on October 23, 2003. Although licensed specifically for use in infant botulism due to Toxin Types A and B, it may have a role in the treatment of bioterrorism victims resulting from exposures to these Toxin Types, as well as to Toxin Types C, D, and E. Antitoxin and/or Botulism Immune Globulin may halt progression of symptoms, but are unlikely to reverse them.

Ricin

Ricin is a protein derived from the castor bean plant, which can be ground into a powder for inhalation, ingestion, or injection. Children can be exposed to toxic amounts of ricin by eating or chewing on castor beans. Severe crampy diarrhea along with nausea, vomiting, CNS depression, shock, and seizures may occur. In children these symptoms may progress quickly and life-threatening effects can be seen immediately. Benzodiazepines are the drugs of choice for seizures and are widely used. Hemolytic anemia and renal failure may develop.

Treatment

Children are managed with supportive therapy (keep patient comfortable, fluids, oxygen, and pain medications), and gut decontamination with activated charcoal is utilized with ricin ingestion (Table 22.4).

TABLE 22.4. Recommended Therapy and Prophylaxis in Children for Additional Select Diseases Associated with Bioterrorism

Disease	Therapy or prophylaxis	Treatment,[a] agent, and dosage
Smallpox	Therapy	Supportive care
	Prophylaxis	Vaccination may be effective if given within the first several days after exposure.
Plague	Therapy	Gentamicin 2.5 mg/kg IV q 8 h *or* Streptomycin 15 mg/kg IM q 12 h (max 2 g/d, although only available for compassionate usage and in limited supply) *or* Doxycycline 2.2 mg/kg IV q 12 h (max 200 mg/d) *or* Ciprofloxacin[b] 15 mg/kg IV q 12 h *or* Levofloxacin 10–15 mg/kg IV q 24 h *or* Chloramphenicol[c] 25 m/kg 6q h (max 4 g/d)
	Prophylaxis	Doxycycline 2.2 mg/kg PO q 12 h *or* Ciprofloxacin[b] 20 mg/kg PO q 12 h
Tularemia	Therapy	Same as for plague
Botulism	Therapy	Supportive care, antitoxin and/or botulism immune globulin may halt progression of symptoms but are unlikely to reverse them
Viral hemorrhagic fevers	Therapy	Supportive care, ribavirin may be beneficial in select cases[d]
Brucellosis	Therapy[e]	TMP/SMX 30 mg/kg PO q 12 h and rifampin 15 mg/kg q 24 h or gentamicin 7.5 mg/kg IM q d × 5

From Markenson.[3] This table was created from recommendations developed at the Consensus Conference and in part is based on reviewed reference materials from the AAP, CDC, and Infectious Disease Society of America.

[a] In a mass casualty setting, parenteral therapy might not be possible. In such cases, oral therapy (with analogous agents) may need to be used.

[b] Ofloxacin (and possibly other quinolones) may be acceptable alternatives to ciprofloxacin or levofloxacin; however, they are not approved for use in children.

[c] Concentration should be maintained between 5 and 20 μg/ml. Some experts have recommended that chloramphenicol be used to treat patients with plague meningitis, because chloramphenicol penetrates the blood–brain barrier. Use in children younger than 2 years may be associated with adverse reactions but might be warranted for serious infections.

[d] Ribavirin is recommended for arenavirus or bunyavirus infections, and may be indicated for a viral hemorrhagic fever of an unknown etiology although not FDA approved for these indications. For intravenous therapy use a loading dose: 30 kg IV once (max dose, 2 g), then 16 mg/kg IV q 6 h for 4 days (max dose, 1 g) and then 8 mg/kg IV q 8 h for 6 days (max dose, 500 mg). In a mass casualty setting, it may be necessary to use oral therapy. For oral therapy, use a loading dose of 30 mg/kg PO once, then 15 mg/kg/d PO in two divided doses for 10 days.

[e] For children younger than 8 years. For children older than 8 years, adult regimens are recommended. Oral drugs should be given for 6 weeks. Gentamicin, if used, should be given for the first 5 days of a 6-week course of TMP/SMX (trimethoprim/sulfamethoxazole).

Chemical Agent Exposure and the Pediatric Patient

Classes of chemical agents that have been used or are considered likely candidates for use in a chemical release are listed in Table 22.8 with examples of each class and possible pediatric antidotes and treatments if available.

The availability of adequate antidotes and treatments for children is also problematic. Most treatments and antidotes were developed for military personnel (i.e., adults) who might be victims. Most of these agents have never been tested on children. Although there is ongoing development of new and improved antidotes and treatments to better protect our military and adult population, there is no parallel process in place for developing appropriate agents for use in children.

Pulmonary Agents

Signs and Symptoms

Pulmonary (choking) agents, such as phosgene and chlorine, will have very similar effects in children except that a child may become ill and more symptomatic at a lower exposure. The difference in respiratory anatomy in young children can lead to unexpected upper airway obstruction. Acute signs of exposure will include tearing, eye irritation, respiratory difficulties, wheezing, and stridor with upper airway obstruction. Lower airway effects may be delayed up to 24 h after exposure and nonverbal children may show inappropriate tachypnea and wheezing.

Treatment

Appropriate airway management should include high-flow oxygen via a nonrebreather face mask. Early endotracheal intubation and positive-pressure ventilation may be needed for the patient with depressed airway reflexes and signs of airway narrowing (stridor). Children with bronchospasm can be treated with β2 inhaled agents such as albuterol. Children with stridor may benefit from inhaled epinephrine.

Phosgene Oxime

Phosgene oxime acts as an irritant and produces erythema, itching, and wheals. It causes immediate pain. The skin will blanch and then become rapidly reddened. Eyes will have immediate pain. Nausea and vomiting signify systemic effects.

Treatment of Phosgene Oxime

Phosgene oxide is treated in the same manner as mustard and carries the same problems with children.

Blood Agents

Signs and Symptoms

Inhaled cyanide is a rapidly intoxicating agent. The pediatric population, with their increased metabolic rate, will probably succumb to exposure at lower concentrations. Children may initially show hyperexcitability and tachypnea without cyanosis. Verbal children may complain of headache and nausea. Where ambient concentrations are high, there may be rapid unconsciousness and seizures followed by apnea and death.

Treatment

Initial pre-hospital intervention is unchanged from adult therapy with removal of the child from exposure and placement in a clean atmosphere. The child should receive 100% oxygen by face mask. Use of the cyanide antidote kit is problematic. Although the kit may be lifesaving, the adult dosing of the various agents may be toxic in the child. The pharmacology of the antidote kit is to induce methemoglobinemia with amyl nitrite and sodium nitrite, then enhance cyanide elimination with sodium thiosulfate. The iron moiety in methemoglobin binds cyanide more avidly than the iron in hemoglobin or in the cytochromes. The resultant cyanomethemoglobin then complexes with sodium thiosulfate to form sodium thiocyanate which is eliminated in the urine. However, if the level of induced methemoglobin is too high, then the antidote itself will prevent oxygen utilization by cells and cause toxicity. The amount of sodium nitrite used is weight- and hemoglobin-dependent. Consider use of a lower dose for suspected anemia. Young infants (2 months of age) have a physiologic anemia and require a lower dose of sodium nitrite than their weight would suggest. The same would go for any child with anemia or a condition which would predispose them to lowered hemoglobin levels such as sickle cell anemia. Sodium thiosulfate dosing is also weight-dependent but less critical. Sodium bicarbonate IV at 1 mEquiv./kg can be used to treat metabolic acidosis (Table 22.5).

Blister Agents

Signs and Symptoms

Blister agents include mustard, lewisite, and phosgene oxime. All three are similar and can be addressed together although the literature is limited in children.

Children have thinner, more permeable skin, and an increased surface to mass ratio and because of this, will be much more sensitive to the effects of these blister-

TABLE 22.5. Cyanide Antidote Kit

Sodium nitrate 3% IV to maximum 10 ml	Estimated Hb in g/dl for average child
0.27 ml/kg	10
0.33 ml/kg	12
0.39 ml/kg	14
Sodium thiosulfate 25% IV to maximum 50 ml	
1.65 ml/kg	

From Markenson.[3]

ing agents. As with adults, ambient temperature will influence onset and severity of symptoms with more rapid onset in warmer temperatures. High humidity will worsen severity and blistering will tend to be more prominent in the skin folds and damp areas. The perineum has much thinner skin and, in young children, is frequently damp and enclosed by diapers. This is an area where greater damage may occur. Young children may worsen ocular and facial damage by rubbing their eyes and inadvertently spreading these agents to previously unaffected areas.

Mustard

Mustard agents damage DNA in cells. They do their damage immediately, although onset of symptoms may be delayed for several hours. Initial signs and symptoms will include skin reddening similar to a bad sunburn. This skin will eventually blister. Eyes may itch or burn and redden. Children may cough or complain of difficulty breathing or swallowing and nonverbal children may be inconsolable. Noncardiogenic pulmonary edema may cause a persistent cough and hypoxemia. The faster the onset of signs and symptoms, the worse the prognosis will be, and the more severe the exposure. Nausea and diarrhea are symptoms of significant systemic exposure, and put the child at enhanced risk of dehydration, hypovolemia, and circulatory collapse.

Treatment of Mustard Agents

Treatment of mustard exposure is supportive. The skin needs to be decontaminated to limit further damage. Damage occurs immediately, but delayed irrigation may help symptomatically, as well as prevent further contamination by the child and healthcare worker. The pediatric patient with mustard burns, followed by irrigation, will be at significant risk for hypothermia and should be immediately dried and placed in a warm environment. The blisters are quite fragile and should be protected with warm, dry dressings. Eyes should be irrigated profusely and eyelids should be dressed with a water soluble lubricant to prevent the lids from adhering and healing together. Oxygen is necessary for respiratory difficulty and endotracheal intubation is indicated for respiratory failure. Fluid replacement should be what is used for thermal burns. Analgesia should not be forgotten, and if the respiratory status permits, doses of opioids may be needed.

Nerve Agents

Signs and Symptoms

There is almost no information about pediatric exposure to nerve agents. There is, however, a large body of literature on pediatric exposure to organophosphorus pesticides. Children are more sensitive to equivalent doses of pesticides and have increased absorption through their thinner skin. Because of the child's baseline increased respiratory rate, a child may become symptomatic prior to adults with the same exposure. In addition due to their more rapid respiratory rate and increased minute ventilation they may receive a proportionally larger dose than do adults with a similar exposure. Since these agents are heavier than air, children may be the first to show any signs and symptoms since they are closer to the ground. Altered mental status and seizures may present early in the child due to the immature blood–brain barrier and hypersensitivity of CNS receptors. Because hepatic enzyme systems are more immature in young children, they are more symptomatic and less likely to have endogenous ways to detoxify these agents.

In the child, these effects will lead to various complaints. Eye exposure will cause blurred vision, tearing, and small pupils. Inhaling nerve agents can cause difficulty breathing, wheezing, fluid in the lungs with rales and rhonchi, and cyanosis. The secreting glands will be hyperactive with tearing, sweating, runny nose, drooling, lung secretions, cough, vomiting, diarrhea, and urinary incontinence. If the child is still in diapers, the urinary and fecal incontinence is continual. The child will be weak, possibly floppy, have trouble breathing, may twitch or have fasciculations, and may seize and die.

Treatment

Treatment should be immediate, because once these nerve agents bind to the acetylcholinesterase, the acetylcholinesterase *ages* and eventually becomes irreversible until new enzyme is formed. Clothing may harbor nerve agent and off-gas into the environment, further poisoning the child or caregiver.

Symptomatic children should receive 100% oxygen via a nonrebreather face mask. Other than supportive therapy, as with the adult patient the goal of treatment is to block the effects to acetylcholine excess and regenerate the inactivated enzyme. Atropine will block the effects of acetylcholine at the postsynaptic nerve, but will only work for those effects which are muscarinic. It will not affect seizures, muscle weakness, fasciculations, or respiratory failure (nicotinic effects). Pralidoxime or 2-PAM chloride will regenerate the acetylcholinesterase and improve both nicotinic and muscarinic signs. Benzodiazepines have been shown to reduce seizures and the secondary brain structural damage that may result from poisoning. In a mass casualty situation, these medications will need to be given rapidly to a large number of people, so the IM route will be the predominate route of administration (Table 22.6).

Each Mark-1 kit contains two autoinjectors (0.8 in. needle insertion depth), one each of atropine 2 mg (0.7 ml) and pralidoxime 600 mg (2 ml), to be administered in two separate IM sites. DuoDote provides the same medications, atropine 2.1 mg (0.7 ml) and pralidoxime 600 mg (2 ml), but as a single Autoinjector with the need for only one IM injection; while not approved for pediatric use, they should be used as initial treatment in circumstances for children with severe, life-threatening nerve agent toxicity for whom IV treatment is not possible or available or for whom more precise IM (mg/kg) dosing would be logistically impossible (especially pre-hospital). Suggested dosing guidelines are offered; note potential

TABLE 22.6. Pediatric Dosing for Nerve Agent Antidotes

Drug	Dosing
Atropine	0.05–0.1 mg/kg ETT, IV, or IM repeated every 2–5 min as necessary
Pralidoxime	25–50 mg/kg IV or IM repeated in 1 h
Diazepam	0.05–03 mg/kg IV to a max of 10 mg/dose
	0.3–0.5 mg/kg PR to a max of 20 mg/dose

From Markenson.[3]
Other benzodiazepines such as lorazepam (0.1 mg/kg maximum 4 mg/dose) or midazolam (0.1–0.2 mg/kg maximum 10 mg/dose) may be used IM or IV.

TABLE 22.7. Autoinjector Usage

Approximate age	Approximate weight	Number of autoinjectors (each type)	Atropine dosage range (mg/kg)	Pralidoxime dosage range (mg/kg)
3–7 years	13–25 kg	1	0.08–0.13	24–46
8–14 years	26–50 kg	2	0.08–0.13	24–46
>14 years	>51 kg	3	0.11 or less	35 or less

From Markenson.[3]
This table lists usage of the Mark-1 kit or DuoDote only down to age 3 years based on adherence to recommended dosages for atropine and pralidoxime. However, if an adult Mark-1 kit or DuoDote is the only available source of atropine and pralidoxime after a bona fide nerve agent exposure, it should be administered to even the youngest child.

excess of initial atropine and pralidoxime dosage for age/weight, although within general guidelines for recommended total over first 60–90 minutes of therapy for severe exposures.

Based on the above doses, one can use the Mark 1 kit or DuoDote for children as young as 3 years and still be within the dosing guidelines (Table 22.6). In addition, research has shown that side effects from higher dosages are mostly theoretical and are rarely seen, with the exception of tachycardia. Thus the potential benefit after bona fide exposure for treatment and operational ability by using the Mark 1 kit and DuoDote for all ages of children far outweigh the risks.

When using adult autoinjectors, appropriate atropine and pralidoxime dosing for children may be estimated as follows. Recently the FDA has approved Atropine Autoinjectors in pediatric dosages. If pediatric autoinjectors are available and it is operationally practical, the standard 2.0 mg atropine in a Mark-I kit may be replaced with a pediatric atropine autoinjector or the pediatric atropine autoinjector may be combined with a pralidoxime autoinjector. With this approach use the table below to determine the number of pralidoxime autoinjectors. This approach is not possible with DuoDote as this is provided as a single unit with both medications (Table 22.7).

Children presenting without symptoms and exposure to aerosols, vapor, or gas can be watched for 4–6 hours, they may be discharged home with their guardian (Table 22.8).

Table 22.8. Recommended treatment and management of chemical agents used in terrorism

Agent	Toxicity	Clinical findings	Onset	Decontamination[a]	Management
Nerve agents					
Tabun, Sarin, Soman, VX	Anticholinesterase: muscarinic, nicotinic, and CNS effects	Vapor: miosis, rhinor-rhea, dyspnea	Vapor: seconds	Vapor: fresh air, remove clothes, wash hair	ABCs Atropineb,c,d: 0.05 mg/kg IV, IM (min 0.1mg, max 5 mg), repeat q2-5 min prn for marked secretions, bronchospasm
		Liquid: Diaphoresis, Vomiting Both: coma, paralysis, seizures, apnea	Liquid: minutes to hours	Liquid: remove clothes, copious washing of skin and hair with soap and water, ocular irrigation	Pralidoximee: 25 mg/kg IV, IM (max 1 g IV; 2 g IM), may repeat within 30-60 min prn, then again q1hr for 1 or 2 doses prn for persistent weakness, high atropine requirement Diazepam: 0.3 mg/kg (max 10 mg) IV; Lorazepam: 0.1 mg/kg IV, IM (max 4 mg); Midazolam: 0.2 mg/kg (max 10 mg) IM prn seizures, or severe exposure
Vesicants					
Mustard	Alkylation	Skin: erythema, vesicles Eye: inflammation Respiratory tract: inflammation, respiratory distress, acute respiratory distress syndrome	Hours	Skin: soap and water Eyes: irrigation (water) Both: major impact only if done within minutes of exposure	Symptomatic care
Lewisite	Arsenical		Immediate pain		Possibly British anti-lewisite (BAL) 3 mg/kg IM q 4–6h for systemic effects of lewisite in severe cases
Pulmonary agents					
Chlorine, phosgene	Liberate HCl, alkylation	Eyes, nose, throat, irritation (especially chlorine)	Minutes	Fresh air Skin: water	Symptomatic care
		Bronchospasm, pulmonary edema (especially phosgene)	Bronchospasm: minutes; pulmonary edema: hours		

Cyanide	Cytochrome oxidase inhibition: cellular anoxia, lactic acidosis	Tachypnea, coma, seizures, apnea	Seconds	Fresh air Skin: soap and water	Airways, breathing, circulatory support; 100% oxygen Sodium bicarbonate prn for metabolic acidosis Sodium nitrite (3%): Dosage (mL/kg) Estimated Hgb (g/dL) For average child 0.27 10 0.33 12 0.39 14 Max 10 mL Sodium thiosulfate (25%) 1.65 mL/kg (max 50 mL)

RIOT control agents

CS, CN (Mace®) capsaicin (pepper spray)	Neuropeptide substance P release, alkylation	Eye: tearing, pain, blepharospasm Nose and throat irritation Pulmonary failure (rare)	Seconds	Fresh air Eye: lavage	Ophthalmics topically, symptomatic care

[a]Decontamination, especially for patients with significant nerve agent or vesicant exposure, should be performed by healthcare providers garbed in adequate personal protective equipment. For emergency department staff, this consists of nonencapsulated, chemically resistant body suit, boots, and gloves with a full-face air purifier mask/hood.

[b]Intraosseous route is likely equivalent to intravenous.

[c]Atropine might have some benefit via endotracheal tube or inhalation, as might aerosolized ipratropium.

(continued)

TABLE 22.8. (continued)

[d] As of September 2004, the FDA has approved pediatric autoinjectors of atropine in 0.25, 0.5, and 1 mg sizes. Recommendations are:

Approximate age	Approximate weight	Autoinjector size
<6 months	<15 lb	0.25 mg
6 months to 4 years	15–40 lb	0.5 mg
5–10 years	41–90 lb	1 mg
>10 years	>90 lb	2 mg (adult size)

[e] Pralidoxime is reconstituted to 50 mg/mL (1 g in 20 mL water) for IV administration, and the total dose infused over 30 minutes, or may be given by continuous infusion (loading dose 25 mg/kg over 30 minutes then 10 mg/kg/hr). For IM use, it might be diluted to a concentration of 300 mg/mL (1 g added to 3 mL water—by analogy to the US Army's Mark-1 autoinjector concentration), to effect a reasonable volume for injection. Pediatric autoinjectors of pralidoxime are not FDA approved or available.

Key: ABCs = airway, breathing and circulatory support; BAL= British Anti-Lewisite; Hgb= hemoglobin concentration; est.= estimated hemoglobin concentration; max = maximum; min = minimum; prn = as needed.

From Markenson, D. Pediatric Emergency Preparedness for Natural Disasters, Terrorism and Public Health Emergencies: A National Consensus Conference. Executive Summary and Final Report 2007.

This table was created from recommendations developed at the Consensus Conference and in part is based on reviewed reference materials from the American Academy of Pediatrics, Centers for Disease Control, FDA and adapted from Henretig FM, Cieslak TJ, Eitzen EM Jr. J Pediatr 2002; 141:311-326. Reprinted with permission from Elsevier.

Radiation Exposure and the Pediatric Patient

Radiation provokes a special fear, but with appropriate understanding and preparation, effective medical care can be provided to exposed victims. To decrease morbidity and mortality from a radiation disaster or terrorist attack, providers should have a basic understanding of radiation illness and treatment principles and how these apply to the pediatric patient.

The optimal management of the child who has sustained significant radiation exposure depends on the following:

- Knowledge of the type and dose of radiation received as well as the presence of concomitant injuries
- Recognition of the manifestations of radiation sickness
- Use of standard medical care
- Decontamination
- Decorporation techniques (removal of contaminated areas)

The first phase of managing pediatric radiation victims is to determine whether topical decontamination is warranted. Simple removal of clothing is responsible for more than 90% of effective decontamination after a chemical or radiation exposure. Initial medical management includes careful assessment of airway, breathing, and circulation, particularly when there is the potential for blast or thermal injury. It is important to remember that most injuries caused by radiologic terrorism will be associated with a blast. Although decontamination is key, most initial therapy will be that of standard trauma management. If warranted, surgical intervention should be performed as soon as possible, ideally within 48 h of irradiation, before wound healing and immunity become impaired. Life saving treatment such as control of hemorrhaging should be administered immediately.

Signs and Symptoms

The signs and symptoms of acute radiation injury in the pediatric population are the same as the adult population and include damage to the gastrointestinal and nervous systems. In general, while the signs and symptoms are the same, the severity of injury in the child may be greater due to their more rapidly replicating tissues. Symptoms in the gastrointestinal system are regularly seen at acute doses greater than 600 rad and result from damage to the epithelial cells lining the intestinal tract. The higher the exposure, the sooner the symptoms of nausea and vomiting develop. Be mindful that even at lower doses (such as 100 rad) nausea and vomiting may be problematic for the pediatric patient because of lower fluid reserves. The presence of these symptoms typically overlaps with the dropping cell count described previously. As a result, sepsis and opportunistic infections complicate the picture. Persistently high fevers and bloody diarrhea despite adequate fluid and electrolyte replacement are ominous signs.

CNS symptoms are seen with acute radiation doses in excess of 1,000 rad, and are probably due to diffuse microvascular leaks within the brain. Damage to these blood vessels results in the loss of fluids and electrolytes. The patient rarely lives long enough to suffer any hematological or gastrointestinal symptoms. There is also an associated cardiovascular collapse with shock in this kind of patient. One unique aspect in the small child and infant is that CNS symptoms may occur sooner and at lower doses than in the adult. This is because the CNS continues to develop until ~2 years of age, including new cell formation.

Long-term consequences and published epidemiologic studies of children exposed to radiation demonstrate that children have a higher susceptibility to cancers than do adults for the same dose of exposure. This is logical since the life expectancy of a child is longer than that for an adult; therefore, a longer time period exists to manifest the cancers seen from radiation exposure. The typical cancers include thyroid and breast cancer and leukemia. These studies include children from the Hiroshima and Nagasaki atomic bombings, the Chernobyl nuclear reactor accident, and atomic bomb testing fallout from the Bikini Islands. The fact that children have higher respiratory rates and live closer to the ground (where radioactive particles may settle) increases their exposure rate when compared to adults.

Treatment

Decontamination for external contaminants should be performed. Airway, breathing, and circulation should be addressed as soon as safely possible. The remainder of care for the radiation-injured child is supportive. The use of antidotes should only be performed in consultation with a specialist familiar with the clinical management of radiation-exposed patients. If there is an anticipated need for surgery (such as injuries from a blast), the operation should be conducted within 48 hours of exposure to reduce the effects of radiation on wound healing and immunity.

There are a multitude of agents which could be used in a radiologic event. Table 22.9 provides a summary of the most likely radiologic agents, their absorption, symptoms, and treatments.

One of the agents used in radiological exposure is potassium iodide following radioiodine exposure. In the past pediatric dosing was difficult due to only an adult preparation being available. Despite this there are dosages for potassium iodide in children and directions for the creation of these dosages from the adult preparations. Recently, the FDA approved a liquid pediatric preparation of KI (ThyroShield™), containing 65 mg of KI per ml. Given this, the liquid preparation should be made widely available and should become the preferred dosing form for young children and the adaptation of the adult preparation in cases where the liquid preparation is not available. If the liquid preparation is not available below are instructions for converting tablets into solution for administration (Tables 22.10–22.12).

Another agent used in certain radiologic exposures is Prussian Blue (Radiogardase®) which was approved by the FDA in 2003 (as 500 mg capsules) for the treatment of internal ^{137}Cs contamination. While treatment is not "time-critical,"

TABLE 22.9. Radionuclides Produced after Radiologic Terrorism or Disaster, Internal Contamination, Toxicity, and Treatment

Element	Respiratory absorption	GI absorption	Skin wound absorption	Primary toxicity	Treatment
Americium	75%	Minimal	Rapid	Skeletal deposition, marrow suppression, hepatic deposition	Chelation with DTPA or EDTA
Cesium	Complete	Complete	Complete	Whole body irradiation	Prussian Blue
Cobalt	High	<5%	Unknown	Whole body irradiation	Supportive
Iodine	High	High	High	Thyroid ablation, carcinoma	Potassium iodide
Phosphorus	High	High	High	Bone, rapidly replicating cells	Aluminum hydroxide
Plutonium	High	Minimal	Limited, may form nodules	Lung, bone, liver	Chelation with DTPA or EDTA
Radium	Unknown	30%	Unknown	Bone marrow suppression, sarcoma	Magnesium sulfate lavage
Strontium	Limited	Moderate	Unknown	Bone	Supportive
Tritium	Minimal	Minimal	Complete	Panmyelocytopenia	Dilution with controlled water intake, diuresis
Tritiated water	Complete	Complete	Complete	Panmyelocytopenia	Dilution with controlled water intake, diuresis
Uranium	High	High to moderate	High absorption, skin irritant	Pulmonary, nephrotoxic	Chelation with DTPA or EDTA, $NaHCO_3$ to alkalinize urine

TABLE 22.10. Guidelines for KI Dose Administration

Patient/age	Exposure, GY (rad)	KI dose (mg)	KI dose (solution)
12–17 years of age	0.05 (5)	65	
4–11 years of age	0.05 (5)	65	1 ml
1 month to 3 years of age	0.05 (5)	32	0.5 ml
Birth to 1 month of age	0.05 (5)	16	0.25 ml
Pregnant/lactating	0.05 (5)	130	

From Markenson.[3] This table was created from recommendations developed at the Consensus Conference and in part is based on reviewed reference materials from the American Academy of Pediatrics, Centers for Disease Control and Prevention, and FDA.
Note: Children/adolescents weighing >70 kg should receive the adult dose (130 mg).

TABLE 22.11. Guidelines for Home Preparation of KI Solution Using 130-mg Tablet: These Guidelines Allow for Preparation of a Pediatric Solution from Tablets When a Pediatric Solution Is Not Available

Put one 130-mg KI tablet in a small bowl and grind into a fine powder with the back of a spoon. The powder should not have any large pieces.
Add 4 tsp (20 ml) of water to the KI powder. Use a spoon to mix them together until the KI powder is dissolved in the water.
Add 4 tsp (20 ml) of milk, juice, soda, or syrup (e.g., raspberry) to the KI and water mixture. Potassium iodide mixed with any of the recommended drinks will keep for up to 7 days in the refrigerator.
The resulting mixture is 16.25 mg of KI per teaspoon (5 ml).
Age-based dosing guidelines:
  Newborn through 1 month of age = 1 tsp
  1 month through 3 years of age = 2 tsp
  3 years through 17 years of age = 4 tsp
  Children/adolescents weighing more than 70 kg should receive one 130-mg tablet

From Markenson.[3] This table was created from recommendations developed at the Consensus Conference and in part is based on reviewed reference materials from the American Academy of Pediatrics, Centers for Disease Control and Prevention, and FDA.

and as the "dirty bomb" which might be expected to provide the exposure to ^{137}Cs would likely affect only modest numbers of people, stockpiling of large amounts of Prussian Blue in forward locations would not be needed. The dosing recommendations are shown in Table 22.13.

In addition to specific treatments for each of the radiologic agents, in such events while not an immediate need there will be a need for marrow stimulative agents. These treatments will not be part of the initial care but for those with significant exposure they will be needed in the following days to weeks (Table 22.14).

TABLE 22.12. Guidelines for Home Preparation of KI Solution Using 65-mg Tablet

Put one 65-mg KI tablet in a small bowl and grind into a fine powder with the back of a spoon. The powder should not have any large pieces.

Add 4 tsp (20 ml) of water to the KI powder. Use a spoon to mix them together until the KI powder is dissolved in the water.

Add 4 tsp (20 ml) of milk, juice, soda, or syrup (e.g., raspberry) to the KI and water mixture. Potassium iodide mixed with any of the recommended drinks will keep for up to 7 days in the refrigerator.

The resulting mixture is 8.125 mg of KI per teaspoon (5 ml).

Age-based dosing guidelines:

  Newborn through 1 month of age = 2 tsp

  1 month through 3 years of age = 4 tsp

  4 years through 17 years of age = 8 tsp or one 65-mg tablet children/adolescents weighing more than 70 kg should receive two 65-mg tablets

From Markenson.[3] This table was created from recommendations developed at the Consensus Conference and in part is based on reviewed reference materials from the American Academy of Pediatrics, Centers for Disease Control and Prevention, and FDA.

TABLE 22.13. Prussian Blue Dosing: Prussian Blue (Radiogardase®) was Approved by the FDA in 2003 (as 500-mg Capsules) for the Treatment of Internal 137Cs contamination. Dosing instructions are as follows.

Age	Dose
Adults and adolescents	3 g (6 capsules[a]) PO tid
Children 2–12 year old	1 g (2 capsules[a]) PO tid

From Markenson.[3]

[a]Capsules may be opened and the contents mixed with food or beverages.

TABLE 22.14. Marrow Stimulative Agents

Agent	Action	Dosage[a]
Epoetin alpha[b] (Epogen, Procrit)	Induces erythropoiesis	150 units/kg/dose
Filgrastim (Neupogen)	Granulocyte colony stimulating factor (GCSF)	2.5–5 µg/kg/d (dosages of 20 µg/kg/d may be needed in selected patients)
Sargramostim (Leukine)	Colony stimulating factor (AMCSF)	5–10 µg/kg/d (dosages of 30 µg/kg/d may be needed in selected patients)

From Markenson.[3] [a]Dosage derived from Medical Management of Radiological Casualties, Armed Forces Radiobiology Research Institute, 1999, and accepted dosages for pediatric oncology and pediatric congenital neutropenia and erythropenia patients.

[b]Epoetin alpha may also be useful to reduce the overall requirements for blood transfusion in any mass casualty incident.

Conclusion

One of the first steps in addressing emergency preparedness for children is to reinforce the notion that they have unique vulnerabilities and needs which must be integrated in to all levels of planning. But, addressing these particular needs is difficult due to the enormous gaps in the understanding of how disasters and weapons of terror affect children medically and psychologically. A clear research agenda is being developed to examine these and other crucial areas of concern. The fact is that reliable data on children is scant, and planners must often rely on clinical experience and extrapolation from adult studies. These both have significant limitations. While testing of new medications and therapeutics is rarely done in children, it has not been done at all for antidotes or preventive agents for terrorist events. Funding is needed to conduct research that addresses vaccines, resistance, antidotes, pediatric dosing recommendations, resilience, and mental health considerations. Disaster and terrorism preparedness must become an integral part of the scope of academic pediatric activities, including both education and research.

It should also be pointed out that there is significant potential for inequitable distribution of information and resources with respect to terrorism and disaster preparedness. Just as traditional health and public health resources are often relatively unavailable or inaccessible in underserved communities, it would not be unreasonable to expect the same patterns in the distribution of resources for these new challenges. Pediatricians need to be vigilant about such possibilities and be prepared to advocate appropriately for underserved communities, as well as for children in general.

Suggested Resources for Further Information

- Burklow, T., Yu, C., and Madsen, J. (2003). Industrial Chemicals: Terrorist Weapons of Opportunity. *Pediatric Annals, 32:4,* 230–234.
- *Children More Vulnerable Than Adults in the Event of a Chemical Spill or Chemical Weapons Attack.* (2003). Cedars Sinai Medical Center Online. Retrieved August 1, 2005, from http://www.csmc.edu/pdf/Pediatrics-ChemicalWeapons&Kids.pdf.
- Henretig, F., Mechem, C., and Jew, R. (2002). Potential Use of Autoinjector-Packaged Antidotes for Treatment of Pediatric Nerve Agent Toxicity. *Annals of Emergency Medicine, 40:4,* 405–408.
- JumpSTART Pediatric Multiple Casualty Incident Triage. (2005). Retrieved August 1, 2005, from http://jumpstarttriage.com.
- Markenson, D. and Redlener, I. (2005). *Pediatric Preparedness for Disasters and Terrorism: A National Consensus Conference: Executive Summary.*
- Pediatric Expert Advisory Panel. (2004). *Atropine Use in Children after Nerve Agent Exposure: Info Brief.* New York: National Center for Disaster Preparedness.
- Rotenberg, J. (2003). Diagnosis and Management of Nerve Agent Exposure. *Pediatric Annals, 32:4,* 242–251.
- Rotenberg, J. and Newmark, J. (2003). Nerve Agent Attacks on Children: Diagnosis and Management, *Pediatrics, 112,* 648–658.

- Rotenberg, J., Burklow, T., and Selaniko, J. (2003). Weapons of Mass Destruction: The Decontamination of Children. *Pediatric Annals, 32:4,* 260–268.

American Academy of Pediatrics
(www.aap.org/terrorism)
Publications and media

- Balk SJ, Miller RW. FDA issues KI recommendations. *AAP News.* 2002;20(3):99
- *Feelings Need Check Ups Too* (CD ROM). (2004).
- Committee on Environmental Health. Radiation disasters and children. *Pediatrics.* 2003;111:1455–1466.
- Committee on Infectious Diseases. Smallpox vaccine. *Pediatrics.* 2002;110: 841–845.
- Committee on Pediatric Emergency Medicine. Pediatricians' liability during disasters. *Pediatrics.* 2000;106:1492–1493.
- Committee on Pediatric Emergency Medicine and Committee on Infectious Diseases. Chemical-biological terrorism and its impact on children. *Pediatrics.* 2000;105:662–670.
- Committee on Psychosocial Aspects of Child and Family Health. How pediatricians can respond to the psychosocial implications of disasters. *Pediatrics.* 1999;103:521–523.
- Committee on Psychosocial Aspects of Child and Family Health. The pediatrician and child bereavement. *Pediatrics.* 2000;105:445–447.

Informational documents

- Child with a Suspected Anthrax Exposure or Infection (http://www.aap.org/advocacy/releases/anthraxsusp.htm)
- Anthrax/Bioterrorism Q&A (http://www.aap.org/advocacy/releases/anthraxqa.htm)
- AAP Offers Advice on Communicating With Children About Disasters (http://www.aap.org/terrorism/topics/psychosocial_aspects.html)
- AAP Responds to Questions About Smallpox and Anthrax (http://www.aap.org/advocacy/releases/smlpoxanthrax1.htm)
- AAP Experts Address Smallpox Questions (http://aapnews.aappublications.org/cgi/content/full/e200164v1)
- Family Readiness Kit: Preparing to Handle Disasters (http://www.aap.org/family/frk/frkit.htm)
- Responding to Children's Emotional Needs During Times of Crisis: An Important Role for Pediatricians (http://www.aap.org/terrorism//topics/parents.pdf)
- Smallpox: Frequently Asked Questions – Parent Handout (http://www.aap.org/advocacy/releases/smallpoxfaq.htm)
- Terrorism: A Family Disaster Plan (http://www.aap.org/advocacy/releases/famdisplan.pdf)
- The Youngest Victims: Disaster Preparedness to Meet Children's Needs (http://www.aap.org/terrorism/topics/PhysiciansSheet.pdf)

American College of Emergency Physicians
(www.acep.org)

American Hospital Association
(www.aha.org)

American Red Cross
(www.redcross.org)

Centers for Disease Control and Prevention
(www.bt.cdc.gov)

Children's Health Fund
(www.childrenshealthfund.org)
- The 9/11 terror attacks: emotional consequences persist for children and their families. *Contemp Pediatr.* 2002;19:43–59.

Emergency Medical Services for Children (www.emsc-nrc.com)

Federal Emergency Management Agency (www.fema.gov)

Infectious Diseases Society of America (www.idsociety.org)

Program for Pediatric Preparedness, National Center for Disaster Preparedness (www.pediatricpreparedness.com)

- Executive Summary From Pediatric Preparedness for Disasters and Terrorism: A National Consensus Conference, 2003
- Report of Pediatric Preparedness for Disasters and Terrorism: A National Consensus Conference, 2003

Report of the National Advisory Committee on Children and Terrorism, Department of Health and Human Services
(www.bt.cdc.gov/children)

References

1. Redlener I, Markenson D. Disaster and terrorism preparedness: What pediatricians need to know. Advances in Pediatrics. 2003;50:1–37.
2. Chemical-biological terrorism and its impact on children. Pediatrics. 2002;105:662–670.
3. Markenson D. Pediatric Emergency Preparedness for Natural Disasters, Terrorism and Public Health Emergencies: A National Consensus Conference. Executive Summary and Final Report 2007.

Part V
Aftermath and Ethical Considerations

23
Forensic Investigation of Suicide Bombings

JEHUDA HISS and TZIPI KAHANA

Since the late 1980s and throughout the early 2000s, Palestinian Muslim fundamentalist groups have chosen suicide terrorism as a means of expressing their dissent against Israel, taking the lives of hundreds of civilians, military personnel, and perpetrators.

The first intifada (uprising), comprised a series of violent incidents between the years 1987 and 1993, when the Oslo accords were signed and the Palestinian National Authority was established. This period, also known as the "War of Rocks," was characterized by few suicide attacks. The majority of suicide bombings occurred later, from 1993 onwards. In the 22 suicide terrorist bombings that took place in Israel between the years 1994 and 1998, 141 victims and 23 perpetrators were killed. The second wave of suicide terror, known as the "Al-Aqsa Intifada," took place between 2000 and 2006. In 87 suicide bombings, the lives of 581 victims and 91 perpetrators were taken. In 58 other incidents, 65 perpetrators perished.[1] A majority of the victims and all the perpetrators have been examined at the National Centre of Forensic Medicine, the only forensic medical facility in Israel.

The forensic investigation of terrorist suicide bombing attacks has three main objectives: ascertaining the identity of the victims and perpetrators, clarifying the cause of their death, and reconstructing the event. With these three purposes in mind, a diverse group of forensic experts works in close collaboration to provide answers to the next of kin of the victims, the investigating agencies (i.e., the police, military, and legal system), and the medical profession.

The planning of mass disaster management procedures is paramount to accomplishing the tasks at hand. Predesignated personnel, equipment, forms, and facilities are imperative, along with the combined functioning of all the authorities in charge.[2] The experience gained in Israel in the last two decades by all the agencies involved in the recovery, treatment, and identification of victims from terrorist bombings has generated the management policy currently in effect in Israel.

Scene Investigation

The investigation at the scene is carried out by police Scene of Crime Officers (SOCOs) and Bomb Squad Examiners. Their main aim is to collect all relevant data on the exploded device before any other technical personnel enter the area.[3,4]

S.C. Shapira et al. (eds.), *Essentials of Terror Medicine*,
DOI: 10.1007/978-0-387-09412-0_23, Springer Science+Business Media, LLC 2009

At times, an initial explosion has been followed by another one intended to increase the number of casualties among the gathering crowd and emergency teams summoned to the location of the incident; so the cordoned area may be entered only after the bomb squad sappers give their clearance.

Medical teams direct the wounded to the preselected local trauma centers, while police or military personnel collect and preserve evidence from the scene. Photo-documentation of the exact position of all bodies and body parts, and their spatial relation to the personal effects scattered in the area, is a pivotal clue to the identification of the victims and the reconstruction of the explosion. The remains are sequentially numbered (Fig. 23.1), labeled, collected into marked body bags, and gathered in one central location in the vicinity of the scene.[5] From there they are transported to a predesignated forensic medical facility for further examination.

Collection of all body fragments and blood-soaked objects, and delivering them to the forensic teams for identification, is usually performed by professional teams. In Israel, orthodox Jews recruited and trained by the police are in charge of this task.

While the bodies are being located, recovered, and documented at the scene by the forensic field crews, the medico-legal facility for the incoming casualties is prepared.

The bodies are usually examined in the regional medical examiner's office. If there are space constraints, any adequate construction with sufficient electric power to accommodate refrigerated containers, running water, easy road access, and communication capability, may be used as a temporary morgue.[6] In addition, there

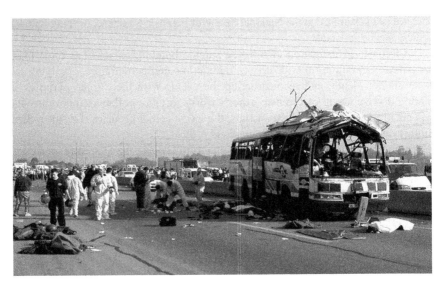

FIG. 23.1. Scene of Crime Officers (SOCOs) collecting evidence and documenting the location of the bodies and body parts prior to their removal to the forensic facility.

should be sufficient space for long-term stay of the working teams. The location of, and equipment at, the temporary morgue should be preplanned and tested, to be ready for immediate action.

Family Assistance and Information Center

Activation of an emergency multiline telephone number in an Information Center (IC) is an essential step that mitigates public anxiety and provides assistance to the next of kin. In the IC, data regarding the missing victims (wounded and killed) are collected.[7]

Establishing the minimum number of victims is one of the most important tasks of the investigation; this information is essential to the rescue teams searching the rubble, to the law enforcement agency investigating the incident, and to the IC that receives dozens of calls, many of them unrelated to the event. The medical centers admitting the wounded are instructed to update the investigating units regarding the names of the victims; thus, when a missing person is reported to the IC as wounded, his next of kin can be directed to the appropriate hospital.[8]

The IC serves also as a family assistance facility for "walk-in" relatives searching for victims of the bombing. The IC should be staffed by local police investigators, social workers, religious leaders, and psychologists. The main objective of the IC is to obtain and catalog antemortem data from individuals searching for missing persons, while at the same time providing them with psychological and social assistance. The relevant information regarding physiognomic characteristics, medical data, clothing, and other identifying features of the missing person, is recorded on antemortem forms, which are similar to postmortem forms, where the same information regarding the bodies is noted.

Some of the data necessary for positive identification is obtained through information provided by the next of kin. Individuals with a criminal record or those who had served in military, police, or fire departments have fingerprint records; fingerprints can also be obtained from the personal effects of individuals presumed to be dead. Dental and general medical records can be located through data given at the IC. Personal effects bearing traces of DNA of the missing individual, including dry samples from military repositories and criminal databases, swabs from the inner aspect of the cheek, or blood samples of close relatives (parents, siblings, and offspring), are collected.[9]

Thanatological Examination

The aim of the thanatological examination is twofold: description of the bodies, for gathering data leading to positive identification, and evaluation of various injuries sustained.

(a) Collection of Individualizing Characteristics

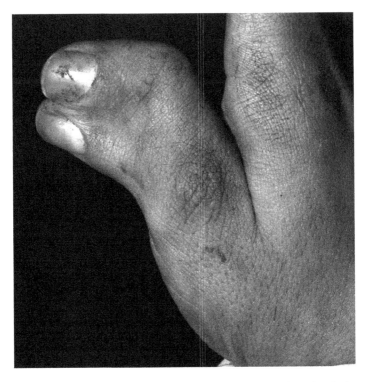

FIG. 23.2. Individualizing characteristics like polydactyly of the right thumb documented during thanatological examination of a victim and contrasted with data obtained from the next of kin at the Information Center (IC).

Particular signs to be contrasted with the data obtained at the IC are gathered by forensic experts from various fields. Medical examiners document all signs of surgical intervention, acquired or congenital pathology (Fig. 23.2), cutaneous nevi, tattoos, and body piercing, as well as sample tissues for DNA profile.[10] This examination is complemented by radiography as required by the medical examiner.[11,12]

Dental examination is performed by odontologists or anthropologists familiar with forensic techniques.[13] The examination includes preparation of a dental chart, taking at least two bitewing or four periapical radiographs and, if there are no time constraints, photographs of the dentition for quality control.[14]

Identification technicians from the police take fingerprints, utilizing a variety of techniques, depending on the condition of the body [15,16] to obtain a ten-print card of each corpse as well as palm prints (Fig. 23.3).

Police field investigators are in charge of photographing the clothing and personal belongings found in association with the bodies, as these data are useful in obtaining presumptive identifications. Access to the property removed from the bodies, such as wallets, cellular phones, and keys, is permitted only through the

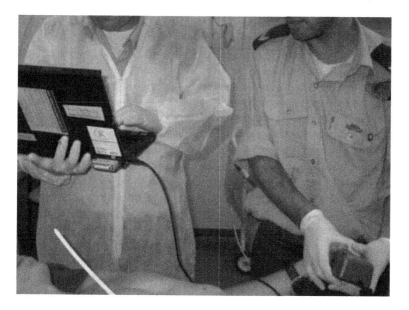

FIG. 23.3. Portable fingerprinting scanner utilized for fingerprinting the deceased.

officer in charge. As a rule, jewelry is not removed from the body throughout the examination, to avoid misplacement of valuables. The property is returned to the next of kin upon release of the identified body. When possible, the facial tissues are restored, to spare the families' feelings while viewing the body.[17]

After the complete and partially complete bodies have been processed, the forensic teams often must deal with dozens and sometimes hundreds of body parts, occasionally transported from the scene days after the attack and usually in a poor state of preservation. The forensic pathologists and anthropologists classify all parts, describe and photograph them, and finally take tissue samples from body fragments for DNA analysis. Anatomic reconstruction of the shattered bodies can be accomplished through physical matching of the torn parts.[10,18] Those segments that cannot be approximately matched by gross anatomic morphology are analyzed at the tissue level.

(b) Documentation of Injuries and Reconstruction of the Event

Clarification of the cause of death and reconstruction of the event is another major objective of the medico-legal examination.[19] Six main physical phenomena, with a great variety of concomitant injuries, result from explosions: Complete disruption of the body, explosive injuries, penetrating wounds from flying missiles, internal lacerations and hemorrhages from the blast wave, burns from thermal effects, and, finally, blunt injuries from fallen masonry and similar materials.[20]

Those individuals in close proximity to the explosive device, that is, the perpetrator and victims within a radius of less than 1 m, are literally blown to pieces, causing complete dissipation of the body and a dispersion of tissues as far as 200 m. Tissue fragments from the perpetrator are blown in a centrifugal fashion toward the wounded. In suicide bombings, it is recommended to take blood (when available) or muscle samples of the bomber for hepatitis B and C and human immunodeficiency virus (HIV) testing.[21] Remnants of the explosive device and encasing container are also dispersed in a radial fashion and sometimes un-detonated parts of the contrivance are found within the body cavities of the victims.

Shrapnel wounds result from metallic objects added to the explosive device. Screws, nails, pieces of wire, and ball bearings are some of the fragments commonly used by the perpetrators, and their wounding capacity depends on their weight, velocity, ballistic shape, and spread (Fig. 23.4).[22] Although spherical pellets have poor ballistic characteristics compared with ordinary bullets, they are favored by the perpetrators for their ability to penetrate large target areas and to increase the extent of wounding. Devastating injuries such as comminuted fractures or lacerations of internal organs are produced when a large number of shrapnel pieces penetrate the skin and disperse throughout the body.

The blast produced by the detonation is a wave of air under very high pressure that emanates in a radial fashion from an explosive source at the speed of sound, and is followed by a wave of air under negative pressure.

There are four mechanisms of trauma produced by the blast: primary (direct effect of pressure), secondary (effects of projectiles), tertiary (effect of wind and

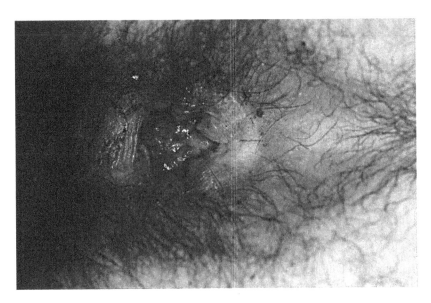

Fig. 23.4. Cranial photograph of a victim with metallic shrapnel, embedded in the explosive material.

motion of air), and quarternary (burns, asphyxia, and exposure to toxic inhalants). (For more information on blast injury types, see Chap. 11 and Table 19.1.)

Data Reconciliation

Comparing and contrasting the data compiled for identification purposes is known as reconciliation. At this stage, experts from various fields (i.e., fingerprints, dental, medical, and DNA analysis) search for consistencies between antemortem and postmortem records.[23]

Depending on the magnitude of the event, this task requires the implementation of a computerized system for effective data comparison. There are various systems dedicated to specific forensic fields, such as Automatic Fingerprint Identification Systems, computerized dental comparison, and DNA profile matching. For an effective reconciliation strategy, a system that consolidates all or most of the data fields is recommended.[24]

Once a potential link between antemortem and postmortem records is established, further investigation of this link, known as data mining, is essential. When a valid reason for comparison between a particular antemortem file and a postmortem file is established, the forensic expert requests the original documents for matching. Prior to issuing a positive identification based on any specific field, the expert should submit the potential match to professionals in other fields who can supply additional methods of identification for the same individual.

For the process of positive identification to be successful, quality control procedures should be mandatory at all stages; in the reconciliation step, a board of experts headed by a senior medical examiner should review all the pertinent information before issuing a death certificate and releasing the body for burial.[25]

Reconstruction of the Event

Forensic scientists should be familiar with the basic concepts related to explosive devices, to conduct an effective and comprehensive investigation. The distribution and nature of the injuries of the victims indicate their location in relation to the epicenter of the explosion. The ability to discern the human bombers, based on the premise that proximity to the bomb directly corresponds to severity of injuries (Fig. 23.5) and the identification of the explosive device from the recovered trace evidence, are crucial for the investigator.[26]

Most explosive devices are similar, constructed on the same technical principles. The attacks are perpetrated either by suicide bombers carrying the device strapped to their bodies, or by bombs placed in public areas. The bomb usually consists of a small and simple switch, often battery operated, for the detonation of the explosives, although many terrorist cells utilize cellular phones for wireless detonation.

Four patterns have been detected in the *modus operandi* of the suicide bombers: When the device is strapped to the perpetrator's body (strapped human bomb – SHB) it could be detonated either within an enclosed space (SHB1) or in an open

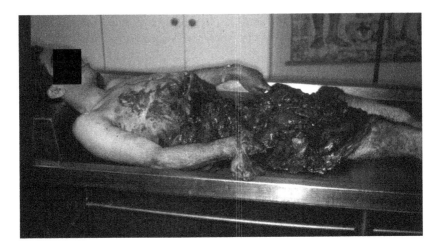

FɪG. 23.5. Typical injuries encountered on the body of the perpetrator carrying a strapped human bomb (SHB) and on victims standing in his immediate proximity.

space (SHB2). When the device is transported in a car and detonated by the driver (vehicular human bomb – VHB), the detonation can occur either in the vicinity of an enclosed space (VHB1) or in an open area (VHB2).[5]

The quantities of explosives used in the bombs often vary from 700 g (SHB) to 50 kg (VHB), being either the commercial or homemade type. The explosive device can be encased in a metallic container such as a pipe, wrapped in cloth (SHB), or affixed to domestic medium-sized gas containers (VHB).

Conclusion

In Israel, the only forensic institution authorized to conduct thanatologic investigations is located in Tel Aviv and carries out all the medico-legal necroscopies and identifications of sudden unexpected deaths (circa 2,500 annual examinations).[27]

The purpose of the forensic investigation of suicide bombings is manifold: to establish the minimum number of casualties, identify the victims and perpetrators, and clarify the causes of death, and *modus operandi* of the terrorists. This undertaking is accomplished by medico-legal inspection, gathering evidence about the victims and perpetrators, collecting data at the scene of the event, and examining it in various forensic laboratories.[9]

In forensic sciences, recognition of the deceased by family members or friends falls within the realm of presumptive identification. Under Jewish Law (the Halacha), visual identification in itself is acceptable, provided the face or a unique external body feature is completely or partially preserved in such a way as to comply with the Halacha.[28] Although visual recognition of relatively well-preserved facial morphology is implemented in the daily forensic work for identification of corpses, the practice is not recommended in mass fatality situations.[29] Even though viewing the remains helps the family to accept the sudden and unexpected death of their loved ones, positive identification by scientific means is advocated in mass casualty situations.

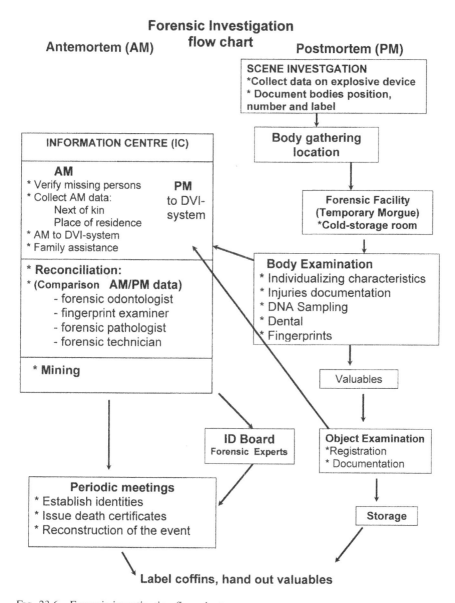

FIG. 23.6. Forensic investigation flow chart.

The release of the remains to the family should be in accordance with various administrative policies, depending on the country's laws: (a) Bodies and body fragments are buried only after all human remains are positively identified; (b) bodies that have been identified and all the body fragments associated with the individual are released to the family; (c) as soon as a body fragment, sufficient to determine the death of an individual, has been positively identified, the part is released for burial. In this last possibility, the family should be informed at the time of initial burial that there could be more body parts to be buried at a later time. The Jewish faith requires interment of the deceased on the same day of death or as soon as possible; so in Israel the most frequent policy is to release body parts immediately after identification.

Documentation of the different types of injuries to the victims of explosions contributes to establishing the cause and manner of death for possible legal action, and to improving the awareness of the medical staff in treating the wounded of similar attacks.[30]

Despite the tight security measures at border posts and on roads beyond the "green line" (the border between the Palestinian Authority and the State of Israel), Palestinian radical groups have continued efforts to launch terrorist attacks. The reconstruction of each event and the interpretation of the *modus operandi* are instrumental in devising effective preventive measures[5] (Fig. 23.6).

References

1. 2000–2006: Major terror attacks. *Israel Ministry of Foreign Affairs.* http://www.mfa.gov. il. Accessed August 15, 2007.
2. Wagner GN, Froede RC. Medicolegal investigation of mass disaster. In: Spitz WU, Ed. *Spitz and Fisher's Medicolegal Investigation of Death.* 4th ed. Springfield, Illinois: Charles C Thomas; 2006: 966–993.
3. Meikle P. Bomb-scene management. In: Siegel JA, Saukko PJ, Knupfer GC, Eds. *Encyclopedia of Forensic Sciences.* San Diego: Academic Press; 2000: 745–750.
4. Glattstein B, Landau E, Zeichner A. Identification of match head residues in post-explosion debris. *J Forensic Sci.* 1991;36:1360–1367.
5. Hiss J, Kahana T. Trauma and identification of victims of suicidal terrorism in Israel. *Mil Med.* 2000;165:889–893.
6. Jensen RA. *Mass Fatality and Casualty Incidents.* Boca Raton, FL: CRC Press; 1999: ix–xii.
7. Levinson J, Granot H. Information centers. In: *Transportation Disaster Response Handbook.* San Diego: Academic Press; 2002: 87–88.
8. Hiss J, Freund M, Motro U, Kahana T. The forensic pathology of terrorism in Israel – Two years of suicide bombing. In: Shemer J, Shoenfeld Y, Eds. *Terror and Medicine. Medical Aspects of Biological, Chemical and Radiological Terrorism.* Lengerish: Pabst Science Publishers; 2003: 446–455.
9. Kahana T, Freund M, Hiss J. Suicidal terrorist bombings in Israel – Identification of human remains. *J Forensic Sci.* 1997;42:260–264.
10. Hiss J, Freund M, Motro U, Kahana T. The medicolegal investigation of the El Aqsah Intifada. *Isr Med Assoc J.* 2002;4:549–553.

11. Vogel H. Explosives. In: Brogdon BG, Vogel H, McDowell JD, Eds. *A Radiologic Atlas of Abuse, Torture, Terrorism, and Inflicted Trauma*. Boca Raton: CRC Press; 2003: 141–150.

12. Kahana T, Goldin L, Hiss J. Personal identification based on radiographic vertebral features. *Am J Forensic Med Pathol*. 2002;23:36–41.

13. James H. Thai Tsunami victim identification – Overview to date. *J Forensic Odontostomatol*. 2005;23:1–18.

14. Clement JC. Role and techniques in forensic odontology. In: Payne-James J, Busutil A, Smock W, Eds. *Forensic Medicine: Clinical and Pathological Aspects*. San Francisco: Greenwich Medical Media; 2003: 689–703.

15. Kahana T, Grande A, Tancredo D, Penalver J, Hiss J. Fingerprinting the deceased: Traditional and new techniques. *J Forensic Sci*. 2001;46:908–912.

16. Valck E. Major incident response: Collecting ante-mortem data. *Forensic Sci Int*. 2006;159(Suppl 1):S15–S19.

17. *Home Office Guidance on Dealing with Fatalities in Emergencies*. Viewing by the bereaved. London: Home Office Communication Directorate; 2004: 40.

18. Kahana T, Fulginiti L, Birkby W, Hiss J. Role of and techniques in forensic anthropology. In: Payne-James J, Busutil A, Smock W, Eds. *Forensic Medicine: Clinical and Pathological Aspects*. San Francisco: Greenwich Medical Media; 2003: 663–676.

19. Laposata EA. Collection of trace evidence from bombing victims at autopsy. *J Forensic Sci*. 1985;30:789–797.

20. Hiss J, Kahana T. Modern war wounds. In: Mason JK, Purdue BN, Eds. *The Pathology of Trauma*. 3rd ed. London: Arnold, 2000: 89–102.

21. Braverman I, Wexler D, Oren M. A novel mode of infection with Hepatitis B: Penetrating bone fragments due to explosion of suicide bomber. *Isr Med Assoc J*. 2002;4:528–529.

22. Saukko P, Knight B. Gunshot and explosion deaths. In: Knight B, Saukko P, Eds. *Knight's Forensic Pathology*. 3rd ed. London: Arnold; 2004: 245–280.

23. Marshal TK. Violence and civil disturbance. In: Mason JK, Ed. 2nd ed. *The Pathology of Trauma*. London: Edward Arnold; 1993: 71–85.

24. Al-Amad SH, Clement JG, McCullough MJ, Morales A, Hill AJ. Evaluation of two dental identification computer systems DAVID and WinID3. *J Forensic Odontostomatol*. 2007;25:23–29.

25. Nilsen R, Rygnestad T, Kjus S. *Evaluation report on the DVI operation in South East Asia*. Oslo: National Criminal Investigation Service; 2006: 31–48.

26. Hiss J, Kahana T. Suicide bombers in Israel. *Am J Forensic Med Pathol*. 1998;19:63–66.

27. Hiss J, Kahana T, Arensburg B. Forensic medicine in Israel. *Am J Forensic Med Pathol*. 1997;18:154–157.

28. *Chatam Sopher*. Tel Aviv: A Talmud Publisher; 1978: 340.

29. Mayer HJ. The Kaprun cable car disaster – Aspects of forensic organization following a mass fatality with 155 victims. *Forensic Sci Int*. 2003;138:1–7.

30. Dolinak D, Matshes E. Explosive injury. In: Dolinak D. Matshes E, Lew E, Eds. *Forensic Pathology, Principles and Practice*. Amsterdam: Elsevier; 2005: 134–135.

24
Psychological Effects of Terror Attacks

SARA A. FREEDMAN

> *Terrorism is about psychology ... [it] is about imagining the monster under our beds or*
> *lurking in dark closets – the faceless, omnipotent enemy who might be ... our neighbor*
> *.... The power of terrorism lies precisely in its pervasive ambiguity, in its invasion of our*
> *minds.*[1]

The statistical chance of being killed by terrorism in the United States in 2001 was significantly lower than dying as a result of a motor vehicle accident. Yet in the same year there was a 6.5% decrease in air travel, 20% of which occurred in the last 3 months of the year, following 9/11.[2] The sarin gas attacks in Tokyo in 1995 resulted in 12 deaths, and another 1,000 people directly exposed: however, 5,000 presented themselves at hospital with physical symptoms.[3] Following the anthrax scare in 2001, some individuals complained of burning sensations following opening mail, which did not contain toxic substances.[3] Scud attacks in Israel resulted in more anxiety-related symptoms than physical injuries.[4] These actual physical symptoms suffered by individuals not actually exposed to a terrorist attack have led some authors to label these reactions as "mass idiopathic illness."[5] Terrorism results in widespread anxiety, and subsequent behavior change, the extent of which is far greater than is warranted from the actual objective danger, and also far more extreme than irrational fears that are found following other traumatic events. These wide-ranging psychological effects in the general population are, it is suggested, unique to terrorism.[2]

However, similar to experiencing a car crash, rape, or interpersonal violence, exposure to terrorism also results in the development of psychopathology: estimates among the New York populace following 9/11, for example, showed rates of posttraumatic stress disorder (PTSD) of 4%.[6]

This chapter will examine the short- and long-term psychological effects of exposure to terrorism, both on an individual level and a community level. It will describe the differential effects of ongoing terrorism and describe interventions for terrorism-related psychopathology. Since PTSD is one of the most commonly found consequences of traumatic events, there will be an emphasis on PTSD research; however, other disorders that often present posttrauma will also be discussed.

S.C. Shapira et al. (eds.), *Essentials of Terror Medicine*,
DOI: 10.1007/978-0-387-09412-0_24, Springer Science+Business Media, LLC 2009

PTSD: General Background

Traumatic Events

It has been long established that while most people are exposed during their lifetime to potentially traumatic events,[7] the vast majority of individuals cope well with these. A significant minority, however, develop psychopathology as a direct result of exposure to the traumatic event, most often PTSD.[7]

PTSD is unique in the psychiatric literature in that it has a defined etiology. In its initial conceptualization in DSM-III,[8] PTSD was assumed to be a normal reaction to an abnormal event. This implied that almost anyone who had experienced such an unusual event, such as war, would be likely to display symptoms of PTSD. Research studies have shown that in fact PTSD occurs after more common, albeit difficult, events, such as car accidents. Moreover, the disorder actually appears in a relatively small percentage of people exposed to a traumatic event.[9]

According to DSM-IV,[10] the traumatic event in PTSD is defined as follows: "the person must have experienced an event that objectively was traumatic (it involved a threat to personal integrity), and subjectively was experienced at the time as traumatic (the person felt fear, horror, or helplessness)." Thus, the current definition reflects a need for both objective and subjective severity when defining an event as traumatic. This definition is clear when an individual has directly experienced an event such as war, terrorism, or violence. It becomes more complex when considering events such as the sudden, difficult end of a relationship, or watching the Twin Towers collapse on television, while sitting in Los Angeles.

Symptoms

Symptoms occurring soon after the traumatic event that last for 2 weeks are known as acute stress disorder (ASD).[11] These symptoms include reexperiencing, avoidance and arousal, and in addition some symptoms of dissociation, such as depersonalization. Although ASD is a good predictor of PTSD, not all people who develop PTSD fulfilled criteria for ASD.[12] When symptoms have lasted for 1 month, then a diagnosis of PTSD can be made. PTSD symptoms lasting 3 months or longer are considered chronic.

PTSD is composed of three major symptom groups: intrusion, avoidance, and arousal.[10] *Intrusion* involves reexperiencing the event, and this can occur through spontaneous intrusive thoughts or images, nightmares, and flashbacks, all of which cause distress when they occur. In addition, individuals may react with distress to reminders of the event, or suffer physiological reactivity to reminders. *Avoidance* includes actively avoiding reminders of the traumatic event: attempting not to think about it, feel it, or remember it, as well as behavior changes (e.g., not driving after a car crash). Avoidance also includes traumatic amnesia (not being able to remember important aspects of the event) and feelings of detachment. *Arousal* includes symptoms such as irritability, sleep problems, startle response, and hyper vigilance to danger. In order for a diagnosis of PTSD to be made, one symptom of intrusion, three avoidance symptoms, and two arousal symptoms must be present.[10]

Development of PTSD

A number of studies have shown that the majority of people exposed to a traumatic event experience initial PTSD symptoms, which wane over time. For instance, a study of rape victims[13] showed that at 12 days posttrauma, 94% of their sample could be said to have PTSD. This number had dropped to 65% at 35 days, and to 47% at 3 months. Similar results have been shown by other researchers.[14-16] There is some indication that this natural decline in symptoms is mostly found in the first 6 months following a traumatic event, and that after 1 year, very little change is seen.[7] This pattern of symptoms suggests that early on after a traumatic event, manifestations of anxiety are natural, and may even be indicative of a necessary process of accepting the traumatic event.[17] This process is characterized by a reduction in this anxiety over time; when it persists, then psychopathology is indicated.

Prevalence

Potentially traumatic events are experienced at least once, and often more frequently, by the majority of individuals. Epidemiological studies estimate that 70%[18] to nearly 90%[19] of people have experienced at least one trauma in their lifetime.

Exposure to a traumatic event does not usually result in any long-lasting psychological effects. Epidemiological studies show that the lifetime risk of developing PTSD as a result of exposure to any type of traumatic event is estimated between 7.8%[7] and 9.2%.[20] This risk varies greatly depending on the type of trauma, from 2.3% following a car crash, to 49% following rape.[19] In addition to PTSD, other types of psychopathology are also seen: for example, major depressive disorder, specific phobia.[19]

Prospective research studies examining the development of PTSD following traumatic events show that the levels of PTSD decrease by 50% between 1 and 3 months postevent.[14] Six months following a traumatic event, 20% of individuals will have chronic PTSD. This estimate again varies according to the type of event: for example, rape 48%,[20] motor vehicle accidents 18.7%.[21]

Who Develops PTSD?

Given that the majority of individuals do not develop any long-term pathology, it is an important clinical question as to how to identify those individuals most at risk. There is a large literature examining those factors that might predict the likelihood of PTSD developing. The results of the studies are not consistent, with many factors having been identified as significant predictors. However, one meta-analysis[22] showed that psychiatric history, in self and family, and early abuse, were robust risk factors, with female gender, lower social economic status, and general previous adversity, negatively affecting some trauma populations.

Terrorist Attacks: PTSD and Beyond

Research studies examining psychological symptoms following terrorist attacks have increased steadily over the past decade, particularly relating to 9/11 and the Al Aqsa Intifada (the Palestinian uprising beginning in 2000). These studies include epidemiological studies that have examined whole populations following an attack. These samples have different amounts of "exposure" to the event. Some are based on convenience samples, others on randomly chosen samples that are representative of the general population. In addition, there are smaller studies that have examined specific populations, generally those directly affected by a terrorist attack (Table 24.1).

9/11

The events of 9/11 resulted in nearly 3,000 fatalities. The number of exposed individuals is difficult to estimate, since the studies described below document PTSD symptoms in those minimally exposed to the events. In addition, a large number of people were bereaved, as well as vicariously exposed to the terrorist attacks through their work roles. The major studies examining the psychological effects of 9/11 are summarized here.

A web-based study[23] examined stress reactions from a few days following the attacks, and followed up sub-samples at 2 and 6 months. Acute stress reaction was found in 8.9% of the sample, with 17% showing PTSD symptoms at 2 months, and 5.8% at 6 months. Another web-based survey[6] examined levels of PTSD 1–2 months post 9/11 in both the New York City areas, and nationally. This study found higher levels of PTSD in New York. The levels of distress found outside of New York were not significantly higher than would be expected under normal circumstances.

In a telephone survey, carried out between 3 and 5 days after 9/11, 560 people were interviewed across the United States.[24] A high proportion (44%) reported experiencing one or more substantial symptom of stress. One thousand and eight individuals living in Manhattan were interviewed in a telephone survey carried out 1–2 months following 9/11.[25] The results indicated that 7.5% of the respondents fulfilled criteria for PTSD, 9.7% for depression, and 3.7% for both disorders. Finally, levels of PTSD in 930 primary care patients were assessed 7–16 months following 9/11. 10.2% of this group had PTSD.[26]

One study[27] has examined the levels of complicated grief among those bereaved as a result of 9/11. This web-based survey, that took place between 2.5 and 3.5 years after the attack, found that 43% had complicated grief. This was related to losing a child, being female, and having watched the attacks live on television. A telephone survey[28] one and a half years after 9/11 found that of those who had

TABLE 24.1. Studies of PTSD following terrorist attacks

Study	Terrorist attack	Population	Time posttrauma	Method	N	% PTSD	% MDD
Bleich et al. (2003)[32]	Ongoing Israel	Random	During	Telephone interview	512	9.2	
Bleich et al. (2005)[33]	Ongoing Israel	ER patients	During	Telephone interview	702	9	
Shalev et al. (2004)[35]	Ongoing Israel	Convenience sample	During	Questionnaire	167 (high exposure)	9.58	
Kaplan et al. (2005)[34]	Ongoing Israel	Random sample	During	Questionnaire	89 (low exposure) 107 (high exposure) 103 (medium exposure) 104 (high exposure)	6.74 10 10 11	
Somer et al. (2005)[36]	Ongoing Israel	Random	During	Telephone interview	327	5.2	
Kutz and Dekel (2006)[38]	Suicide bombing in mall	Directly exposed	4 months	Telephone interview	54	24	
Gil and Caspi (2006)[39]	Bus Bomb	ER patients	6 months	Interview	185	17	
Shalev and Freedman (2005)[21]	Various terrorist attacks	ER patients	4 months			38	
Gidron et al. (2004)[78]	Ongoing Israel	General population	During	Questionnaires	149	10.1	
Dolberg et al. (2007)[37]	Ongoing Israel	ER patients	3–9 months 30 months	Questionnaires	129	15.5 (3–9 months) 35 (30 months)	
Conejo-Galindo et al. (2007)[43]	Madrid	Injured survivors	1, 6, and 12 months	Interview	56	35.7 (1 month) 34.1 (6 months) 28.6 (12 months)	28.6 (1 month) 22.1 (6 months) 28.6 (12 months)
Gabriel et al. (2007)[42]	Madrid	Injured survivors and local population	5–12 weeks	Interview	96 67	44 (injured survivors) 12.3 (local population)	31.5 12.3
Fraguas et al. (2006)[41]	Madrid	ER patients	1 and 6 months	Interview	56	41.1 (1 month) 40.9 (6 months)	

(continued)

TABLE 24.1. (continued)

Study	Terrorist attack	Population	Time posttrauma	Method	N	% PTSD	% MDD
Miguel-Tobal et al. (2006)[40]	Madrid	Random sample	1–3 months	Telephone interview	1,589	2.3	8.0
North et al. (2005)[79]	Nairobi	Directly exposed	8–10 months	Interview	227	25.8 (men) 35.1 (women)	11.6 (men) 15.5 (women)
North et al. (2005)[79]	Oklahoma City	Directly exposed	6 months	Interview	182	19.5 (men) 34.0 (women)	8.0 (men) 17.0 (women)
Verger et al. (2004)[44]	Various bombs	Directly exposed	2 years post	Interview	196	31.1	
Jehel et al. (2003)[45]	Bomb Paris	Directly exposed	6–32 months	Interview	32	39 25	
Neria et al. (2006)[26]	9/11	Primary care patients, NY	7–16 months	Questionnaire	930	10.2	
Schlenger et al. (2002)[6]	9/11	Web-based epidemiological	1–2 months	Web-based	2,273	11.2 (New York) 4.0 (rest of United States)	
Galea et al. (2002)[25]	9/11	Random digit dialing, Manhattan	1–2 months	Telephone interview	1,008	7.5	
Silver et al. (2002)[23]	9/11	Random, national	9–32 days, 2 months, 6 months	Web-based 2% direct exposure	2,729, 933, 787	8.9 17% – 2 months 5.8% – 6 months	
Schuster et al. (2001)[24]	9/11	Random digit dialing, national	3–5 days	Telephone interview	560	44 – substantial stress	
Perrin et al. (2007)[50]	9/11	Rescue and recovery	2–3 years	Questionnaire	28,962	12.4	
Rubin et al. (2005)[29]	London 7/7	Random digit dialing, London	11–13 days	Telephone interview	1,010	31 – substantial stress	
Rubin et al. (2007)[30]	London 7/7	Random digit dialing, London	7 months	Telephone interview	574	11 – substantial stress	

been bereaved, 44% had complicated grief. This was related to the loss of a family member as opposed to an acquaintance.

London Bombing, July 7, 2005

In these bomb attacks on London, 52 people were killed, and more than 700 injured. One set of studies has thus far been published on the effects of these attacks. In a telephone survey of 1,010 people, using the same methods as described above,[26] 31% of individuals had one or more substantial stress symptoms; this number had reduced to 11% at a 7-month follow-up.[29,30]

Israel

Most of the research from Israel has been carried out during the period of 2001–2006. These terror attacks resulted in 1,139 Israeli fatalities and 6,700 injured. The number of attacks in 2001 reflected a greater than 300% increase relative to the previous year.[31]

A telephone survey of adults across Israel was carried out at two time points – after 19 months of ongoing terrorism[32] and after 44 months.[33] In the first survey, 16.4% had been directly exposed to a terrorist attack, with another 37.3% indirectly exposed (via family member or friend). Nine percent of this sample had PTSD, and this rate remained consistent (9.4%) at the second time point.

In a questionnaire survey, PTSD symptoms among individuals from three different areas of Israel were assessed.[34] These areas differed greatly in terms of direct exposure to terrorist attacks. The results found no significant differences in the incidence of PTSD (10%), although those with less exposure showed significantly higher levels of acute stress symptoms.

Another questionnaire survey[35] also compared rates of PTSD in different geographical areas, with different exposure to terrorist attacks. In the group from the high exposure area, 9.6% showed PTSD, whereas in the low exposure group, 6.7% showed PTSD.

A telephone survey of 327 adults examined psychological effects of terror exposure[36]; this was a random sample, but there was over-sampling for areas of the country most affected, and unaffected, by terrorist attacks. Ten percent of the sample had directly been exposed to an attack, with a further 27% claiming they had just missed an attack (took the previous bus, left late for work, etc.). 44.5% knew someone who had been injured in an attack. Probable PTSD was found in 5.2% of this sample.

In a study carried out over 2 years,[37] 129 survivors of terrorist attacks who presented to the ER were followed up: 15.5% had PTSD at 3–9 months posttrauma. Of the 54 individuals who were followed up at 30 months, 35% had PTSD.

Three prospective studies have examined the development of PTSD following exposure to a terrorist attack. In the first, patients brought to the ER following a bomb in a mall were interviewed via telephone within a month of the event, and then again at 4 months.[38] 24% had ASD at the first interview, and these individuals were three times more likely to have developed PTSD at the 4-month interview. A convenience sample of students was interviewed 2 weeks before a suicide attack on a bus, and then 1 week, 1 month, and 6 month postevent.[39] 17% of the students had PTSD at 6 months. A prospective study,[23] that included survivors of various terrorist attacks, as well as other traumatic events followed patients from the ER for 4 months. Levels of PTSD at 4 months post-trauma were 17% for motor vehicle accidents, and 38% for terrorist attacks. Survivors of terrorist attacks were more symptomatic at each time point post-trauma, although the development of PTSD, and decline in symptoms, was similar regardless of traumatic event type.

Madrid

In March 2004, ten bombs on commuter trains resulted in 192 fatalities and 2,000 injured. In a large-scale telephone survey[40] 1–2 months following the Madrid bombings, 2.3% of individuals had PTSD, and 8% depression. In a study of those directly affected,[41] 41.1% of patients brought to the ER showed PTSD at 1 month, and this had not declined significantly at 6 months (40.9). In a separate study of injured survivors,[42] they showed higher rates of PTSD (31.5%) than the local population (12.3%), 5–12 weeks following the attacks. In another study of injured survivors,[43] PTSD rates were 35.7 at 1 month, 34.1 at 6 months, and 28.6 at 1 year.

France

In a study carried out around 2 ½ years following terrorist attacks during 1995–1996 in France,[44] 31% of directly exposed individuals had PTSD. Following one of these attacks, a bomb in Paris in 1996, 39% of directly exposed individuals had PTSD at 6 months and 25% at 3 years.[45]

Oklahoma

In the terrorist attack in Oklahoma City in 1995, 168 people were killed, with more than 800 injured. In a study[46] carried out 6 months following the attack, 182 directly exposed survivors were interviewed. This study showed that 15% of those exposed had PTSD regarding another event *before* the attacks, and 43% had suffered from some type of pre-event psychiatric disorder. PTSD resulting from the terrorist attack was present in 34.3% of the survivors. Twenty-six percent of those had had PTSD prior to the terror attack. This study also examined depression: 12.6% developed depression following that attack, and 44% of these had suffered from depression even before the attack. This study also showed that women were almost twice as likely to develop PTSD than men (women: 44%; men 23%). Another study[47] examined community reactions following the attack that showed that proximity to the attack was related to higher levels of distress.

Nairobi

In 1998, the US Embassy in Nairobi was bombed, resulting in 211 deaths. In one study[46] carried out 8–10 months after the bombing, 227 directly exposed individuals were interviewed. PTSD was found in 33.7% of the men, and 48.8% of the women. In addition, 15% of the men and 24% of the women were suffering from depression. Six months after the attack, a random sample of 2,883 individuals was studied.[48] The majority (60%) had been directly exposed to the bombing, and a quarter of the whole sample had PTSD.

Predictors of PTSD Following a Terrorist Attack

When examining the general conclusions of all these studies, there is a reasonable agreement regarding predictors of distress following exposure to a terrorist attack. Proximity to the attack, and direct exposure, predicts PTSD levels in almost all studies. In addition, active coping was related to lower levels of PTSD.[30] PTSD was also associated with ethnicity (Hispanic vs. White) having two or more life stressors in the year preceding the attacks, loss of possessions due to the attacks, and experiencing a panic attack during or soon after the attacks.[26] In addition, previous psychiatric illness and female gender were associated with PTSD in a number of studies.[24] These predictors do not differ from those found to predict PTSD after other trauma types.

Secondary PTSD

It has long been documented that those who work with survivors of traumatic events may also be affected by the event via this interaction. Although there is no official recognition of this phenomenon, it has been described frequently, and has been called vicarious, or secondary, PTSD.

A number of studies have examined the psychological effects of working with victims of terrorist attacks. In one study of hospital physicians in Israel, who had different levels of exposure in working with terror victims,[49] 15% were shown to suffer from PTSD. This PTSD was, however, related to the doctors' exposure to terrorism *outside* their working environment. In an extremely large-scale study,[50] 28,962 personnel who worked in rescue and recovery following 9/11 were interviewed 2–3 years after the event. Of these, 12.1% had PTSD. Workers who had no previous experience in working with disaster, as well as those who worked for longer, and started work earlier, were all at higher risk of PTSD.

Another study[51] from 9/11 showed that among social workers, compassion fatigue was highest in those who had worked directly with 9/11 survivors, and experienced less support at work.

Not all studies have shown any increased levels of distress however: in a study of 87 body handlers from Israel,[52] only two had PTSD. In a sample of 3,055 Red Cross volunteers who were surveyed a year after 9/11,[53] no differences in levels of distress were found between high and low exposure. Overall, the level of symptoms among workers was low, and tended to be non-related to the actual work. It is possible that a combination of factors protect these people: choice over the work they do, and the opportunity to actively help victims.

Resilience

As has been described above, the large majority of individuals exposed to a terrorist attack do not develop any long-lasting psychological effects, and might be in fact described as "resilient." One of the studies described above[36] was analyzed regarding the prediction of those who had no more than one symptom of PTSD in the first half year following 9/11. These individuals had low levels of depression, and were less likely to smoke or use marijuana. Various factors were identified as being predictive: being male, being older than 65, being Asian, and not having completed high school. In addition, more social support, less income loss, and less experience of traumatic events both prior to and subsequent to September 11 were related to resilience. In another study[54] comparing residents of three different communities in Israel, those who had both strong religious and ideological beliefs, and were living in a cohesive community, were significantly less likely to develop PTSD. These results suggest that resilience is not simply the opposite of PTSD, but rather has its own profile. The suggestion that community cohesiveness is a protection during trauma has a theoretical basis.[55] These results also implicate early interventions, in that they suggest that psychological interventions alone may not be sufficient to help, but that a myriad of social- and community-based interventions may be as necessary.[36]

Ongoing Attacks

There is a logical assertion that exposure to many terrorist attacks will take a greater psychological toll than exposure to an isolated incident. Research, however, suggests otherwise. In one study,[23] terrorist survivors during a period of isolated incidents were compared with those during the Al Aqsa Intifada: no significant differences in rates of PTSD were found. Additionally, two epidemiological studies in Israel during this intifada suggest that as time goes on, rates of PTSD remain the same, while less depression and functional impairment are found.[34,35]

General Findings

Taken together, these studies show a fairly consistent picture. Terrorist attacks result in widespread symptoms of anxiety in the general population that reduce considerably over time. Anxiety symptoms are also related to the mass idiopathic illness symptoms described earlier: these physical symptoms are more likely to be found in those with higher levels of exposure and PTSD.[56] Less distress following a terrorist attack was related to active coping. There is remarkable consistency regarding incidence: ~10% of the general population who are in greater proximity to the event have PTSD following a terrorist attack. This number drops to ~4% in the wider population. Among survivors who were directly exposed to the terrorist attack, this number is ~30%.

Thus, the incidence of PTSD following terrorist attacks in those directly affected is far higher than that following other traumatic events, such as car crashes.

Moreover, symptom intensity is far greater, both immediately following the attack and in the months that follow.[21]

It has been suggested[2] that the occurrence of PTSD in those not directly affected by the terrorist attack is an anomaly in terms of PTSD, since there is no objective exposure to danger. These authors suggest that this pattern is unique to terrorist attacks, and can be explained by faulty appraisals of risk. Another perspective on this apparent widespread psychiatric disturbance found following a terrorist attack has also been suggested.[35] These authors calculated rates of PTSD twice – once using symptoms as a guide for determining PTSD status, and once using symptoms and whether these symptoms resulted in dysfunction. The latter is a necessary requirement by DSM for a diagnosis of PTSD to be made, but it not generally part of self-report questionnaires. Once dysfunction is taken into account, the levels of PTSD drop considerably: from 26.95% to 9.58% in directly exposed individuals, and from 21.35% to 6.74% in non-directly exposed. This suggests that while *symptoms* of PTSD may be very common in the aftermath of a terrorist attack, this should not be confounded with *psychopathology*. Many people feel scared, and change their behavior, and sleep less well: that may be a natural response to threat, and not only does not constitute a psychiatric problem, may even be considered a positive result. These "symptoms" may protect the individual from actual exposure to danger, elicit social support, and indicate natural processing of difficult life events. Only when symptoms are combined with a change in the ability to function, do they constitute a pathological reaction. Two studies also show[34,57] that most people who have "PTSD" see no need to seek therapy as a result of their symptoms. This reinforces the idea that suffering from terror-related stress "symptoms" does not necessarily constitute a problem, which warrants psychiatric intervention.

Interventions

The case vignette below illustrates some of the challenges in intervention that commonly need to be addressed in survivors of terrorist attacks: timing of intervention, normalcy of response, context of response, and mass casualties.

Composite Case Vignette

J, a 45-year-old woman, was driving with her sister to work when a bomb went off in the bus in front of her. She was not physically hurt, although was evacuated to hospital due to psychological shock. From her car, she was able to see into the bus, and witnessed many grotesque images: body parts, burning flesh, and injured survivors. Her windscreen was covered with body parts and blood. When she was brought into the ER, she saw injured survivors being treated. While in the ER, she was unable to communicate, as she was overwhelmed with the images she had seen. J became very agitated, as she could not stop those intrusive images: she was shaking, crying, and feeling faint. Following discharge from the ER, J's symptoms continued to cause great distress. Her sister, however, experienced a few days of anxiety, which quickly abated. J's family (who was also very upset for a few days) expected her to also return to "normal" within a few days. J found herself unable to control the intrusive images, and also suffered from nightmares about the attack. As a result, she avoided all reminders of the event: she would not watch TV or open a newspaper, as she was scared she would see a report of another attack; she would not drive in her car; she was unable to retrace the route she had taken that day; she would not touch the clothes or bag she had worn on the day. She would not sleep at night in the dark. In addition, she was extremely anxious regarding her family, and would not let her teenage children go out after dark. She was constantly on the look out for danger, and would jump at the slightest noise. Her children were unable to invite friends round, or play music. J became easily irritated, and this caused friction between her and her husband.

Targets of Intervention and Mass Casualties

As is discussed above, PTSD symptoms are a common reaction immediately following a traumatic event. In the case of a terrorist attack, some symptoms are common not only in those who are directly exposed, but also in the general population. These symptoms tend to decrease over time, although in the case of ongoing attacks, they may persist. Even when they do not disappear, these symptoms are often not associated with a change in functioning, and most people do not feel they are in need of psychological therapy.

This picture means that correctly targeting interventions can be difficult. How can the "real" patients be identified? In the case described above, should intervention be offered to J? J and her sister? All the family members? It would be easy to look at help-seeking, and assume that those in real need will seek out the interventions that they need. Recent studies have, however, suggested that many PTSD patients actively ignore treatment, even when it is available to them.[58] This leaves a public health conundrum since the PTSD cases and non-cases will look very similar, particularly in the early stages following a terrorist attack. Some authors have suggested that one approach to this problem may be education regarding PTSD via natural community resources, such as schools and churches.[59] Education regarding appropriate responses, and where to seek help, might be useful in normalizing anxiety reactions, identifying patients, and persuading them to get help. In reference to J, this level of intervention may have helped her family place J's reactions in context. Other authors have identified primary care physicians as potential conduits in assessing and referring patients with PTSD.[28] Outreach has been examined – although costly, it seems effective in identifying target populations.[60]

In a world with unlimited resources, then all survivors of a terrorist attack should be followed up, and offered treatment if symptoms do not abate. One study that has examined this, suggests even with systematic outreach, uptake of interventions in the first weeks following a traumatic event tends to be quite low: of 100 individuals coming to an ER following a trauma, only around 5 will come to therapy within 4 weeks.[61] This indicates that when planning services, especially around a mass casualty event, expectations should be that existing psychiatric services, unless already over-burdened, should be able to manage the patient-flow.

When resources are more limited, or when the sheer numbers of potentially exposed people make this approach untenable, then providing survivors with education regarding their symptoms, guidelines that enable them to self-monitor, and interventions available once they feel they need help, may be the most appropriate response.

Timing

Although the time divisions presented here are somewhat artificial, they give a framework within which to describe different phases of intervention. In reality, there will be overlap between them.

ER/Immediate Response

In the immediate aftermath of a terrorist attack, the priority will be to ensure patients' safety and access to medical help. Within this context, however, psychological intervention can be helpful and necessary.

Patients arriving at an ER following a terrorist attack generally present with a wide variety of psychological reactions. While some are calm and already utilizing active coping strategies such as telephoning relatives to reassure them,[62] others may be extremely distressed. This distress cannot be easily classified, as it fits no "disorder" or profile. It often includes anxiety symptoms: crying, shaking, and agitation. It can also manifest as dissociation: patients feel as if they are not "there," but are watching themselves, or have such vivid intrusive images of the attack that they are not aware of their immediate surroundings. These symptoms may fluctuate, even while the patient is being treated in the ER.

As mentioned above, symptoms of PTSD are extremely common in the immediate aftermath of a traumatic event, and should not be considered necessarily pathological. These are usually part of the natural reaction to the event, and form the first step toward spontaneous recovery. Again, the first challenge for intervention, even the ER, is determining the difference between "normal" symptoms and pathological ones. While some approaches assume that any sign of anxiety needs to be "treated," others are more circumspect, and define a target population at this stage of posttrauma as only those with full PTSD.[63] The literature on this issue is complex: while some studies have shown early intervention in the form of "debriefing" to be a positive experience for the patient,[64] controlled studies have suggested that one-off, group or individual sessions of debriefing at best do no good, and at worst may be harmful.[65] The former studies have normally included in treatment all survivors, whereas the latter have taken only those who, for example, have a diagnosis of ASD.[66]

No research exists as to the effects of interventions in the ER that are not defined as debriefing. Despite this paucity of data, there exists an anecdotal literature gleaned from clinical experience.[67,68]

The main aims of intervention in the ER – often named psychological first aid – are to stop the traumatic event for the patient and allow her to regain control over her emotional state. The first aim seems perhaps unnecessary – once the patient is in the ER, is it not clear that the terrorist attack is over? Clinical experience shows that this issue can be very important. Patients can be confused as to what exactly happened, are unable to locate relatives or friends, and are unsure of the medical procedures they will undergo. Providing this orienting information while reiterating the message that they are now in a safe place is often extremely helpful in ending the traumatic event.

Various strategies are helpful in regaining control. Relaxation techniques can be used, giving the patient conscious control of breathing. In addition, orienting techniques are helpful in patients who are dissociative. These range from repeating information to the patient (who you are, where you are, what happened) to encouraging them to walk around. Medication can be used: again the literature is divided, with some studies showing that the use of SSRIs at this time to be unhelpful.[69] Providing information regarding natural reactions to a traumatic event is usually well received, and can help to "normalize" the patient's reaction. Many ERs, in the aftermath of a terrorist attack, give out printed information regarding these reactions, along with a contact number in case of need.

Patients will normally be discharged once they are able to control their emotions, and are beginning to be able to reflect, even if only a little, on their experience. At this stage, patients are normally able to view the event as having finished.

ASD and PTSD Treatment

In the first 4 weeks following a traumatic event, many patients will have ASD.[10] Several studies have examined psychological interventions with patients at this time point. These studies have all examined cognitive behavior therapy (CBT). These interventions have for the most part, been short (around five sessions). The research shows that CBT is helpful both in treating the current symptoms, as well as in preventing the chronic PTSD from developing.[65,70] A recent study[61] showed that although early intervention with CBT was beneficial, and prevented PTSD, this was the only case for those with full PTSD. Patients who had fewer symptoms showed a similar reduction in symptoms as those in a wait list control. This reiterates the need to target interventions to those who will most benefit from them.

Effective treatment for chronic PTSD includes different types of CBT. Both exposure-based and cognitive restructuring have been shown to be effective treatments for PTSD.

In what way should interventions for PTSD following a terrorist attack differ from traditional treatment for PTSD? PTSD is normally conceptualized as excessive fear, where there is a feeling of current threat, even though none exists.[71] This is a useful way to understand most traumatic events and the resultant PTSD, but a sense of current threat when there are threatened or real terrorist attacks is realistic and even helpful. In this situation, it cannot be "treated," and so our understanding of PTSD and its treatment must also change.

Clinical work with terror attack survivors has given rise to three major challenges in this treatment.[72] First, in many countries (e.g., Israel) media coverage of attacks is explicit, showing live pictures, and in-depth interviews, of the terrorist attack. It is extremely difficult to avoid this exposure. In addition, exposure via other people is relatively high: A number of studies have shown that watching TV coverage of terrorist attacks contributes to the severity of PTSD.[73] Thus, treatment of PTSD must take into account this reexposure. Second, many terrorist attack survivors witness grotesque images, which are unique to this type of event.

Third, terrorist attacks result in changes in the behavior in the general population. As mentioned earlier, a large proportion of Americans stopped flying immediately following the attacks on 9/11, and changes in many area of daily living were seen in Israel during the Al Aqsa Intifada. These changes in behavior may reflect genuine safety behaviors, or may be an exaggerated response to a terrorist attack. In either event, they represent avoidance in the general population.

At this time, four studies have examined CBT for PTSD resulting from a terrorist attack. Two related studies of survivors of the Omagh bombing[74,75] have shown that CBT is effective, even when carried out by therapists with no prior experience with this type of therapy. Workers at 9/11 were treated using CBT, which was effective.[76] Lastly, a computer-generated version of CBT was more effective than supportive counselling.[77]

These studies indicate that terror-related PTSD is a treatable entity, in much the same way as PTSD following other traumatic events. Some uncontrolled reports[67] have indicated that, especially with ongoing attacks, PTSD following a terror attack may present unique challenges to treatment.

These reports suggest that traditional CBT must be slightly modified in order to cope with these challenges. First, with patients who avoid situations which are objectively dangerous, and are therefore avoided by those without PTSD, then these situations can be approached differently. Avoidance can be carried out using pictures and computer graphics, thus enabling patients to habituate to their irrational fears. In the context of ongoing attacks, they are likely to remain with adaptive fear and concomitant avoidance. Indirect exposure, via the media, should be limited as far as possible. In terms of the grotesqueness of the images, our experience has shown that patients who find it hard to describe verbally their intrusive images, are often helped by pictures and other "props." With one patient, who was covered with body parts following a bomb attack, and found it extremely difficult to talk about these, real pieces of meat were used in the therapy sessions, to help her describe the indescribable. With another patient, an anatomy book was extremely helpful: he was able to use the pictures of limbs to describe what he had seen.

In a case such as J's, in vivo exposure to objectively safe situations, such as the clothes worn on the day of the attack, can be carried out easily. Exposure to the site of the attack may have to be modified. CBT carried out both early after the attack (within 1 month) or once the PTSD has become chronic, has been effective with many cases such as J's.[61]

Conclusion

Terrorism results in widespread anxiety responses in both those in close proximity to the attack, as well as those with no direct exposure. This anxiety tends to be temporary for most people. In situations where terrorist attacks are ongoing, then these responses may continue, but tend to be adaptive coping. A small proportion of individuals, usually those with more direct exposure to the attack, are likely to develop psychopathology. This will most likely be PTSD, although a significant proportion will develop depression. Terrorist-related PTSD can be treated successfully, even during a period of ongoing attacks.

Terrorism is effective in part because of the anxiety it creates. Understanding this anxiety is an integral part of withstanding it.

References

1. Zimbardo PG. The political psychology of terrorist alarms 2002 [last verified on 26 March 2006]. In: http://www.zimbardo.com/current.html.
2. Marshall RD, Bryant RA, Amsel L, Suh EJ, Cook JM, Neria Y. The psychology of ongoing threat: relative risk appraisal, the September 11 attacks, and terrorism-related fears. *Am Psychol.* 2007;62(4):304–16.
3. Bartholomew RE, Wessely S. Protean nature of mass sociogenic illness: from possessed nuns to chemical and biological terrorism fears. *Br J Psychiatry.* 2002;180:300–6.
4. Bleich A, Dycian A, Koslowsky M, Solomon Z, Wiener M. Psychiatric implications of missile attacks on a civilian population. Israeli lessons from the Persian Gulf War. *JAMA.* 1992;268(5):613–5.
5. Engel CC, Locke S, Reissman DB, DeMartino R, Kutz I, McDonald M, Barsky AJ. Terrorism, trauma, and mass casualty triage: how might we solve the latest mind-body problem? *Biosecur Bioterror.* 2007;5(2):155–63.
6. Schlenger WE, Caddell JM, Ebert L, Jordan BK, Rourke KM, Wilson D, Thalji L, Dennis JM, Fairbank JA, Kulka RA. Psychological reactions to terrorist attacks: findings from the National Study of Americans' Reactions to September 11. *JAMA.* 2002;288(5):581–8.
7. Kessler PC, Sonnega A, Bromet E, Hughes M, Nelson CB. Posttraumatic stress disorder in the National Comorbidity Survey. *Arch Gen Psychiatry.* 1995;52:1048–60.
8. *Diagnostic and Statistical Manual of Mental Disorders. 3rd ed. Revised.* Washington, DC: American Psychiatric Association; 1980.
9. Yehuda R, McFarlane AC. Conflict between current knowledge about posttraumatic stress disorder and its original conceptual basis. *Am J Psychiatry.* 1995;152(12):1705–13.
10. *Diagnostic and Statistical Manual of Mental Disorders. 4th ed.* Washington, DC: American Psychiatric Association; 1994.
11. Harvey AG, Bryant RA. Acute stress disorder: a synthesis and critique. *Psychol Bull.* 2002;128(6):886–902.
12. Harvey AG, Bryant RA. The relationship between acute stress disorder and posttraumatic stress disorder: a 2-year prospective evaluation. *J Consult Clin Psychol.* 1999;67:985–8.
13. Rothbaum BO, Foa EB, Riggs DS, Murdock T, Walsh W. A prospective examination of posttraumatic stress disorder in rape victims. *J Trauma Stress.* 1992;5:455–75.

14. Freedman SC, Brandes D, Peri T, Shalev AY. (1999). Predictors of chronic post-traumatic stress disorder. *Br J Psychiatry*. 174:353–9.

15. Feinstein A, Dolan R. Predictors of post-traumatic stress disorder following physical trauma: an examination of the stressor criterion. *Psychol Med*. 1991;21(1):85–91.

16. Blanchard EB, Hickling EJ, Barton KA, Taylor AE, Loos WR, Jones-Alexander J. One-year prospective follow-up of motor vehicle accident victims. *Behav Res Ther*. 1996;34(10):775–86.

17. Rachman S. Emotional processing. *Behav Res Ther*. 1980;18(1):51–60.

18. Resnick HS, Kilpatrick DG, Dansky BS, Saunders BE, Best CL. Prevalence of civilian trauma and posttraumatic stress disorder in a representative national survey of women. *J Consult Clin Psychol*. 1993;61:984–91.

19. Breslau N, Davis GC, Andreski P, Peterson E. Traumatic events and posttraumatic stress disorder in an urban population of young adults. *Arch Gen Psychiatry*. 1991;48:216–22.

20. Foa EB. Trauma and women: course, predictors, and treatment. *J Clin Psychiatry*. 1997;58(Suppl 9):25–8.

21. Shalev AY, Freedman SA. PTSD resulting from terrorist attacks. *Am J Psychiatry*. 2005;162:1188–91.

22. Brewin CR, Andrews B, Valentine JD. Meta-analysis of risk factors for posttraumatic stress disorder in trauma-exposed adults. *J Consult Clin Psychol*. 2000;68(5):748–66.

23. Silver RC, Holman EA, McIntosh DN, Poulin M, Gil-Rivas V. Nationwide longitudinal study of psychological responses to September 11. *JAMA*. 2002;288:1235–44.

24. Schuster MA, Stein BD, Jaycox L, Collins R, et al. A national survey of stress reactions after the September 11, 2001, terrorist. *N Engl J Med*. 2001;345(20):1507.

25. Galea S, Ahern J, Resnick H, Kilpatrick D, Bucuvalas M, Gold J, Vlahov D. Psychological sequelae of the September 11 terrorist attacks in New York City. *N Engl J Med*. 2002;346(13):982–7.

26. Neria Y, Gross R, Olfson M, Gameroff MJ, Wickramaratne P, Das A, Pilowsky D, Feder A, Blanco C, Marshall RD, Lantigua R, Shea S, Weissman MM. Posttraumatic stress disorder in primary care one year after the 9/11 attacks. *Gen Hosp Psychiatry*. 2006;28(3):213–22.

27. Neria Y, Gross R, Litz B, Maguen S, Insel B, Seirmarco G, Rosenfeld H, Suh EJ, Kishon R, Cook J, Marshall RD. Prevalence and psychological correlates of complicated grief among bereaved adults 2.5–3.5 years after September 11th attacks. *J Trauma Stress*. 2007;20(3):251–62.

28. Shear KM, Jackson CT, Essock SM, Donahue SA, Felton CJ. Screening for complicated grief among Project Liberty service recipients 18 months after September 11, 2001. *Psychiatry Serv*. 2006;57(9):1291–7.

29. Rubin GJ, Brewin CR, Greenberg N, Simpson J, Wessely S. Psychological and behavioural reactions to the bombings in London on 7 July 2005: cross sectional survey of a representative sample of Londoners. *BMJ*. 2005;331(7517):606.

30. Rubin GJ, Brewin CR, Greenberg N, Hughes JH, Simpson J, Wessely S. Enduring consequences of terrorism: 7-month follow-up survey of reactions to the bombings in London on 7 July 2005. *Br J Psychiatry*. 2007;190:350–6.

31. http://www.mfa.gov.il/MFA/Terrorism-+Obstacle+to+Peace/Palestinian+terror+since+2000/Victims+of+Palestinian+Violence+and+Terrorism+sinc.htm).

32. Bleich A, Gelkopf M, Solomon Z. Exposure to terrorism, stress-related mental health symptoms, and coping behaviors among a nationally representative sample in Israel. *JAMA*. 2003;290:612–20.

33. Bleich A, Gelkopf M, Melamed Y, Solomon Z. Mental health and resiliency following 44 months of terrorism: a survey of an Israeli national representative sample. *BMC Med.* 2006;4:21.
34. Kaplan Z, Matar MA, Kamin R, Sadan T, Cohen H. Stress-related responses after 3 years of exposure to terror in Israel: are ideological-religious factors associated with resilience? *J Clin Psychiatry.* 2005;66(9):1146–54.
35. Shalev AY, Tuval R, Frenkiel-Fishman S, Hadar H, Eth S. Psychological responses to continuous terror: a study of two communities in Israel. *Am J Psychiatry.* 2006;163(4):667–73.
36. Somer E, Ruvio A, Soref E, Sever I. Terrorism, distress and coping: high versus low impact regions and direct versus indirect civilian exposure. *Anxiety Stress Coping.* 2005;18(3):165–82.
37. Dolberg OT, Barkai G, Leor A, Rapoport H, Bloch M, Schreiber S. Injured civilian survivors of suicide bomb attacks: from partial PTSD to recovery or to traumatisation. Where is the turning point? *World J Biol Psychiatry.* 2007;26:1–8.
38. Kutz I, Dekel R. Follow-up of victims of one terrorist attack in Israel: ASD, PTSD and the perceived threat of Iraqi missile attacks. *Pers Indiv Diff.* 2006;40(8):1579–89.
39. Gil S, Caspi Y. Personality traits, coping style, and perceived threat as predictors of posttraumatic stress disorder after exposure to a terrorist attack: a prospective study. Students. *Psychosom Med.* 2006;68(6):904–9.
40. Miguel-Tobal JJ, Cano-Vindel A, Gonzalez-Ordi H, Iruarrizaga I, Rudenstine S, Vlahov D, Galea S. PTSD and depression after the Madrid March 11 train bombings. *J Trauma Stress.* 2006;19(1):69–80.
41. Fraguas D, Teran S, Conejo-Galindo J, Medina O, Sainz Corton E, Ferrando L, Gabriel R, Arango C. Posttraumatic stress disorder in victims of the March 11 attacks in Madrid admitted to a hospital emergency room: 6-month follow-up. *Eur Psychiatry.* 2006;21(3):143–51.
42. Gabriel R, Ferrando L, Corton ES, Mingote C, Garcia-Camba E, Liria AF, Galea S. Psychopathological consequences after a terrorist attack: an epidemiological study among victims, the general population, and police officers. *Eur Psychiatry.* 2007;22(6):339–46.
43. Conejo-Galindo J, Medina O, Fraguas D, Teran S, Sainz-Corton E, Arango C. Psychopathological sequelae of the 11 March terrorist attacks in Madrid: an epidemiological study of victims treated in a hospital. *Eur Arch Psychiatry Clin Neurosci.* 2007;258(1):28–34.
44. Verger P, Dab W, Lamping DL, Loze JY, Deschaseaux-Voinet C, Abenhaim L, Rouillon F. The psychological impact of terrorism: an epidemiologic study of posttraumatic stress disorder and associated factors in victims of the 1995–1996 bombings in France. *Am J Psychiatry.* 2004;161(8):1384–9.
45. Jehel L, Paterniti S, Brunet A, Duchet C, Guelfi JD. Prediction of the occurrence and intensity of post-traumatic stress disorder in victims 32 months after bomb attack. *Eur Psychiatry.* 2003;18(4):172–6.
46. North CS, Nixon SJ, Shariat S, et al. Psychiatric disorders among survivors of the Oklahoma City bombing. *JAMA.* 1999;282:755–62.
47. Sprang G. Post-disaster stress following the Oklahoma City Bombing: an examination of three community groups. *J Interpers Violence.* 1999;14:169–83.
48. Njenga FG, Nicholls PJ, Nyamai C, Kigamwa P, Davidson JR. Post-traumatic stress after terrorist attack: psychological reactions following the US embassy bombing in Nairobi: naturalistic study. *Br J Psychiatry.* 2004;185:328–33.
49. Weiniger C, Shalev AY, Ofek H, Freedman SA, Weissmann C, Einav S. Post traumatic stress disorder among hospital physicians exposed to terror. *J Clin Psychiatry.* 2006;67(6): 890–6.

50. Perrin MA, DiGrande L, Wheeler K, Thorpe L, Farfel M, Brackbill R. Differences in PTSD prevalence and associated risk factors among World Trade Center disaster rescue and recovery workers. *Am J Psychiatry.* 2007;164(9):1385–94.
51. Boscarino JA, Figley CR, Adams RE. Compassion fatigue following the September 11 terrorist attacks: a study of secondary trauma among New York City social workers. *Int J Emerg Ment Health.* 2004, Spring;6(2):57–66.
52. Solomon Z, Berger R. Coping with the aftermath of terror – resilience of ZAKA body handlers. *J Aggress Maltreat Trauma.* 2005;10(1–2):593–604.
53. Long ME, Meyer DL, Jacobs GA. Psychological distress among American Red Cross disaster workers responding to the terrorist attacks of September 11, 2001. *Psychiatry Res.* 2007;149(1–3):303–8.
54. Kaplan Z, Matar MA, Kamin R, Sadan T, Cohen H. Stress-related responses after 3 years of exposure to terror in Israel: are ideological-religious factors associated with resilience? *J Clin Psychiatry.* 2005;66(9):1146–54.
55. Hobfoll S, Canetti-Nisim D, Johnson R. Exposure to terrorism, stress-related mental health symptoms, and defensive coping among Jews and Arabs in Israel. *J Consult Clin Psychol.* 2006;74(2):207–18.
56. Davidson J, Hughes D, Blazer D, George L. Post-traumatic stress disorder in the community: an epidemiological study. *Psychol Med.* 1991;21(3):713–21.
57. Levav I, Novikov I, Grinshpoon A, Rosenblum J, Ponizovsky A. Health services utilization in Jerusalem under terrorism. *Am J Psychiatry.* 2006;163(8):1355–61.
58. Hoge CW, Castro CA, Messer SC, McGurk D, Cotting DI, Koffman R. LCombat duty in Iraq and Afghanistan, mental health problems and barrier to care. *N Engl J Med.* 2004;351(1):13–22.
59. Friedman MJ, Hamblen JL, Foa EB, Charney DS. Fighting the psychological war on terrorism. *Psychiatry.* 2004;67(2):123–36.
60. Shalev AY, Freedman SA, Israeli-Shalev Y, Frenkiel S, Adessky R. Treatment of trauma survivors with acute stress disorder: achievements of systematic outreach. In Wessely S, Krasnow VN. (Eds.). *Psychological Responses to the New Terrorism: A NATO-Russia Dialogue.* 2005.
61. Shalev AY, Freedman SA, Adessky R, Errera Y, Peleg T, Israeli-Shalev Y, et al. Prevention of PTSD by early treatment: a randomized controlled trial. The Jerusalem Trauma Outreach and Prevention Study (J-TOPS). Poster Presentation, American College of Neuropsychopharmacology, 46th Annual Meeting, Boca Raton, December 2007.
62. Shalev AY, Schreiber S, Galai T. Early psychological responses to traumatic injury. *J Traumatic Stress.* 1993;6(4):441–50.
63. Sijbrandij M, Olff M, Reitsma JB, Carlier IV, de Vries MH, Gersons BP. Treatment of acute posttraumatic stress disorder with brief cognitive behavioral therapy: a randomized controlled trial. *Am J Psychiatry.* 2007;164(1):82–90.
64. Lee C, Slade P, Lygo V. The influence of psychological debriefing on emotional adaptation in women following early miscarriage: a preliminary study. *Br J Med Psychol.* 1996;69(Pt 1):47–58.
65. Bisson JI, Jenkins PL, Alexander J, Bannister C. Randomised controlled trial of psychological debriefing for victims of acute burn trauma. *Br J Psychiatry.* 1997;171:78–81.
66. Bryant RA, Moulds ML, Nixon RV. Cognitive behaviour therapy of acute stress disorder: a four-year follow-up. *Behav Res Ther.* 2003;41(4):489–94.
67. Tuval-Mashiach R, Freedman SA, Bargai N, Boker R, Hadar H, Shalev AY. Coping with trauma: narrative and cognitive perspectives. *Psychiatry.* 2004;67(3):280–93.

68. Adessky R, Freedman SA. Treating survivors of terrorism while adversity continues. *J Aggress Maltreat Trauma*. 2005;10(1/2):443–54.

69. Mooney P, Oakley J, Ferriter M, Travers R. Sertraline as a treatment for PTSD: a systematic review and meta-analysis. *Ir J Psychol Med*. 2004;21(3):100–3.

70. Foa EB, Zoellner LA, Feeny NC. An evaluation of three brief programs for facilitating recovery after assault. *J Trauma Stress*. 2006;19(1):29–43.

71. Ehlers A, Clark DM. A cognitive model of posttraumatic stress disorder. *Behav Res Ther*. 2000;38(4):319–45.

72. Freedman SA, Tuval-Mashiach R. Mental health issues and implications of living under ongoing terrorist threats. In Schein LA, Spitz HI, Burlingame GM, Muskin PR. (Eds.). *Psychological Effects of Catastrophic Disasters: Group Approaches to Treatment*. NY: Haworth Press; 2006.

73. Ahern J, Galea S, Resnick H, Kilpatrick D, Bucuvalas M, Vlahov D. Television images and psychological symptoms after the September 11 terrorist attacks. *Psychiatry*. 2002;65:289–300.

74. Gillespie K, Duffy M, Hackmann A, Clark DM. Community based cognitive therapy in the treatment of posttraumatic stress disorder following the Omagh bomb. *Behav Res Ther*. 2002;40(4):345–57.

75. Duffy M, Gillespie K, Clark DM. Post-traumatic stress disorder in the context of terrorism and other civil conflict in Northern Ireland: randomised controlled trial. *BMJ*. 2007;334(7604):1147.

76. Difede J, Malta LS, Best S, Henn-Haase C, Metzler T, Bryant R, Marmar C. A randomized controlled clinical treatment trial for World Trade Center attack-related PTSD in disaster workers. *J Nerv Ment Dis*. 2007;195(10):861–5.

77. Litz BT, Engel CC, Bryant RA, Papa A. A randomized, controlled proof-of-concept trial of an Internet-based, therapist-assisted self-management treatment for posttraumatic stress disorder. *Am J Psychiatry*. 2007;164(11):1676–83.

78. Gidron Y, Gal R, Zahavi S. Bus commuters' coping strategies anxiety from terrorism; an example of the Israeli Experience. *J Trauma Stress*. 1999;12(1):185–92.

79. North CS, Pfefferbaum B, Narayanan P, Thielman S, McCoy G, Dumont C, Kawasaki A, Ryosho N, Kim YS, Spitznagel EL. Comparison of post-disaster psychiatric disorders after terrorist bombings in Nairobi and Oklahoma City. *Br J Psychiatry*. 2005, June;186:487–93.

25
Ethics and Terror Medicine

Leonard A. Cole

The field of medicine has long been defined not only by diagnostic and treatment techniques but also by standards of behavior. The Hippocratic Oath was introduced about the same time as the concept of case histories and prognosis, in ancient Greece, fifth century BCE. Despite vast changes in medicine through the ages, the oath's core message continues to resonate: that a physician has a special responsibility to perform honorably. Forms of the Hippocratic Oath are still recited during graduation ceremonies at medical schools, many in the United States, though the classical version has been altered to suit contemporary values.[1] For example, passages in the early oath that prohibited the practice of abortion or euthanasia now are commonly omitted. The shifting text is a reflection of attempts to accommodate medical ethics to new findings, experiences, and values.

The relationship of ethics to terror medicine is an expression of this dynamic process. Recognition of terror medicine as a distinctive discipline emerged during the wave of Palestinian attacks against Israelis between 2000 and 2006. But ethical questions concerning this new field also draw from preceding moral understandings about the rights of patients, the responsibilities of medical caregivers, and other bioethical issues. An overview of these matters can suitably begin with the Nazi medical experiments during World War II.

Changing Attitudes Since World War II

In the early 1940s, German doctors and scientists performed experiments on Jews and other concentration camp inmates, which commonly resulted in disfigurement and agonizing death. After the war, the allied powers conducted a series of trials in Nuremberg, Germany, which found several Nazi leaders guilty of crimes against humanity and other nefarious activities. One of the trials led to the conviction of German doctors for their inhumane research on involuntary subjects. Subsequent information that Japanese doctors had also experimented on involuntary subjects was ignored by the United States with the advent of international political realignments prompted by the Cold War.[2] But the Nuremberg verdict, in 1947, included a code affirming that "voluntary consent" – later commonly understood to mean "informed consent" – be required of any subject of human research. The

S.C. Shapira et al. (eds.), *Essentials of Terror Medicine*,
DOI: 10.1007/978-0-387-09412-0_25, Springer Science+Business Media, LLC 2009

Nuremberg Code also proved to be a forerunner of enhanced sensitivity in general to the rights of patients and the responsibilities of physicians.[3] Prior to this period, in the United States and elsewhere, medical doctors were often viewed as an insular and exclusive fraternity.

The American Medical Association (AMA), since its inception in 1847, has periodically issued codes of medical ethics. An early twentieth century version noted the responsibility of physicians to their patients, but recited at greater length "the duties of physicians to each other and to the profession."[4] Thus, no less important than the care of patients was the felt need to nurture the privileged status of the profession. This sense of paternalism was also reflected in the code's admonition that doctors ordinarily not give patients complete information about their condition.

By the 1950s, the notion of elitism as an ethical principle had diminished and the AMA's 1958 principles of ethics made no mention of doctors' obligations to each other.[5] Subsequent cultural changes in the general society further eroded paternalistic attitudes in favor of the rights of the individual. During the 1970s, the field of bioethics grew in response to information about pre- and postwar experiments on unwitting human subjects by agencies of the US government. The Public Health Service had dispensed placebos to syphilitic black men in Alabama in order to observe the course of their untreated disease.[6] The Central Intelligence Agency had secretly dropped mind-altering drugs in the drinks of citizens to watch their reactions.[7] The Atomic Energy Commission had sponsored experiments in which unwitting hospital patients were injected with plutonium.[8,9] These experiments clearly violated the informed consent precept of the Nuremberg Code, though they had ended by the time the public learned about them. Still, the belated revelations prompted outrage and generated strengthened legal and institutional safeguards to protect human subjects.

At the same time, in the world of medicine, the notion of patient self-determination had gained further traction. In 1980, the AMA issued a revised code of ethics that for the first time included an admonition that a physician must "respect the rights of patients."[10] This ideal was becoming firmly entrenched as a matter of principle no less than the earlier notion of medical paternalism once was. The trend was abetted by the burgeoning recognition of the AIDS crisis, as civil libertarians joined with homosexual rights activists to press for protection of privacy in the public health sphere. They successfully rejected efforts toward enforced testing for HIV and for several years even blocked a requirement in the interest of public health that physicians report people with HIV infection.[11] Critics who worried that a boundless primacy of individual rights could harm the general welfare, seemed to be a dwindling minority. But the simmering tension between individual and community rights resurfaced over the issue of terrorism.

Until the end of the twentieth century, neither medical ethics nor bioethics was focused on terrorism. Ethicists, particularly in the United States, were contending with other matters, many of which were born of biomedical technological advances. Some of these issues, including embryonic stem-cell research, organ transplantation, and physician-assisted suicide, continue to be subjects of intense national debate. But the attacks on September 11, 2001, and the subsequent release of anthrax spores in the US mail also heightened concerns about national security. Resulting policies about ethnic profiling, wiretapping, and other intrusions into privacy and individual liberty have been contentious. Concerns about terrorism have also prompted debates about the limits of scientific inquiry. For example, the recent synthesis of the poliovirus suggests that potential bioagents like the smallpox virus could be fabricated as well. The scientific community remains divided about whether such research should be prohibited, or publication about it restricted, in the name of national security.[12]

In the medical and bioethical arenas, terrorism has also highlighted areas of tension between the rights of individuals and needs of the larger society. Striving for balance between individual liberties and public security is a perennial challenge in every civic society. But the anticipation of numerous casualties from terrorism or other disasters has generated particular concern about the propriety of medically connected coercion in mass casualty events.[13] Four prominent examples include the relationship of ethics to quarantine, vaccination, triage, and the responsibilities of healthcare workers.

Quarantine

Through most of the twentieth century, the right of government officials to impose quarantine for health purposes, though periodically challenged, was generally accepted and upheld in the courts of law.[14] But in recent decades, reflecting the cultural shift toward individual rights, many bioethicists began to view quarantine as an inappropriate infringement.

Then, following the 9/11 and anthrax attacks, the Center for Law and the Public's Health at Georgetown and Johns Hopkins Universities produced a draft of model legislation for states to deal with bioterrorist and other public health emergencies. Titled a Model State Emergency Health Powers Act (MSEHPA), it would empower state and local officials during a public health emergency to appropriate property and require medical tests, vaccinations, and quarantine without due process.[15]

The MSEHPA drew criticism from several bioethicists, none more withering than from George Annas, who described its provisions as draconian. "The model act seems to have been drafted for a different age; it is more appropriate for the United States of the 19th century than for the United States of the 21st century. Today, all adults have the constitutional right to refuse examination and treatment, and such a refusal should not result in involuntary confinement simply on the whim of a public health official."[16]

Two principal authors of the act, James Hodge and Lawrence Gostin, rejected the notion that "respecting individual civil liberties was an overriding good." Rather, they held that "restraints of civil liberties may be justified by the compelling need to protect public health."[17]

Soon after, the issue was tested by real-life experience. In 2002, severe acute respiratory syndrome (SARS) was recognized as a potentially fatal communicable disease caused by a previously unknown virus. An outbreak of SARS began in Canada in February 2003, and by April some 350 people had been infected, 20 of whom had died. Canadian authorities then instituted a quarantine of about 15,000 thousand residents of Toronto, the center of the outbreak.[18] This was the first imposition of widespread quarantine measures in North America in more than 50 years. Quarantined persons were instructed not to leave their homes or have visitors, to wash their hands frequently, wear masks when near other household members, take their temperature twice daily, and not share personal items like towels or drinking cups. The median duration of quarantine was 10 days. In a survey soon after their quarantine ended, some 30% of respondents revealed symptoms of depression or posttraumatic stress disorder. More than half felt they received inadequate information about home infection control measures. But only 15% believed they should not have been placed in quarantine.[19]

By the time of the last recorded Canadian case, in July, 44 victims had died and the effectiveness of the quarantine remained unclear. But soon after, a preliminary study for the Toronto Board of Health concluded that while quarantine did not eliminate SARS, "it was effective in reducing transmission by about 50% for the closest community contacts."[20]

Following the Canadian experience, Ross Upshur, a medical ethicist, noted the divide between those who consider quarantine an unwarranted diminution of personal liberty, and those who deem it important for disease control. Still, in the midst of the outbreak and afterwards, few Canadians objected to the government's decision. Upshur expressed the prevailing view that public health officers should err on the side of safety rather than risk exposure to a preventable disease.[21]

Confinement during the Canadian experience was for a limited duration. Moreover, potential management complications were not evident, such as issues concerning the availability of food for the confined individuals and provision of care for their children. Under similar conditions, the implications for future manmade or naturally occurring disease outbreaks seem hardly in doubt. Despite objections to imposed quarantine by some academic ethicists, the public would apparently accept such a measure for a prescribed period if health authorities deemed it necessary.

Vaccination

The history of vaccinations began with the understanding that people who survived certain diseases became immune to contracting those diseases again. This phenomenon was long recognized in the case of smallpox, where fatality rates from virulent strains could reach 50%. Efforts to protect against smallpox led to crude inoculation practices in several ancient societies. In India, as long ago as 1,000 BCE, the skin of healthy individuals would be cut open for the placement of pus or scabs from people with a mild form of the disease. The procedure, known as variolation, caused an infection that killed perhaps 1% of recipients and made the others very sick. But after recovery they too were no longer susceptible to smallpox reinfection. Variations of the procedure were later practiced in Tibet, China, and eventually in Europe during the eighteenth century.[22]

In the late-1700s, the English physician Edward Jenner found that milkmaids who had contracted cowpox, a relatively innocuous disease, were also immune to smallpox. In 1796, he conducted an experiment that today would doubtless have put him in jail. Jenner made an incision in the arm of an 8-year-old boy and injected into it fluid from a cowpox pustule of an infected milkmaid. The boy's arm developed a rash and blisters but left only a small scar. Jenner then injected the boy with pus from a smallpox case, but it produced no symptoms. The experiment demonstrated the protective effect of cowpox infection against smallpox. In time, the genetic make-up of both causative agents – the variola virus (smallpox) and the vaccinia virus (cowpox) – were found to be similar.

Nearly a century after Jenner's experiment, the French chemist Louis Pasteur produced an effective vaccine from the actual agent that could cause a disease. In 1881, he showed that livestock could be protected from contracting anthrax if injected with an attenuated form of the anthrax bacterium. This opened the way to the development of vaccines against a range of diseases from cholera and plague to polio. In the course of the twentieth century, vaccinations dramatically reduced the incidence of many health nemeses. Indeed, a global vaccination program against smallpox eradicated the disease in 1979.[23]

Compulsory vaccination in the United States and elsewhere extends back to the nineteenth century. Currently every state has a law requiring children to be vaccinated against certain diseases, including diphtheria, measles, rubella, and polio, before enrolling in school. These are among 26 vaccine-preventable diseases for which vaccines are available, according to the Centers for Disease Control and Prevention (CDC).[24]

But many states permit exemptions for medical, religious, or philosophical reasons.[25] In recent decades, questions about the safety of some vaccines have prompted more people to seek exemptions for themselves and their children. The trend was accelerated following a 1998 report that suggested a possible link between autism and the vaccine for measles, mumps, and rubella (MMR). A survey in the United Kingdom indicated that before the controversial report was issued, 92% of children there received the MMR vaccine, but 5 years later the figure had fallen to 79%.[26] The trend has generated concern among public health authorities, who question the validity of the purported linkage and have strongly reaffirmed the value of childhood immunizations.

Studies have ascribed childhood outbreaks of measles in Philadelphia and whooping cough (pertussis) in Boulder, Colorado, to low vaccination rates in the affected communities.[27] Diphtheria cases in Russia increased from 900 in 1989 to 50,000 in 1994, also attributable to a drop in vaccination rates. Moreover, polio, measles, and childhood meningitis (from *Haemophilus influenza* type b bacteria) have been nearly eliminated wherever vaccination rates against them are high.

Most dramatically, before smallpox was eradicated by immunization, in 1979, it had killed 300 million people in the twentieth century.[28] Still, after the Gulf War began in 2003, the safety of vaccinations again became an issue. Fears of an Iraqi attack with smallpox and anthrax agents prompted a policy of vaccinating military personnel against these diseases. When some troops suffered serious side effects from either vaccine, the program was suspended. Ironically, the biological threat from Iraq later proved to be nonexistent – its biological weapons had evidently been destroyed years earlier.

Even healthcare workers who respect the protective value of vaccinations have placed a higher priority on the right to refuse. Thus, the Washington State Nurses Association in 2004 filed suit to prevent a Seattle hospital from mandating flu vaccinations for its personnel. The nurses association sidestepped the contention that an inoculated staff would improve patient safety. Rather the group stated that it supported flu vaccinations, but that the approach to compliance must be through education and not threats.[29]

Subsequently, many medical leaders ramped up efforts to underscore the value of immunization. In 2007, the Sabin Vaccine Institute released a statement that strongly supported vaccination programs. Signed by more than 100 leading physicians and medical administrators, and endorsed by the AMA, the statement described "immunization as the safest, most effective way to control and eradicate infectious diseases."[30] Whether such efforts will alleviate the concerns of skeptics remains unclear.

In fact, people have refused vaccinations even in the face of dire disease threats. During the global campaign to wipe out smallpox in the 1960s and 1970s, some people in countries where the disease was endemic had to be forcibly inoculated. In 1976, few Americans heeded government warnings to seek vaccination against an anticipated swine flu outbreak. In the end, the epidemic never materialized and several people who were vaccinated suffered serious side effects.

The jetliner and anthrax attacks in the United States in 2001 also raised concerns that terrorists might seek to use smallpox as a biological weapon. The following year, President George W. Bush announced a plan to vaccinate 500,000 US healthcare workers, and later up to 10 million firefighters, police, and emergency responders for smallpox.[31] But hundreds of hospitals and thousands of medical personnel refused to comply. By the end of 2004, fewer than 40,000 people had been vaccinated and the program was abandoned.[32] Reluctance was attributed to failure of the government to provide adequate information, though concern about side effects of the vaccine also played a part. (Smallpox vaccinations can cause one or two deaths and a few dozen serious illnesses per million.)

Unlike quarantine, vaccinations are invasive and carry a risk, however minimal, of undesirable effects. Thus, compulsory vaccinations are likely to draw more resistance than quarantine. Still the public health benefits of vaccination are indisputable, and they far outweigh the small risk of untoward effects. Resistance to implementing a massive vaccination or prophylactic drug program occurs when a prospective disease outbreak is perceived as unlikely. In this situation, the public is less willing to cooperate than if an outbreak was already evident. An actual outbreak would enhance acceptance of medications as evidenced by public reactions during the anthrax attacks in 2001. Following the first confirmed death from inhalation anthrax, physicians and pharmacists were overwhelmed by demands from the general population for ciprofloxacin and other antibiotics. The challenge is to find a balance in public health policy that can overcome complacency in advance of a possible outbreak, and avoid frenzied overreaction when the outbreak is in progress.

Triage

The usual connotation of triage, French for "sorting," derives from military medicine. It encompasses a quick assessment and dividing of casualties on the battlefield according to the severity of injury. The concept emerged in the French army during the early 1800s, when the most severely injured were identified and then evacuated for care without regard to rank.[33] Triage has been employed increasingly in American hospitals in recent decades as emergency departments experienced overcrowding. The expanded patient load is attributable in part to the Emergency Medical Treatment and Active Labor Act (EMTLA) of 1986. The EMTLA requires that any patient who arrives at a hospital emergency department must receive a medical screening examination and be provided with emergency care.[34] Treating all patients according to need, and irrespective of insurance or economic status, echoes the early French army approach to triage that disregarded rank.

Toward the end of the twentieth century, the threat of terrorism involving weapons of mass destruction became a growing public health concern. A recognized weakness was the absence of guidelines for emergency physicians in the event of a massive biological, chemical, or radiological attack. In such a setting, "triage may bear little resemblance to the standard approach to civilian triage," according to a study on terrorism and ethics. Since treatment might necessarily be denied to some, physicians should not have to make individual triage decisions. Rather, protocols should be formulated based on bioethical decision-making.[35]

This concern was intensified in the United States by the 2001 terror attacks, which prompted a gathering of some 40 experts in the fields of bioethics, emergency medicine, health law, and policy. Their meeting was convened by agencies in the Department of Health and Human Services, including the Agency for Health Care Preparedness. The conferees spotlighted the novel challenges posed by mass casualties from "an act of bioterrorism or other … medical emergency involving thousands or even tens of thousands of victims." Their deliberations resulted in a 2005 report titled *Altered Standards of Care in Mass Casualty Events*.[36]

The report proposed sharp deviations from commonly understood ethical conduct. Thus, in mass casualty events, providers may have to reuse disposable supplies, may not have time to obtain informed consent, and could discharge hospital inpatients even if "certain lifesaving efforts may have to be discontinued."

Regarding triage, traditional protocols to provide care to the sickest and most injured would not apply. Instead, triage efforts would focus on maximizing the numbers of lives saved. That means giving priority to individuals whose chances of survival are best, and not to the sickest or most injured whose care would require disproportionate attention and scarce supplies.[37]

The World Medical Association (WMA) had listed some of these recommendations in a 1994 statement on medical ethics in disaster situations. In 2006, the WMA produced a revised advisory on triage that included separating patients into five categories and then treating them in a hierarchical order. The highest priority would be for patients who could be saved but whose lives are in immediate danger. Next, patients whose lives are not in immediate danger but need urgent care. Third, injured patients who require minor treatment. Fourth, individuals who are psychologically traumatized, but not physically injured. Last, "patients whose condition exceeds the available therapeutic resources, who suffer from extremely severe injuries ... and cannot be saved in the specific circumstances of time and place, or complex surgical cases ... which would take too long."[38]

At about the same time, Ontario health officials along with other medical and ethics specialists, authored a study on the effects of a massive outbreak of a communicable disease. Models of an influenza pandemic indicated that hospital admissions for infected patients could peak at more than 1,800 per day over a 6-week period. Available resources would be inadequate to address everyone's needs. Limits on care would have to be imposed, which, as the study indicated, is a concept foreign to medical systems in developed countries.

The study proposed a triage protocol based on numerical scores. A person's score would derive from an aggregation of measurements including those of respiratory function, blood pressure, cardiac condition, neurological responses, organ failure, and age. Depending on the score, a patient would be placed in a category designated by color. Red category patients are the highest priority. These include sick individuals who are more likely to recover if they receive intensive care, though unlikely to recover without such care. Yellow signifies intermediate priority, for very sick patients who may or may not benefit from critical care. They could receive such care if resources are available, though not at the expense of the needs of people in the red category. People in the two remaining color categories would not receive critical care at all. Green covers persons well enough to be treated without intensive intervention. Blue signifies patients who are so ill they should not receive critical care, only palliative measures.[39]

How effective this protocol would be in the event of a disease outbreak, whether of deliberate or natural origin, is uncertain. But the study underscores the need to reconfigure traditional understandings of ethics. The authors acknowledge that under normal circumstances, all patients should have a claim to the health care they need. But when faced with bioterrorism or other large-scale disaster, individual rights and needs may be restricted in the interest of the larger community. Certain terrorist acts may generate unique ethical challenges. For example, a terrorist who unintentionally survives a suicide bombing may be critically wounded, as are the people he targeted. Although some of his victims may be less severely injured than the terrorist, would treating them first be morally acceptable? If so, does this mean by extension that in a mass casualty event, some should receive priority treatment apart from severity of injury, but rather based on their age or perceived value to society? Existing ethical codes of healthcare organizations provide little guidance about such questions. The AMA and other health organizations should consider these matters and provide guidance to their constituents.

Healthcare Workers

Do physicians and other healthcare workers have a responsibility to treat patients when their own health and lives could be endangered? The current AMA code says physicians have a duty to provide care in emergencies and that responsibility to the patient should be the paramount consideration.[40] The code of the American Dental Association affirms that dentists should regard the benefit of the patient as their primary goal.[41] The American Nurses Association explicitly addresses ethical obligations during a disaster event including a nurse's obligation to protect self with appropriate gear.[42] But as with other healthcare groups, the nurses association's ethics protocols are silent on the matter of refusing to give care in the interest of personal safety.

A review of studies in the United States, Canada, Israel, and other Asian countries showed that many healthcare workers would not report to work that might risk their own and their families' safety or health.[43–45] A survey of US emergency medical technicians indicated variations of willingness to report to work according to the nature of the disaster. Seventy-four percent of the respondents indicated they would show up in the event of a terrorist attack involving chemical or radioactive agents. The number fell to 65% for a smallpox outbreak.[46] Another study, which included physicians and nurses as well as emergency technicians, found that commitment to work in a disaster scene was as high as 84% and as low as 18%, depending on the perceived danger.[47] But the basic finding of these studies was consistent: in the event of a terrorist or disaster incident, absenteeism among healthcare workers could be substantial, as projected by the workers themselves.

The attitudes expressed in the surveys have been mirrored by actual experience. In the 1980s, when the outbreak of HIV/AIDS began in the United States, several physicians, dentists, and nurses refused to treat patients for fear of becoming infected and transmitting the disease to their families. Many remained hesitant even after the CDC issued assurances that transmission was unlikely if infection control precautions were taken, such as using latex gloves. During the bioterror attacks after 9/11, when anthrax was released through the US postal system, fearful pathologists were reluctant to perform an autopsy on the first confirmed anthrax victim.[48]

The behavior of health professionals was similar during the 2003 outbreak of SARS in Toronto. Many doctors refused to treat patients who were infected with the virus and some resigned from their hospitals rather than face pressure to treat them. The shortage of available physicians prompted the Canadian government to offer temporary medical licenses and two thousand dollars (Canadian) per day to doctors from the United States who would come to help. About 300 US physicians accepted the offer.[49] In the end, some healthcare workers who tended to SARS patients became infected, though the vast majority did not. Infection control measures generally provided adequate protection.

Still, the notion of an absolute duty of care without regard to the well-being of self and family is ethically untenable. Of course, by entering the medical profession a doctor agrees to accept elevated risks, such as increased exposure to patients with infectious disease. But refusal to render treatment in certain dangerous environments is not invariably immoral. Daniel Sokol, a British medical ethicist, recounts the experience of a physician who visited the Congo during the 1995 Ebola epidemic. The doctor came upon 30 dying patients amid rotting corpses in a hospital that had been abandoned by the staff. The Ebola virus is highly virulent, communicable, and unresponsive to treatment. In the absence of any remaining palliative medication and of equipment to protect oneself, should the last physician have stayed to offer inevitably futile care? Sokol's conclusion, that abandonment in this case was justifiable, seems defensible.[50] The ultimate challenge is to establish ethical criteria that allow for refusal to work in a dangerous environment. Ignoring the matter, as is now the case with ethical codes of healthcare organizations, invites poorly informed and unwarranted behavior among practitioners.

Israel, Terrorism, Ethics

Besides giving rise to the field of terror medicine, the surge of Palestinian attacks against Israelis generated new ethical dilemmas not only to health workers but also to the general population. In 2005, when a suspicious young man approached a shopping mall in the northern Israeli city of Netanya, passersby alerted a nearby policewoman. The man ignored the officer's calls to stop. She drew her gun and began to run after him but was reluctant to shoot amid the crowd of people. At the mall entrance, a security guard tried to apprehend the man, who then detonated a bagful of explosives, killing the guard and four others.[51,52]

Should the police officer have fired her gun despite the possibility of hitting bystanders? What if the man turned out not to have been a terrorist? Shooting the culprit could have saved innocent lives, though the officer's restraint can hardly be condemned. The incident exemplifies excruciating moral dilemmas posed by the threat of terrorism.

Other moral choices are more directly related to health and wellbeing. At a forum of the United Nations, a Palestinian spokesman condemned Israel for establishing checkpoints, which delayed ill and pregnant Palestinian women from reaching hospitals. An Israeli representative replied that Israel sought to accommodate people with medical needs, though careful screening was necessary. Between 2000 and 2006, Israeli authorities thwarted suicide attacks by more than

50 Palestinian women. But eight women had succeeded in blowing themselves up and killing scores of Israelis.[53] In fact, in 2002, a young Palestinian woman acknowledged a plan to disguise herself as a pregnant woman and carry out a suicide attack amid a crowd. She was apprehended before putting the plan into action.[54] Later, in June 2005, another woman was found to have explosives under her trousers when she tried to enter Israel from Gaza, an adjacent Palestinian territory. She previously had been treated at Israel's Soroka Hospital in Beer Sheva for burns from a cooking accident in her Gaza home. Now, by her own account, she had hoped to return to the hospital and kill dozens of people there.[55]

An additional threat to healthcare workers arose with the discovery of weapons and gunmen in some Palestinian ambulances. As a result, all vehicles, including Israeli ambulances, are searched at the perimeter of a hospital's grounds before they are permitted to reach the entryway. The Israeli Supreme Court rejected a petition by Physicians for Human Rights, which had protested the practice of stopping and searching Palestinian ambulances. Although international law recognizes the neutrality of ambulances and medical personnel, the Court held that the Israeli practice was justified by the actions of Palestinian belligerents.[56]

Ordinarily, impeding pregnant women or ambulances from traveling freely should be impermissible. But behavioral codes that normally apply must be reevaluated in the face of a competing moral claim, in this case on behalf of potential victims of terrorism. Michael Gross, an Israeli medical ethicist, laments the upending of traditional medical neutrality, but notes that international law and custom provide no alternative solution to the insurgent behavior.[57] While the medical community and others in Israel have had to face these issues as part of their daily lives, they may seem less pressing elsewhere. Still they merit consideration not only as theoretical exercises, but as templates for policy wherever the threat of terrorism exists.

Not every preparedness or protective measure employed by the Israelis is applicable in other societies, but many are. For example, to minimize absenteeism during terror alerts, hospital workers should be assured of priority care for themselves, as is the case in Israel. Along with other first responders they would be quick to receive vaccinations in the event of a biological attack. Work attendance would be further encouraged during prolonged conflict by providing 24-hour onsite nursery care and kindergarten for children whose parents toil elsewhere in the hospital. Numerous other lessons as well can be learned from the Israeli experience.[58]

Table 25.1 lists examples of ethical challenges associated with terror medicine. As noted, some items pertain exclusively to terror incidents, and some may apply as well to other disaster events.

Conclusion

Incidents of terrorism in recent years have altered approaches to medical care and raised a host of issues concerning medical ethics. The threat of bioterrorism and natural disease outbreaks has revived debates about the propriety of compulsory quarantine and vaccination, and altered priorities during triage. Other challenges

TABLE 25.1. Twelve ethical challenges associated with terror medicine[a]

---

1. Delaying and searching someone who is in apparent need of medical attention, but who may be a suicide bomber concealing explosives.
2. Stopping ambulances for inspection before they reach a hospital though they may be transporting people in urgent need of care.
3. Expecting responders to rush to an attack scene despite the risk of additional bombs being detonated at that location following the initial attack.
4. Dealing with hospital personnel who are reluctant to part with their frightened children and other family members during an extended attack.
5. Dealing with hospital personnel who do not report to work for fear of harm to themselves or their families from exposure to a biological agent.
6. Treating a critically injured terrorist before (or after) less severely injured victims are treated.
7. Deciding when to reuse disposable supplies such as needles, latex glove, and protective masks.
8. Deciding when to disregard the doctrine of informed consent.
9. When resources are scarce, determining which victims should receive priority attention and which should receive no care.
10. Determining if and when quarantine should be compulsory.
11. Determining if and when vaccinations or prophylactic antibiotics should be compulsory.
12. Determining when treatment may be delayed by not delivering a patient to the nearest hospital – gauged by conditions such as severity of injury and overcrowding.

---

[a]The first six challenges are exclusive to terrorist threats/incidents, and the remaining six apply to both terrorist and other types of disaster events

have a briefer history, such as dealing with an apparently pregnant woman in need of care, but who may actually be a suicide bomber. Terrorism has also recast the role of the emergency responder who traditionally rushes to the scene of an incident. Nearly simultaneous bombings in the same vicinity have occurred in Israel, and with increasing frequency in Iraq and Afghanistan. A responder must wonder whether a second and third attack might quickly follow the first at the same location. If a responder hesitates to enter the scene is he morally irresponsible?

Such questions were hardly considered in the past. But in this era of heightened terrorist threats, ethicists are presented with new issues to contemplate. As the health and medical consequences of terrorism have given rise to the field of terror medicine, so have their moral implications generated concern with an associated new dimension, terror ethics.

References

1. Markel H. "I swear by Apollo" – on taking the Hippocratic oath. *New Engl J Med.* 2004; 350: 2026–9.
2. Harris SH. *Factories of Death: Japanese Biological Warfare 1932–45 and the American Cover Up*. New York: Routledge; 1994.
3. Annas GJ, Grodin MA. *The Nazi Doctors and the Nuremberg Code: Human Rights in Human Experimentation*. New York: Oxford University Press; 1995.
4. American Medical Association. *Principles of Medical Ethics*, House of Delegates, May 1903, Chap. 2.

5. American Medical Association. *Principles of Medical Ethics*, House of Delegates, June 1958.

6. Jones JH. *Bad Blood: The Tuskegee Syphilis Experiment*. New York: Free Press; 1993.

7. Marks JD. *The Search for the Manchurian Candidate: The CIA and Mind Control*. New York: Norton; 1991.

8. Advisory Committee on Human Radiation Experiments. *The Human Radiation Experiments*. New York: Oxford University Press; 1996.

9. Welsome, E. *The Plutonium Files: America's Secret Medical Experiments During the Cold War*. New York: Delta; 2000.

10. American Medical Association. *Principles of Medical Ethics*, House of Delegates, June 1980.

11. Bayer R, Colgrove J. Rights and dangers: bioterrorism and the ideologies of public health. In: Moreno JD, ed. *In the Wake of Terror: Medicine and Morality in a Time of Crisis*. Cambridge, MA: MIT Press; 2003: 54.

12. Committee on Research Standards and Practices to Prevent the Destructive Application of Biotechnology. National Institute of Medicine. *Biotechnology Research in an Age of Terrorism*. Washington, DC: National Academies Press; 2004.

13. Trotter G. *The Ethics of Coercion in Mass Casualty Medicine*. Baltimore, MD: Johns Hopkins University Press; 2007.

14. Bayer, Colgrove, 52–3.

15. *The Model State Emergency Health Powers Act*, Draft for Discussion Prepared by the Center for Law and the Public's Health at Georgetown and Johns Hopkins Universities, for the Centers for Disease Control and Prevention, December 21, 2001. http://www.publichealthlaw.net/MSEHPA/MSEHPA2.pdf. Accessed July 30, 2007.

16. Annas GJ. Bioterrorism, public health, and civil liberties. *New Engl J Med*. 2002; 345: 1337–42.

17. Lawrence O. Gostin and James, Jr. Protecting the Public's Health in an Era of Bioterrorism. In: *In the Wake of Terror: Medicine and Morality in a Time of Crisis*. Jonathan D. Moreno, editor. Basic Bioethics Series. Massachusetts: The MIT Press, 2003.

18. Makarenko J. Severe acute respiratory syndrome (SARS) outbreak in Canada. *Mapleleafweb*, April 20, 2005. http://www.mapleleafweb.com/old/education/spotlight/issue_31/index.html?q=education/spotlight/issue_31/index.html. Accessed August 3, 2007.

19. Hawryluck L, Gold WL, Robinson S, et al. SARS control and psychological effects of quarantine, Toronto, Canada. *Emerg Infect Dis*. 2004; 10: 1206–12.

20. McKeown D. Medical Officer of Health. *Preliminary Results of SARS-Related Public Health Research*. Toronto Staff Report to the Board of Health, November 23, 2005. http://www.toronto.ca/legdocs/2005/agendas/committees/hl/hl051128/it002.pdf. Accessed August 9, 2007.

21. Upshur R. The ethics of quarantine. *AMA-Med. Soc*. 2003; 5: 1–4.

22. Tucker, JB. *Scourge: The Once and Future threat of Smallpox*. New York: Atlantic Monthly Press; 2001: 5–22.

23. Fenner F., ed. *Smallpox and Its Eradication*. Geneva: World Health Organization; 1988.

24. U.S. Centers for Disease Control and Prevention. http://www.cdc.gov/vaccines/vpd-vac/vpd-list.htm. Accessed September 17, 2007.

25. Welborn AW. Mandatory vaccinations: precedent and current law. Report for Congress by the Congressional Research Service. January 2005. http://www.fas.org/sgp/crs/RS21414.pdf. Accessed September 17, 2007.

26. Figes K. A shot in the dark. *Guardian.* August 13, 2003. http://www.fas.org/sgp/crs/RS21414.pdf. Accessed, September 20, 2007.

27. Berlinger N. Parental resistance to childhood immunizations: clinical, ethical and policy considerations. *AMA J Ethics.* 2006; 8(10): 681–4.

28. Open Statement on Vaccines. The Sabin Vaccine Institute. 2007. http://www.sabin.org/programs/open_vaccine/index.html. Accessed September 20, 2007.

29. Robeznieks A. Washington state nurses sue hospital over mandatory flu vaccination rule. *amednews.com,* October 18, 2004. http://www.ama-assn.org/amednews/2004/10/18/prse1018.htm. Accessed September 20, 2007.

30. Open Statement on Vaccines.

31. Cohen C, Curley A. Source: Bush to announce plan for smallpox vaccinations. CNN.com. November 27, 2002. http://archives.cnn.com/2002/HEALTH/conditions/11/26/smallpox.vaccine/index.html. Accessed September 23, 2007.

32. Baciu A, Anason AP, Stratton K, Strom B, eds. *The Smallpox Vaccination Program: Public Health in an Age of Terrorism.* Institute of Medicine. Washington, DC: National Academies Press; 2005.

33. Answers.com. *The American Heritage Dictionary.* http://www.answers.com/topic/triage?cat=health. Accessed July 21, 2007.

34. Emergency Medical Treatment and Active Labor Act, 42 U.S.C. § 1395dd, 1986.

35. Pesik N, Keim ME, Iserson KV. Terrorism and the ethics of emergency medical care. *Ann Emerg Med.* 2001; 37(6): 642–6.

36. *Altered Standards of Care in Mass Casualty Events: Bioterrorism and Other Public Health Emergencies.* AHRQ Publication No. 05-0043. Rockville, MD: Agency for Healthcare Research and Quality, April 2005.

37. Health and medical care delivery in a mass casualty event. In: *Altered Standards of Care in Mass Casualty Events,* Chap. 2.

38. World Medical Association Statement on Medical Ethics in the Event of Disasters, Revised by the WMA General Assembly, Adopted 1994, Revised 2006. http://www.wma.net/e/policy/d7.htm. Accessed August 10, 2007.

39. Christian MD, Hawryluck L, Wax RS, et al. Development of a triage protocol for critical care during an influenza epidemic. *Can Med Assoc J.* 2006; 17(11): 377–81.

40. American Medical Association. *Principles of Medical Ethics,* House of Delegates, June 2001.

41. American Dental Association. *Principles of Ethics and Professional Conduct.* Revised January 2005. http://www.ada.org/prof/prac/law/code/preamble.asp. Accessed August 13, 2007.

42. American Nurses Association. Position Statement on Work Release During a Disaster. Adopted by the Board of Directors, June 2002.

43. Smith E. Emergency health care workers' willingness to work during major emergencies and disasters. *Aust J Emerg Manage.* 2007; 22(2): 21–4.

44. Imai T, Takahashi K, Hoshuyama, T, et al. SARS risk perceptions in healthcare workers, Japan. *Emerg Infect Dis.* 2005; 11(3): 404–10.

45. Ho SM, Kwong-Lo RS, Mak CW, Wong, JS. Fear of severe acute respiratory syndrome (SARS) among health care workers," *J Consult Clin Psychol.* 2005; 73(2): 344–9.

46. DiMaggio C, Markenson D, Loo GT, Redlener I. The willingness of U.S. emergency medical technicians to respond to terrorist incidents. *Biosecur Bioterr Biodefense Strat Pract Sci.* 2005; 3(4): 331–7.

47. Syett JL, Benitez JG, Livingston WH, Davis EA. Will emergency health care providers respond to mass casualty incidents? *Prehospital Emerg Care.* 2007; 11(1): 49–54.

48. Cole LA. *The Anthrax Letters: A Medical Detective Story.* Washington, DC: Joseph Henry Press/National Academies Press; 2003: 134.

49. Altman LK. The doctor's world; behind the mask, the fear of SARS," *New York Times,* June 24, 2003: F-1.

50. Sokol DK. Virulent epidemics and scope of healthcare workers' duty of care. *Emerging Infectious Dis* [serial on the Internet]. 2006 Aug. Available from http://www.cdc.gov/ncidod/EID/vol12no08/06-0360.htm. Accessed September 5, 2007.

51. Myre G. Palestinian bomber kills himself and 5 others near Israel mall. *New York Times,* Dec. 6, 2005, A-6.

52. Israel Ministry of Foreign Affairs. http://www.mfa.gov.il/MFA/MFAArchive/2000_2009/2005/Suicide%20bombing%20at%20Sharon%20Mall%20in%20Netanya%205-Dec-2005. Accessed April 16, 2006.

53. U.N. Economic and Social Council, Commission on the Status of Women, New York, March 3, 2006. http://domino.un.org/UNISPAL.NSF/eed216406b50bf6485256ce100 72f637/53ce29e4c796b8868525712900527f92!OpenDocument. Accessed August 18, 2007.

54. Israel Ministry of Foreign Affairs. A woman terrorist, en route to carry out a suicide attack, arrested in Tulkarm. April 11, 2002. http://www.israel-mfa.gov.il/MFA/Government/Communiques/2002/A%20woman%20terrorist-%20en%20route%20to%20carry%20out%20a%20suicide. Accessed August 20, 2007.

55. Descent from patient to suicide bomber. MSNBC-TV report, June 23, 2005. http://www.msnbc.msn.com/id/8330374. Accessed August 15, 2007.

56. Israel Ministry of Foreign Affairs. Palestinian misuse of medical services and ambulances for terrorist activities. October 13, 2004. http://www.israel-mfa.gov.il/MFA/Government/Law/Legal+Issues+and+Rulings/Palestinian%20Misuse%20of%20Medical%20Services%20and%20Ambulances%20for%20Terrorist%20Activities%20 13-Oct-2004. Accessed August 25, 2007.

57. Gross ML. *Bioethics and Armed Conflict: Moral Dilemmas of Medicine and War.* Cambridge, MA: MIT Press; 2006.

58. Cole LA. *Terror: How Israel Has Coped and What America Can Learn.* Bloomington, IN: Indiana University Press; 2007.

Index

A

Aarabi, B., 329
Abdominal and brain injuries, 157–158
Advanced biological warfare (ABW)
  agent, 196
Advanced Research Projects Agency
  (ARPA) ARPAnet concept, 257
Advanced trauma life support (ATLS)
  guidelines, 279
  protocols, 339
Agent-based modeling, 88
Aharonson-Daniel, L., 156
Al-Aqsa intifada, 299, 301, 393
Alert levels, 103
  preparedness procedures, 104
*Altered Standards of Care in Mass Casualty
  Events,* 431
American Burn Association, 70
American Medical Association (AMA)
  and codes
    medical ethics, 426
    physicians and healthcare workers,
      433–434
Amirjamshidi, A., 313
Ammonium nitrate fuel oil (ANFO)
  high-energy explosives, 31
Annas, G., 427
Anthrax attacks, 196
  Bacillus anthracis spores and
    aerosolization, 198
  and children, 370–371
  cutaneous anthrax, 199
  gastrointestinal anthrax, 199, 201
  inhalational anthrax, 199–201
  mail anthrax attacks, in USA, 90
  treatment and prophylaxis, 202
  in United States, 9

Argentine Israeli Mutual Association
  building in Buenos Aires car
  bombing, 34
Armed Forces Radiobiology Research
  Institute (AFRRI), 70
Aschkenasy-Steuer, G., 161
Atomic Energy Commission, experiments
  with citizens, 426
Atropine drug, 231
Attack execution, 21

B

Balloon angioplasty, 325
Ben Taub General Hospital, system
  dynamics model of disaster plan,
  87, 91
Bentley, G., 337
Bioethics development and pre-and postwar
  experiments on unwitting human
  subjects, 426
Biological attacks, 19
  warfare agent, 150
  weapons system, 196
*Biotechnology Research in an Age of
  Terrorism,* 138
Blood agents, 375, 376
Blunt trauma, 274–275
Bomb blast
  blast lung injury (BLI), 178–179
  blast wave, 31
  brain swelling, 315
  injuries
    air transportation, 326–327
    auditory, 280–281
    clinical patterns of, 318
    craniofacial, 321–324
    CT scan for, 319–321

Bomb blast (*cont.*)
  explosion, 31
  head, 315
  penetrating missiles, 272–273
  reconstruction, 327
  rehabilitation, 330–332
  pathophysiology, 177–178
  physics, 175–177
Bossi, P., 196, 201, 206, 208, 211–213, 216
Botulism
  botulinum toxin, 207
  and children, 373
  clinical features and diagnosis, 209
  Clostridium botulinum, groups of, 208
  treatment
    investigational pentavalent (A–E)
      botulinum toxoid vaccine, 209
Bowyer, G. W., 289, 292
Brain trauma foundation guidelines, 326
Brandvold, B., 313
Braverman, I., 159
Bregman, D., 90
Bromobenzylcyanide (CA), riot control
  agent, 235
Brown, A. A., 338
Burn injuries. *See also* Terrorism
  acute lung injuries, 305
  burn wound management, 308–310
    burn wound sepsis, 307
  case report, 303–304
  hemodynamic support, 305–306
  infections, 306–307
  management of casualties, 303
Business continuity management (BCM), 54
  international standards in, 55

C
Candida sepsis, 303–304
Capsaicin (pepper spray), riot control
  agent, 235
Casualty collection area (CCA), 185
CBRN (Chemical, Biological, Radiological,
  and Nuclear) terrorism, 18
Centennial Olympics bombing
  in Atlanta, 177
Centers for Disease Control (CDC)
  and Prevention
  bioagent categories, 197–198
  bioterrorism and, 195
    pediatric age group, 198

CHEMPACK project, 232
  study, on terrorism preparedness, 59
  vaccinations, 429
Central Intelligence Agency, experiments
  with citizens, 426
Chemical terror attacks, 19, 150
  chemical agent
    children exposure and, 374–375
    in terrorism, recommended treatment
      and management of, 380–382
  chemical attack by Japanese cult Aum
    Shinrikyo in Tokyo, 16
  decontamination after, 228, 230
  hospital issues, 230
    blood agent, 232–233
    incapacitating agent, 234
    nerve agent and insecticides, 231–232
    patients, management of, 235
    pulmonary/choking agent, 233–234
    riot control agent/tear gas, 235
    vesicants/blister agent, 233
  hot zone, 228–229
  outcome, 235–237
  pre-hospital management of, 228
  symptom-based algorithm for, 236
Chen, A. Y., 354
Childhood outbreaks, 429
Chloroacetophenone, riot control
  agent, 235
Chlorobenzylidenemalononitrile (CS)
  and chloropicrin (PS), riot control
  agent, 235
Christie, P. M., 89
Civil Contingencies Act 2004, 54
Civilian trauma victims, 274–275
Clinicians, role in MCI management, 61
Coagulopathy, 319
Cochrane, Thomas, 62
"Code Orange," 70, 72
Cohen, J. T., 280
Collaborative Multi-Agency Exercise
  (CMAX), 73
Combined blast injuries, 181
Common relevant operational picture
  (CROP), technology tools, 141
Communication system, in disaster
  response, 115–116, 130
Computer modeling and simulation, use in
  terror medicine, 79
  concept of, 80

limitations of, 83–84
modeling
  cycle, 81–83
  hospital response, 90–91
modeling tools, for disaster response, 86
  agent-based modeling, 88
  discrete-event simulation (DES), 86–87
  system dynamics, 88
need of, 80–81
pre-hospital phase, 89–90
published reports on, 88
types of models, 83
Concrete extortion attacks threats, 20
Congo-Crimean hemorrhagic fever,
  (CCHF), 213
Conventional terror, 149–150
weapons, in MCI, 62
Counter-terrorism
avian influenza viruses threat, 142–143
medical operations, command and
  control
    biological warfare scenario and,
     135–136
    new technologies and, 137–139
    technologic dilemma and security,
     136–137
technology landscape
  challenges and opportunities, 139–140
  information sharing environments,
    140–141
  limitations, 141–142
  measures of effectiveness and
    performance (MOEs and MOPs), 140
Coupland, R. M., 290, 291
Craniectomy, 329
Critical casualties service line, 84
Critical incident stress management
  (CISM), 129
Crush injury (CI), 337–339
active treatment for, 340
crush syndrome (CS), 341–342
  etiology, 342
  prevention plan, 343
hospital issues
  fasciotomy/debridement, 340
  mechanisms of, 341
  vascular and neural injury, 341
pre-hospital treatment, 339
protocol for preventing acute renal
  failure in, 344

Cyanides
blood agent, 232–233
cyanide antidote kit, 376
cyanide-laced Tylenol® capsules, 223
cyanogen chloride (CK), 233
Cyber-terrorism, 95
computer security in future, 265–267
cybernetics and modern information
  technology, 256–257
health and hospital services, 261–262
  means of protection, 263
  sources of threats, 262
Internet security and privacy, 259
  reliability of service and
    data storage, 260
nodes on net, 258–259
technology developments and, 258
terrorist targets and weapons, 255–256

D
De Boer, J., 88–89
Debriefing after, terror attacks, 107–108
Decision-makers threatening, 20
Defense and Veterans Brain Injury Center
  (DVBIC) in USA, 327
Deflagration, 175. See also Bomb blast
Deterministic model, 83
Detonation, 175. See also Bomb blast
Dibenzoxazepine (CR) and
  diphenylaminearsine (DM), riot
  control agent, 235
Direct economic damage, 21
Dirty bomb, 30
Disaster management, 59
  medical director(s), 113–114
  simulation, 80
Discrete event simulation (DES) model, 86–87
  of pre-hospital response, 89–90
Dobson, J. E., 347–348
Dynamite high-energy explosives, 31

E
Eardrum perforation, 31
Eastern Equine Encephalomyelitis (EEE)
  as threat agent, 197
Elitism as ethical principle, 426
Emergency medical services (EMS), 30, 59,
  61, 87, 89, 98–100
activities of, 35–36
commander, 36

Emergency medical services (EMS) (*cont.*)
    emergency response framework, 112
    emergency room, Code Red, 70
    trained personnel, 37
Emergency Medical Treatment and Active
        Labor Act (EMTLA) of 1986, 431
Emergency operations plans, of hospitals.
        See Hospital emergency operations
        plans
Emergency system for advanced
        registration of volunteer health
        professionals program
        (ESAR-P), 131
ER *One* Institute, 65, 70
"Error-tolerant design", in hospital disaster
        planning, 85
Explosive disasters, 172
    caused by ammonium nitrate
        (fertilizer), 174

F

Federal Bureau of Investigation's (FBI)
        National Infrastructure Protection
        Center (NIPC), 266
Federal Emergency Management Agency
        (FEMA), 70, 112
Forrester, J. W., 88
Fragment and projectile wounds, 292
Frykberg, E. R., 32, 178, 184, 347, 348

G

Gas masks, use in World War I, 62, 63
Geiger counter. *See* Geiger-Mueller tube
        radiation detector
Geiger-Mueller tube radiation detector, 247
General extortion attacks threats, 20
George Washington University School of
        Medicine, 64
German doctors and inhumane research on
        involuntary subjects, 425
Glasgow coma scale score (GCS), 315
Global jihadi terrorism, 16
Global war on terror (GWOT), 133
    and cold war, 134
Gofrit, O. N., 314
Gostin, L., 427
Great Hashin-Awaji earthquake, 89
Ground zero hospital, 186
Gunshot injuries, 354–355

H

Hackers, 262. *See also* Cyber-terrorism
Hadassah University Hospital, Israel
        bombing, 65
Hadden, W. A., 356
Halifax and Texas City disasters, 175
Hanoch, J., 271, 354
Hantavirus as threat agent, 197
Hazard vulnerability assessment (HVA), 115
HAZMAT hazardous materials, 40
Healthcare system and threat
    agent of attack, rapid detection and
        identification, 23
    casualties transfer, 22–23
    consequences of, 56–57
    coordination in, during terror attack,
        98–99
    cyber-terrorism against, 25
    direct attack on, 24
    forestalling panic, 24
    injuries, types of, 22
    medical teams, protection of, 24
    medication and medical instruments, 23
    number of casualties, 22
    primary care facilities, 53–54
    quick containment of attack area, 23
    relatives of victims, 23
    sequential conventional and
        unconventional attacks against, 24–25
    as victim of, 54
Heering, S. L., 352
Helsinki Area Disaster Plan, 35
Helsinki, Finland terrorist bombing, 177
HHH (hypertension, hypervolemia,
        hemodilution) therapy, 326
High-energy explosives, 31
Hippocratic Oath, 425
Hiroshima and Nagasaki, use of MCI
        weapons in, 62–63
Hirshberg, Asher, 75
Hodge, J., 427
Holmes, S., 356
Homeland Security Act of 2002, 112
Hospital emergency operations plans, 117
    Acts on preparation for, 111–113
    administrators role, in MCI, 61
    alternate care site planning, 125
    casualty family center, 130
    casualty flow planning, 126–127

commitment, 113–114
communication systems, 115–116
community volunteers, registration of, 130–131
disaster response, system characteristic of, 84–85
employee education, 130
evacuation planning, 125–126
finance/administration section, 123
hazard vulnerability assessment, 115
hospital incident command system (HICS), 59, 119–120
incident command system (ICS), 119–121
logistics section, 122–123
medical controller, role of, 127–128
mitigation, 118
morgue, temporary, 128–129
operations section, role of, 121–122
patient care documentation, 129
patient flow, 127–128
performance improvement exercises, 131
planning committee, role of, 114–115
planning section, function of, 122
preparedness, 118
    structural, in high-risk metropolitan areas, 105
recovery, 119
response plan, 118–119
safety and security, 117
staffing alterations, 126
sustainability planning, 124–125
triage, 123–124
Hupert, N., 90
Hydrogen cyanide (AC), 233
Hypovolemia, 305

I
Immediate attack zone, 99
Improvized explosive device (IED), 313
Incident command system (ICS), 119, 121
    incident commander, 120
InfluSim, 90. *See also* Hospital emergency operations plans
Information Reform and Terrorism Prevention Act of 2004, 140
Injuries
    abdominal and brain, 157–158
    arrival and patterns, 151–152
    body regions injured, 156–157
    distribution of type of injury by body region, 158
    gunshot wounds, 153–154
    injury severity score (ISS) of casualties, 301, 303
    intubation in ED, 162
    lung and chest, 157
    mass casualty event (MCE) networks, 161
    mechanisms, 152–153
    operating rooms, utilization of, 163–164
    orthopedic, 158
    patient care and service utilization, 161
    patients entering surgery, 164
    penetrating missiles, 272–273
    perpetrator bone fragment, 159
    pre-hospital issues, 159–160
    preparedness for mass arrival in hospital, 160–161
    profiles of, 154
    psychological effects, 159
    severity, 155–156
    shifting patterns of hospital utilization, 163
    shrapnel wounds, 153
    thoracotomies in ED, 162
    ultrasound scanning and diagnostic imaging, 162–163
Inoue, H., 89
Institute for Bioterrorism and Emerging Disease (BEPAST), 65
Intangible threat, 20
Integrative Center for Homeland Security, Texas A&M University, 64
Intelligence information, 95
    flow of, 96
International Atomic Energy Agency (IAEA)
    radioactive materials, security of, 241
International Standard Archival Description (ISAD) Information Sharing and Analysis Center (ISAC), 266
Internet use in terrorism, 256. *See also* Cyber-terrorism
Israeli debriefing method, 107–108
Israeli National Skin Bank, 309
Israeli Sheba Medical Center at Tel Hashomer, suicide attack, 24
Istanbul terrorist bombings, 34

J

Jacob, E., 290
Jeffreys, T. E., 337
Johns Hopkins Bloomberg School of Public
    Health, 64
Joint Commission standards, on disaster
    planning, 113
"Just In Time Training", 68

K

Karayilanoglu, T., 229
Katz, E., 278
Kenar, L., 229
Khobar Towers terrorist truck bombing,
    32, 177
Kluger, Y., 276
Koren, I., 358

L

Laminectomy, 329
Leap-frogging, 124, 186
Levary, R. R., 89
Levi, L., 90
Limited unconventional attack, 18–19
Lin, D. L., 290
Liu, Y., 138
Lobectomy, 323
London bombings, 33
Long-range intelligence, 95
Low-order explosives, 31

M

Madrid train bombings, 33
Mail anthrax attacks, in USA, 90
Markenson, D., 371, 374, 376, 379,
    386–387
Mass-casualty management
    hospital resource utilization, 186–188
    injury patterns, 182–183
    mass casualty incident (MCI), 59 (see
        also Terrorism)
        hospital operations in, 84–85
    pre-hospital casualty handling, 185–186
    triage implications, 183–185
Mass media, role in terrorism, 14, 106–107,
    116
Medical Simulation Center (MSR), Israel, 70
Medical training vehicles, in terror
    medicine, 68–69

Metrorail crash in Washington, DC, 33
Michaelson, M., 340
Military Acute Concussion Evaluation
    (MACE), 327
Model State Emergency Health Powers
    Act (MSEHPA) for bioterrorist and
    public health emergencies, 427
Molotov Cocktail, 31. See also Low-order
    explosives
Multidimensional injuries, 183
Murrah Federal Building in Oklahoma City
    terrorist bombing, 183
Musgrave Park Hospital, Belfast bomb
    blast, 54
Mustard agent
    and children explosure, 377 (see also
        Terrorism)

N

Nahlieli, O., 353
National Academy of Sciences (NAS)
    study on countering bio-terrorism, 137
National Emergency Coordination
    Committee (NECC), 97
National Emergency Medical Coordinating
    Committee (NEMCC), in Israel, 99
    alert level, declaration of, 103–104
    audit and surprise inspections, 103
    exercises and rehearsals, 101–102
    hospital SOP, 101
    patient distribution, to various
        hospitals, 100–101
    SOP preparation, 99–100
    storage and maintenance, of
        equipment, 102
    training to medical, paramedical, and
        administrative teams, 102–103
    unconventional terrorism, training to deal
        with, 103
National incident management system
    (NIMS), 59, 112–113
National interagency genomics sciences
    coordinating committee (NIGSCC),
    recommendations for research on
    bioterrorism, 137
National response plan, 112
National Science Advisory Board for
    Biosecurity (NSABB) of dual-use
    research of concern, 138

Nerve palsy, 293
Nicholls, R. J., 338
Nipah virus as threat agent, 197
Nitroglycerine high-energy explosives, 31
Noncritical casualties service line, 84
Nuclear attacks, 19
Number of direct casualties, 21
Nuremberg verdict, in 1947, 425–426

O

Occam's razor, in modeling, 83
Odhiambo, W. A., 356
Ohboshi, N., 89
Omer, G. E., 293
Online terror medicine education, 65–66
Open-air blast, 175
Operation Bushmaster, 73, 74
Operation Kerkesner, 73
Organizational information protection
        system, 263–264
Organizational operational
        debriefings, 108, 109
Overtriage, 85. *See also* Triage

P

Packet switching concept, 257
Paran, H., 278
Patient flow coordinator, 127
Patient simulators, for MCI, 69–70
Penetrating injuries, 271
    and bombing attacks
        attack setting, 276–277
        auditory injury, 279–281
        gastrointestinal tract injury, 278–279
        management of victims, 274–275
        ocular injury, 281
        scope of injury, 275–276
        suicide terrorism, 273–274
        vascular injury, 281–283
Personal protective equiment (PPE), 60
Phosgene oxime
    and children, 375 (*see also* Terrorism)
Physicians training, for MCI, 60
Pipe bombs, 31
Plague
    and children, 370
    clinical and biological characteristics
        of, 206
    clinical syndromes of, 205

criteria for suspecting deliberate release
        of, 207
    diagnosis, 205
    treatment and postexposure prophylaxis,
        recommendations for, 207, 208
    Yersinia pestis infection, 205
Police and intelligence services, 262. *See
        also* Cyber-terrorism
Postconcussion syndrome, 327–328
Post-traumatic stress disorders (PTSD),
        106, 328
    and ASD Treatment, 418–419
    secondary PTSD, 413
    terrorist attacks
        anxiety in population, 414–415
        ER/immediate response, 417–418
        9/11, events of, 408, 411
        intervention and mass casualties,
            targets of, 416–417
        Israeli terror attacks, 411–412
        London bombing, 411
        Madrid and France bombings, 411
        in Oklahoma City, 412
        predictors of, 413
        prevalence and development
            of, 407
        resilience, 414
        studies of, 409–410
        symptoms, 406–407
        traumatic events, 406
        US Embassy in Nairobi, 412–413
        victim, psychological
            shock, 415–416
Potassium cyanide (KCN), 233
Powers, D. B., 355
Pradiloxime chloride (PAM), 231
Primary blast injuries, 8, 31, 178–180
Professional medical debriefing, 108
Protective service personnel, role in MCI
        management, 61
Public health preparedness and critical
        biological agent categories, 197
Public Information Center
    public information officer
        (PIO), 116, 120
    in terror attacks, 105–106
Pulmonary blast injury, 315. *See also* Bomb
        blast
Pure petroleum-based bombs, 31

Q

Quaternary blast injury, 181–182, 288

R

Radiation Emergency Assistance Center/
    Training Site (REAC/TS), 245
Radiological terror agent, 150–151
    and children
        KI dose administration, 386–387
        marrow stimulative agent, 387
        prussian blue dosing, 387
        radiation exposure, 383–384
        radionuclides and, 385
    decontamination effort, 242
    HAZMAT guidelines, 243
    ionizing radiation, 243
    lymphocyte response, 244
    radiation energy from, 242
    radioactive contamination, 243–245
    response to terrorist event involving
        radioactivity
        patient care, 246–250
        planning for and managing of
            radiation injuries, 245–246, 251
        and recovery, 250
    risk to health care staff, 247
Rational fear, 14. *See also* Terrorism
Red Cross E.X.C.V.F.M. Wound Scores, 289
Reference threat, 96
Reis, N. D., 340
Resource allocation problem, 79
Rhabdomyolysis, 342. *See also* Crush
    injury (CI)
Ricin exposure
    and children, 373 (*see also* Terrorism)
Rift Valley fever (RVF), 213
Rivkind, A. I., 274, 275, 277, 278, 282
Robertson, O. B., 355
Robert T. Stafford Disaster Relief and
    Emergency Assistance Act. *See*
    Stafford Act

S

Safe harbor area, 126
Safety and security issues, in response
    planning, 117
Salvageability, 183. *See also* Triage
Secondary blast injuries, 8, 31, 180, 288
Security procedures

during major incident, 49–50
    and terrorism, 30
Segaller, S., 257
Semtex high-energy explosives, 31
September 11 attacks, 16, 175
Severe acute respiratory syndrome (SARS)
    outbreak in Canada, 428
Shear waves, 175. *See also* Bomb blast
Sheba disaster plan, Israel, 90
Shih, C. L., 89
Shock waves, 175. *See also* Bomb blast
Short-range intelligence, 95
Shuker, S. T., 357
Simulation and Training Environment Lab
        Learning Management System, 65
Simulation model, 34
SiTEL Clinical Simulation Centers, 69
SLUDGE symptoms, 231
Smallpox viral infection, 202
    route of transmission, 203
    variola major
        diagnosis and treatment, 204–205
        hemorrhagic-type smallpox, 204
        ordinary-type smallpox, 203–204
Sodium cyanide (NaCN), 233
Solomon, Z., 159
Spartans boys training, 67
Stafford Act, 112
Standardized patients use, for training, 70
Standard operating procedures (SOP), 97
Stapczynski, J. S., 357–358
Staten, C., 229
Stevenson, M. D., 89
Stochastic model, 83
Stoning and intentional road accidents, 149.
        See also Conventional terror
Strapped human bomb (SHB), 399–400
Stress
    and terrorism, 9
    waves, 177 (*see also* Bomb blast)
Suicide bombing attacks
    data reconciliation, 399
    event, reconstruction of, 399–400
    forensic investigation of, 393
    information center (IC) and family
        assistance, 395
    scene investigation
        scene of crime officers (SOCOs) and
            bomb squad examiners, 393–395

suicide attack phenomenon, 17–18
suicide bomber
  high rates of immediate surgery and
    ICU utilization in, 161
  in Lebanon, Hezbollah group, 273
  Tamil Tigers and, 273
  thanatological examination, 395–396
    documentation of injuries and,
      397–398
    fingerprinting scanner, 397
Surge capacity, 81, 126–127
Su, S., 89
System dynamics approach, 88

T
Tangible threat, 20
Terrorism, 13
  age distribution
    of casualties, 302
    terror and non-trauma/trauma
      casualties, 155
  Al-Aqsa intifada, 299
  Alfred P. Murrah Federal Building in
    Oklahoma City bombing, 32
  asymmetric warfare, 15
  attacks, psychological effects of, 405
    PTSD, 406–411
  big powers in regional disputes,
    intervention of, 15
  Bin Laden's World Islamic Front, 16
  biological/chemical weapons detection, 4
  biological weapons system, 196
  bombing attacks against civilians, 29
  burn injuries
    acute lung injuries, 305
    burn case distribution in first terror
      wave and Al-Aqsa intifada, 301
    burn wound management, 307–310
    hemodynamic support, 305–306
    infections, 306–307
    management of casualties, 303
  chemical attack by Japanese cult Aum
    Shinrikyo in Tokyo, 16
  and children, 365–366
    anthrax, 370–371
    blister agent, 376–377
    botulism, 373
    chemical agent exposure and, 374–375
    chemical/ biological toxins, 367–368

    mental health vulnerabilities, 368
    nerve agent, 377–382
    phosgene oxime, 375
    pulmonary/choking agent, 375
    recommended therapy and
      prophylaxis, 371
    ricin exposure, 373
    smallpox, 372
    tularemia, 370–371
    viral hemorrhagic fever (VHF),
      372–373
  conventional terror, 149–150
    conventional weapons, in MCI, 62
  development of standard operating
    procedures (SOP) for medical
    care, 167
  evaluation
    records and documentation of, 352
    and resuscitation of victims, 351
  failures and impairments related to
    conflicts and, 55
  geographical shift, 15–16
  global jihadi terrorism, 16
  gunshot injuries, 354–355
  healthcare system and threat
    agent of attack, rapid detection and
      identification, 23
    casualties transfer, 22–23
    consequences of, 56–57
    cyber-terrorism against, 25
    direct attack on, 24
    forestalling panic, 24
    injuries, types of, 22
    medical teams, protection of, 24
    medication and medical instruments, 23
    number of casualties, 22
    primary care facilities, 53–54
    quick containment of attack area, 23
    relatives of victims, 23
    sequential conventional and
      unconventional attacks against, 24–25
    as victim of, 54
  injuries
    arrival and patterns, 151–152
    body regions injured, 156–157
    distribution of type of injury by body
      region, 158
    injury severity score (ISS) of
      casualties, 301, 303

Terrorism (*cont.*)
  intubation in ED, 162
  lung and chest, 157
  mass casualty event (MCE)
    networks, 161
  mechanisms, 152–153
  orthopedic, 158
  patient care and service utilization, 161
  patients entering surgery, 164
  perpetrator bone fragment, 159
  pre-hospital issues, 159–160
  preparedness for mass arrival in
    hospital, 160–161
  profiles of, 154
  psychological effects, 159
  shifting patterns of hospital
    utilization, 163
  shrapnel wounds, 153
  thoracotomies in ED, 162
  ultrasound scanning and diagnostic
    imaging, 162–163
  Internet service providers (ISPs) and, 257
  Israel National Trauma Registry
    data on, 300
  in Matsumoto, Japan, accidental
    exposure of unidentified toxic
    material, 4
  maxillofacial injury, 347
    blast injuries, 356–362
    epidemiology, 348–349
  medical and bioethics, 427
    ethical challenges associated with, 436
    Palestinian attacks against Israelis and,
      434–435
    physicians and healthcare workers,
      3–5, 433–434
    quarantine and, 427–428
    triage connotation of, 431–433
    and vaccinations, 428–431
  medical response and phases
    casualty receiving, 46
    of chaos, 45
    consolidation, 46
    definitive care, 46
    equipment, 48–49
    rehabilitation, 46–47
    space and, 47
    staff, 47–48
    surgical procedures, 165
  and medicine
    incident management, 6–7
    injuries and responses, 7–8
    medical community, role of, 3–5
    preparedness, 5–6
    psychological consequences, 8–9
  modern terrorism, 14–15
    beginning of twenty-first century, 16–17
    end of twentieth century, 15–16
    history of, 14–15
    suicide attack phenomenon, 17–18
  mortality from terrorist attacks, 164–165
  National military strategic plan for war
    on, 133–134
  neurosurgical injury, 313
    air transportation, 326–327
    head, neck, and spine, 313–317
    indications for diagnostic angiography
      in, 326
    mild traumatic brain injury
      (TBI), 327–328
    ocular trauma, 326
    outcome data, 328–329
    penetrating spine injury, 329–330
    postoperative intensive care, 326
    prophylactic antibiotics, 324–325
    reconstruction, 327
    rehabilitation, 330–332
    traumatic cerebral vasospasm and
      intracranial vascular injury, 325
  Palestinian women and, 434–435
  pediatric patient and biological agent
    exposure, 369
  and politics, 14
  pre-hospital and hospital pediatric
    preparedness
    decontamination procedures, 368–369
  pre-hospital issues, 349
  protocol, 350
  public's fear of, 15
  repeated terror attacks, 5
  rubber bullets, 355
  stab wounds, 354
  stones injury, 352–353
  suicide attack phenomenon, 17–18
  Tamil Tigers and suicide bombers, 273
  terrorist bombings, 30
    aim of pre-hospital response in, 33
    burns, 181

casualty patterns in, 31–33
deaths from, 32
debriefing, 52–53
decontamination, 40–42
factors with adverse impact on
    casualty outcome, 187
handling of relatives, 51–52
lessons applied in, 173–175
major global events, 174
media relations, 50–51
medical care of victims of, 33–34
medical management, 36–37
patterns of injury and mortality in, 178
psychological sequelae of, 182
record keeping, 42
regional mass casualty plan, 35–36
scene safety, 37
selection of triage site and assigning
    key duties, 37–38
triage and, 36, 38–40
terrorist organizations and, 14
    assault on an installation, 22
    dispersal of hazardous materials, 21
terror medicine, 59–60, 75–77 (*see also*
    Computer modeling and simulation,
    use in terror medicine, Hospital
    emergency operations plans)
    education, 61–66
    exercises and drills, 72–75
    training, 66–72
terror-related stab wounds, 271–272
unconventional terrorism, 18–19
    personal terrorism, 21
    purpose of bargaining and extortion, 20
    scope of damage, 21
Tertiary blast injuries, 8, 31, 181, 288
Threat environment, 134
TNT high-energy explosives, 31
Tokyo sarin attack, 40
Toxic chemicals as chemical
    weapons, 223–227
Triage, 85, 123–124
    algorithm for, 41
    categories and, 38
    color codes, 38–40
    implications of, 183–185
    overtriage, 183
    pre-hospital, 37
    principles of, 36

selection of site, 37–38
triaging hospital, 101, 124
Tularemia
    case definitions, 212
    and children, 370–371
    clinical
        and biological description, 211
        features and diagnosis, 210
        Francisella tularensis, 210
        deliberate release with, 212
        treatment and prophylaxis, 212–213

U
Under-triage, 85. *See also* Triage
Unlimited unconventional terrorism, 19
Upshur, R., 428
Up-To-Date.com, 59
Urban terrorism
    and orthopedic injury
        after care, 294
        fracture fixation, 291–292
        fragment management/removal,
            292–294
        limb evaluation, 289–290
        mechanism of, 287–288
        patient evaluation, 288–289
        soft tissue management,
            290–291
U.S. Army Medical Research
    Institute of Infectious Diseases
    (USAMRIID), 64, 70
US emergency medical technicians
    survey, 433
US Marine barracks in Beirut suicide
    bombing, 181
US military's Critical Care Air Transport
    Team (CCATT), 305

V
Vaccinations, 428
    Centers for Disease Control and
        Prevention (CDC) and, 429
    Jenner's experiment for cowpox infection
        against smallpox, 429
    jetliner and anthrax attacks in
        United States, 430
    programs for, 430
Venezuelan Equine Encephalomyelitis
    (VEE) as threat agent, 197

Viral hemorrhagic fevers (VHFs), 212–213
  in biological warfare, 214
  and children, 372–373
  clinical description of, 215–216
  diagnosis and case definition, 217
  diseases, 214
  treatment and postexposure prophylaxis, 217
  vaccine development against, 218
Virtual simulator, for terror medicine
    training, 70–72, 74

W
Waeckerle, J. F., 229
Wahhabist-Salafist fundamentalist terrorist
    groups, 16

Wang, Z., 357
War of rocks, 393
Water and food sources
    poisoning, 22
Weapons of mass destruction (WMD)
    anxiety and stress, 150–151
Weapons of terror, 62
Weil, Y. A., 158
Western equine encephalomyelitis
    (WEE) viruses as threat
    agent, 197
Whitlock, R., 356
World Medical Association (WMA) on
    medical ethics in disaster
    situations, 432